THE HEALTH
CARE DATA GUIDE

THE HEALTH CARE DATA GUIDE

Learning from Data for Improvement

LLOYD P. PROVOST

SANDRA K. MURRAY

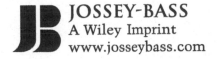

JOSSEY-BASS
A Wiley Imprint
www.josseybass.com

Published by Jossey-Bass
A Wiley Imprint
989 Market Street, San Francisco, CA 94103-1741—www.josseybass.com

Jossey-Bass books and products are available through most bookstores. To contact Jossey-Bass directly call our Customer Care Department within the U.S. at 800-956-7739, outside the U.S. at 317-572-3986, or fax 317-572-4002.

Wiley also publishes its books in a variety of electronic formats and by print-on-demand. Not all content that is available in standard print versions of this book may appear or be packaged in all book formats. If you have purchased a version of this book that did not include media that is referenced by or accompanies a standard print version, you may request this media by visiting http://booksupport.wiley.com. For more information about Wiley products, visit us at www.wiley.com.

Library of Congress Cataloging-in-Publication Data

Provost, Lloyd P.
    The health care data guide: learning from data for improvement / Lloyd P. Provost, Sandra K. Murray.—1st ed.
       p.;   cm.
    Includes bibliographical references and index.
    ISBN 978-0-470-90258-5 (pbk.); ISBN 978-1-118-08588-2 (ebk.);
    ISBN 978-1-118-08610-0 (ebk.); ISBN 978-1-118-08611-7 (ebk.)
       1. Medical care—Quality control—Statistical methods.
       2. Medical care—Quality control—Data processing.   I. Murray, Sandra K. II. Title.
          [DNLM: 1. Process Assessment (Health Care)—methods. 2. Data Interpretation, Statistical.
       3. Quality Assurance, Health Care. 4. Total Quality Management—methods. W 84.41]
    RA399.A3P766   2011
    362.10727—dc23
                                                                          2011017840

FIRST EDITION
PB Printing   10 9 8 7 6 5 4 3

CONTENTS

Contents

FIGURES, TABLES, AND EXHIBITS

FIGURES

TABLES

EXHIBITS

APPENDIX

In memory of Dr. Walter Shewhart,
whose theory of learning provides
the foundation for the science of improvement.

WHO IS THIS BOOK FOR?

This book is designed for those who want to use data to help improve health care. Specifically, this book focuses on developing skills to use data for improvement. Our goal is to help those working in health care to make improvements more readily and have greater confidence that their changes truly are improvements. Using data for improvement is a challenge and source of frustration to many. This book is a good companion to *The Improvement Guide: A Practical Approach to Enhancing Organizational Performance*, 2nd Edition, Langley and others (Jossey-Bass, 2009), which provides a complete guide to improvement. Our first chapter summarizes the messages from *The Improvement Guide* and specific references to *The Improvement Guide* are made throughout this book.

If any of these questions sound familiar, then this book is for you:

- How many measures should I be using with improvement projects?
- What kind of measures do I need? Why should I have outcome, process, and balancing measures for an improvement project?
- What methods do I use to analyze and display my data? How do I choose the correct chart?
- How can I better interpret data from my individual patients?
- How do I tell that these changes I've made are improvements? Do I need to use research methods for improvement projects?
- Why don't I just look at aggregated data before and after my change? Why use a run or Shewhart chart?
- How do I choose the correct Shewhart chart? How do I interpret it? Where do the limits come from? How do I make limits?
- What are 3-sigma limits? Are they different from confidence intervals?
- When do I revise limits on Shewhart control charts?
- I work with rare events (such as infections, falls, or pressure ulcers). What graphs do I use?
- How do we learn from patient satisfaction data?
- How do I best display key organizational data for the board and other senior leaders?

WHY ARE WE WRITING THIS BOOK?

Right now skills related to using data for improvement vary widely among those working to improve health care. We find that, in general, most people are unaware of the difference between approaches to data when used for improvement, for accountability, or for research. This lack of clarity results in paralysis to take action, selecting the incorrect tool, sampling issues, incorrect analysis, and incorrect conclusions related to improvement work. Also, information on the use of some advanced methods that are needed with health care data is not readily available to improvers.

WHAT IS THE BOOK ABOUT?

This book is about using methods and tools, which some people call Statistical Process Control (SPC), to improve health care. SPC is a philosophy, a strategy, and a set of methods for ongoing improvement of processes and systems to yield better outcomes. SPC is data based and has its foundation in Walter Shewhart's theory of variation (differentiating between common and special causes of variation in data) and in W. Edwards Deming's theory of analytic studies. Deming contrasted analytic studies, which focus on prediction, with enumerative studies focused on estimation. SPC uses concepts and assumptions related to analytic, rather than enumerative studies.

We use SPC to evaluate current process performance, search for ideas for improvement, tell if our changes have resulted in evidence of improvement, and track implementation efforts to document sustainability of the improvement. SPC includes a focus on processes, stratification, rational subgrouping, and methods to predict future performance of processes such as stability and capability analysis. SPC incorporates measurement, data collection methods, and planned experimentation. Graphical methods, such as Shewhart charts, run charts, frequency plots, Pareto analysis, scatter diagrams, and flow diagrams are the primary tools used in SPC. The use of SPC in health care requires new thought processes as well as new methods.[1]

What is not included in the book? The book does not attempt to be a stand-alone guide to improving health care, but rather focuses on the use of data in improvement. *The Improvement Guide*, mentioned earlier, provides a more complete description of all aspects of improvement, but with less detail on the methods to learn from data. The important aspects of teamwork and leadership for improvement are also described in other texts.[2] Chapter Twelve does discuss the use of Shewhart charts with "score cards" in leadership and administration.

HOW IS THE BOOK ORGANIZED?

The chapters of the book are organized to allow readers to access the material that best meets their needs. Part I (Chapters 1–6), provides a review of both basic improvement and basic SPC theory and practice. Chapter One is an overview of the improvement process that puts the use of data into perspective and sets up the rest of the book. Chapter Two provides the fundamentals of data for improvement. Chapter Three is stand-alone material that presents the latest approaches to using and analyzing run charts in improvement projects. This material has not previously been available to health care improvers.

[1]Mohammed, M. A., "Using Statistical Process Control to Improve the Quality of Health Care," *Quality and Safety in Health Care*, 2004, *13*, 243–245.
Berwick, Donald M., "Controlling Variation in Health Care: A Consultation with Walter Shewhart," *Medical Care*, December, 1991, *29*(12), 1212–1225.

[2]For example, API-Austin, *Quality as a Business Strategy*, Austin, TX: API-Austin, 1998.

Chapter Four presents Shewhart's theory and the fundamentals of using Shewhart control charts. Chapters Five and Six fully developed Shewhart's method of control charts. The authors have tried to correct numerous misunderstandings and misinformation related to using data for improvement that they have experienced in their consulting practices. The reader interested in a thorough treatment of learning from data in health care improvement will find it in this part of the book.

Part II (Chapters 7–9) addresses more advanced material that the authors feel has not been completely presented in their own or other publications. This part of the book discusses the more advanced Shewhart charts that are useful in health care applications. Situations that arise in health care data such as varying targets, highly skewed data, autocorrelation, very large sample sizes, case-mix adjustment, and other issues are discussed in Chapter Eight. A "Drill Down Approach" for using highly aggregated data in improvement work is presented in Chapter Nine. The experienced reader of this book will go directly to these chapters to find how to deal with the special issues they are facing with their data.

Part III (Chapters 10–12) looks at applications of Shewhart charts in different health care environments. Clinicians might want to start their reading of the book in Chapter Ten, which is about using run charts and Shewhart charts for data from individual patients. Those readers whose work focuses on patient feedback data might start with Chapter Eleven to learn how to summarize, analyze, and report patient reported data. Leaders of improvement in organizations may want to start their study of this book in Chapter Twelve on using Shewhart charts in health care administration and leadership. Chapter Thirteen contains a series of case studies dealing with specific health care situations that illustrate the appropriate application of the theory and methods discussed in the book. These case studies offer an interactive way for the user to evaluate their statistical knowledge and skills and also provide an opportunity for the reader to develop additional skill and confidence in displaying and interpreting data in a meaningful way. Some readers may want to begin their interaction with the book by finding a health care application they are interested in and exploring that case study in Chapter Thirteen.

In addition to the material presented in the book, we have made extensive use of references through footnotes throughout the book. For the data methods and tools, we have included the basic source reference where the concept or method was first presented in the quality improvement literature. Our presentation of the methods tries to stay true to the theory and philosophy of these original authors. These references are usually focused on industrial applications, so we have also included recent references in the health care literature that illustrate applications in health care. These references will allow the reader to explore any of the topics presented in the book in further depth and see how other health care improvers are using the methods.

ACKNOWLEDGMENTS

This book has been a work in progress for the authors for the past twelve years. Most of our consulting and teaching work during this time has been with health care organizations. We learned to work effectively with all types of data generated from health care processes. Many people have helped us develop the approaches and examples presented in the book. We especially thank our clients for their willingness to test the new material and try the methods in their improvement work.

Our colleagues with Associates in Process Improvement (API), and The Institute for Healthcare Improvement have been supportive and provided feedback as they used this material in their teaching and consulting. The first drafts of some of the chapters came from materials developed by API. We wish to thank the following reviewers for their many thoughtful and helpful comments: Yosef Dlugacz, Sheri Fergusson, Rocco Perla, Eric Tom, and David Wayne. Also, we thank Yosef Dlugacz, Maulik Joshi, and Robert Lloyd for their comments on the initial book plan, and we thank our associates and clients who provided many suggestions for improvement of earlier drafts of this material.

We thank our families for their patience and support. We can finally answer their common question: "When are you going to finish that book?"

Lloyd P. Provost is a statistician, advisor, teacher, and author who helps organizations make improvements and foster continuous learning and improvement. He consults and advises through Associates in Process Improvement. His experience includes consulting in data analysis, planning, management systems, planned experimentation, measurement, and other methods for improvement of quality and productivity. He has consulted with clients worldwide in a variety of industries including health care, chemical, manufacturing, engineering, construction, automotive, electronics, food, transportation, professional services, retail, education, and government. Much of his current work is focused on health care improvement in developing countries.

Lloyd has a BS in Statistics from the University of Tennessee and an MS in Statistics from the University of Florida. He is the author of several papers relating to improvement and co-author of a book on planned experimentation (*Quality Improvement Through Planned Experimentation*, 2*nd* edition, McGraw-Hill, 1998) and the Model for Improvement (*The Improvement Guide: A Practical Approach to Enhancing Organizational Performance*, 2*nd* edition, Jossey-Bass, 2009. He was awarded the American Society for Quality's Deming Medal in 2003.

Sandra K. Murray is a principal in Corporate Transformation Concepts, an independent consulting firm formed in 1994. She is an improvement advisor and teacher focusing all of her work in health care. Sandra has extensive background in both quality improvement theory and practice in the areas of using data for improvement, process improvement, and strategic business planning. She concentrates her work in the areas of effectively using process improvement methods to get and sustain results in health care organizations. Sandra has developed and taught numerous courses related to the science of improvement.

Sandra has a BS in Dietetics and Institution Management from Oregon State University and an MA in Management from Webster University, Missouri. She has been an improvement advisor with the Institute for Healthcare Improvement (IHI) since 2002. Sandra has worked with IHI's patient safety efforts, is faculty for IHI's Breakthrough Series College and for IHI's year-long Improvement Advisor Professional Development Program. She is the author of two DVDs on using data for improvement in health care, co-editor of a book related to tools for using data for improvement, and co-author of a recent article published in the *British Medical Journal*.

THE HEALTH
CARE DATA GUIDE

PART

I

USING DATA FOR IMPROVEMENT

## CHAPTER 1

IMPROVEMENT METHODOLOGY

This book is about using data to improve health care[1] and this chapter, a summary of *The Improvement Guide*,[2] describes approaches and methods used to make improvements. It provides a backdrop, setting the stage for understanding and contextualizing the rest of the book. This chapter will:

- Describe the Model for Improvement
- Illustrate use of the Plan, Do, Study, Act Cycle for testing and implementing changes
- Introduce graphical methods to learn from data
- Describe a typical health care improvement project
- Enumerate the methods and tools used to support improvement

How do you make improvements? Historically people have used a trial-and-error approach to improving all aspects of their lives. Typically an idea for an improvement (a change) comes to someone. These ideas are often reactions to problems or difficulties that we all face in life and in our work. So we make the change and then see whether the situation improves. Sometimes we also check to see if anyone complains or if something else stops working because of the change that we made. Because of its sporadic track record on real, sustainable improvement, this natural trial-and-error approach has often been criticized as "jumping to solutions" without sufficient study.

As a response to this criticism, some improvement specialists have turned to extensive study of the problem before a change or trial is attempted. Sometimes this approach leads to a better track record on making sustained improvements, but more often it can lead to never actually making changes. The person with the problem gets bogged down in the study, "paralysis by analysis" sets in, or other problems begin to take priority. Many health care professionals are trained in research methods with strict protocols, rigid data requirements, and large sample sizes. When they begin work on improvement projects, they naturally bring this training to the project. How do we obtain a balance between the trial-and-error approach and extensive study that may never lead to action? How do we find the balance between the goals of formal clinical research and the natural learning and improvement from daily work in health care?

---

[1]Institute of Medicine, *Crossing the Quality Chasm: A New Health System for the 21st Century*, Washington, D.C.: National Academy Press, 2001.

[2]Langley, J. et al., *The Improvement Guide: A Practical Approach to Enhancing Organizational Performance*, 2nd ed., San Francisco: Jossey-Bass, 2009.

This chapter presents a **Model for Improvement**[3] that attempts to provide that balance. The model provides a framework for developing, testing, and implementing changes that lead to improvement. The model can be applied to improving aspects of one's personal endeavors, as well as the improvement of processes, products, and services in health care organizations. The model attempts to balance the desire and rewards from taking action with the wisdom of careful study before taking action. The use of data in this book will frequently be connected to an individual or an improvement team that is using the Model for Improvement to guide their learning and execution.

FUNDAMENTAL QUESTIONS FOR IMPROVEMENT

The Model for Improvement is based on three fundamental questions:

What are we trying to accomplish?

How will we know that a change is an improvement?

What changes can we make that will result in improvement?

The model is also based on a "cycle" for learning and improvement. Variants of this improvement cycle have been called the Shewhart Cycle, Deming Cycle, and PDSA Cycle. The cycle promotes a trial-and-learning approach to improvement efforts. The cycle is used for learning, to develop changes, to test changes, and to implement changes. Figure 1.1 contains a diagram of the basic form of the model.

Why are we promoting the use of this particular approach to improvement? Our experience with the Model for Improvement since its development in the 1980s shows that it:

- Is useful for both process and product improvement
- Is applicable to all types of organizations

FIGURE 1.1 The Model for Improvement

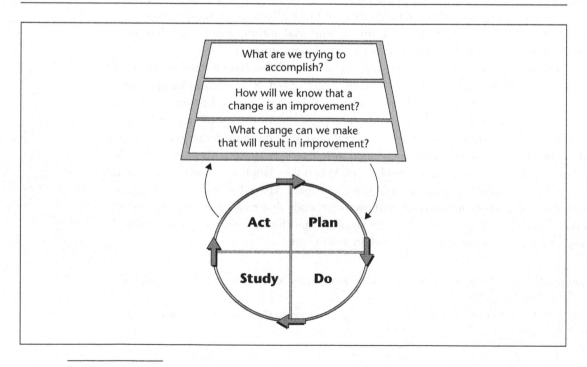

---

[3]Ibid.

- Is applicable to all groups and levels in an organization
- Facilitates the use of teamwork to make improvements
- Provides a framework for the application of statistical tools and methods
- Encourages planning to be based on theory
- Emphasizes and encourages the iterative learning process
- Provides a way to empower people in the organization to take action

This framework is compared to other frameworks used in quality improvement (such as Six Sigma's DMAIC) in Appendix C of *The Improvement Guide*.[4] The use of the Model for Improvement begins with trying to answer the three basic questions.

What Are We Trying to Accomplish?

Before starting to develop any activities, or test or implement changes, participants and other stakeholders in the improvement effort need to agree on *what is to be accomplished*. The use of a well-written **aim statement** can be an effective tool for answering the first question in the Model for Improvement. If there is not a common understanding between people who are depending on the aim statement for guidance, then individuals will naturally try to fill the void of understanding with their personal view of what is to be accomplished. These well-intentioned efforts usually lead to misunderstandings—during team meetings and other activities—that will not achieve the intended accomplishments, ultimately resulting in wasted time, resources, and frustration for everyone involved. The written aim can be a formal document (sometimes called a charter) from a hospital's strategic planning process or it can be a statement written on the whiteboard by a group of nurses and physicians brainstorming more effective care of their patients.

Why take the time to develop an aim statement for an improvement effort? A statement of the aim:

- Provides leaders a mechanism to think through all aspects of the proposed effort
- Aids in selection of the team to make the improvements
- Reduces variation in activities from the original purpose
- Helps in the selection of particular processes or products for study
- Empowers individuals to make changes in health care systems
- Clarifies the magnitude of improvement expected from this project
- Defines the time frame for the improvement work

Individuals or teams can complete improvement efforts. In many health care organizations, teams composed of two to seven people are given assignments to make improvements. The members of the team should be selected from those who are knowledgeable about the processes or services that are likely to be studied, or who have a stake in their performance. A well-thought-out aim statement will aid in the selection of team members.

Without a clear aim statement, it will be easy for a team to become sidetracked and work in areas that are only of minor relevance to the original purpose of the improvement activities. The team will also struggle with the appropriate scope of the activities. The aim statement will help the team focus its efforts and reduce unwanted variations from the original purpose.

Good aim statements are clear, concise, and results oriented. They should be aligned with the goals of the organization sponsoring the improvement to clarify why the work is being done. Teams make better progress when they have unambiguous, specific aims.

---

[4]Ibid.

Setting numerical targets can further define the intent of the charter, create the will for change, and help focus measurements used in the improvement effort. Numerical goals can also be abused and lead to bad practices, so those providing a goal should convince the team that the goal is feasible by:

- Providing the level of support and resources that will be required to achieve the goals
- Observing other organizations that have made similar accomplishments
- Providing some basic ideas that could feasibly result in achieving the goals
- Demonstrating the benefit to the organization if the goals could be achieved

Other guidance given in the aim statement should include anything and everything to keep the team focused (strategies, resources, boundaries, patient populations, time and resource constraints, and so on). The following is an example of an aim statement for a team planning on improving care of asthma patients in a clinic:

AIM STATEMENT

During the next six months, the clinic's practice will be redesigned to obtain a 30% increase in symptom-free days and a 50% reduction in the number of exacerbations reported for the pilot asthma population. At least 90% of patients with persistent asthma will be treated with maintenance anti-inflammatory medication and >80% of patients will have a completed written action plan.

Guidance: All patients with asthma (about 400 in population) of the Neighborhood Health Center will serve as the pilot population for this project. A registry of the asthma patients served by the center should be developed. The clinic should initially focus on patient self-management methods and delivery system design. All physicians in the center will participate.

This is an example of an aim statement for a hospital Emergency Department's team formed to improve patient satisfaction in the ED:

AIM STATEMENT

Redesign Emergency Department processes to increase patient and family satisfaction with their experience in the ED by greater than 30% before June 2010.

Guidance: Focus on all aspects of the emergency department and related services. Emphasize improvements in physical comfort, coordination of care, management of the waiting time, and family involvement. The aim will be measured by the percentage of patients who say they would recommend the ED to a friend. The changes need to work with existing staffing levels.

How Will We Know That a Change Is an Improvement?

Although improvement is about making changes to processes and systems, measurement plays a key role in all improvement efforts. The purpose of measuring here is for learning, not for judgment or comparison. Project teams need measures to give them feedback that the changes they are making are having the desired impact.[5]

---

[5]Lloyd, R., *Quality Health Care: A Guide to Developing and Using Indicators,* Jones and Bartlett, Boston, 2004.

Some measures should focus at the project level (global measures) and be maintained throughout the project. For example, symptom-free days may be an appropriate global measure for a project improving asthma care. Other measures are done on an as-needed basis as part of PDSA Cycles for diagnosis and for assessment of the changes tested. For example, in an asthma project, the percent of patients using appropriate medications might be a useful Cycle measure.

The team in the ED department (aim statement given above) used the following as global measures for their improvement efforts:

- Percentage of patients saying they would recommend the facility to friends on the monthly patient satisfaction survey
- Percentage patients satisfied on specific questions concerning physical comfort, coordination of care, and, family involvement
- Average waiting time for patients visiting the ED

For specific PDSA Cycles, the team planned to use other measures to evaluate the impact of the changes they would test. The Cycle measures would include interviews with providers, staff, and patients affected by tests, and more specific time measures to understand waiting times.

Because improvements are made over time, in order to facilitate learning and communication, measures should be displayed on **run charts** or **Shewhart charts**, which are the major focus of the rest of this book. The time-ordered charts of a set of global measures will provide the primary way to assess the impact of each project team's work. Rather than just doing a before-and-after assessment, feedback from the measures is consistent and ongoing throughout the project. This approach gives teams the opportunity to work on data collection problems and to communicate their progress every month of the project. Key changes made to care systems can be annotated on the charts to begin analysis of the impact of the changes.

What Changes Can We Make That Will Result in Improvement?

Sometimes when confronted with this third question of the Model for Improvement, the answer is obvious. The knowledge to support a specific change has existed for some time, but the conditions, resources, or inclination did not exist to make the change happen. Other times a change that will result in improvement is not known or not apparent. As changes are not readily available, people have a tendency to resort to some common and often ineffective ways of developing change, such as using more of the same (more people, more money, more time, more exhortations, more inspection, more controls, and so forth) or trying to develop the one perfect change.

Developing a change that will help accomplish the project aim usually requires making a fundamental change to the system. In developing changes, it is useful to think about two types of change:

- Changes that are needed to keep the system performing at current levels (first-order change)
- Changes that are needed to improve the system or create a new system (second-order change)

Making first-order changes when they are needed is an important activity, but it should not be confused with implementing second-order changes that prevent problems from occurring. Most improvement efforts require second-order changes because they:

- Require design or redesign of some aspect of the system
- Are necessary for improving a system that does not have many problems
- Fundamentally alter how the system works and what people do in the system
- Often result in improvement of several measures simultaneously
- Have an impact that is felt far into the future

A second-order change can be made by redesigning part of the current system or by designing an entirely new one. Eliminating part or all of the system may be a second-order change. The important notion is not the size of the change but the impact of the change. Big improvements can often be realized by making small changes directed at the right places in the system.

Second-order changes can be developed by critical thinking about the current system, learning from approaches in other organizations, using new technology, applying creative thinking methods, or by using concepts that have worked in other improvement situations. For complex projects, it is often useful to first develop a concept design and then follow with PDSA Cycles to test changes to support the concept.

THE PDSA CYCLE FOR IMPROVEMENT

To help individuals and teams test, adapt, and implement changes, the Model for Improvement uses the **Plan, Do, Study, Act Cycle (PDSA)** as the framework for an efficient trial-and-learning methodology.[6] The cycle begins with a plan and ends with action taken based on the learning gained from the Plan, Do, and Study phases of the cycle. The four steps in the cycle consist of planning the details of the study, test, or implementation and making predictions about the outcomes (Plan), conducting the plan and collecting data (Do), comparing the predictions to the data collected (Study), and taking action based on the new knowledge (Act). Figure 1.2 describes the activities for each step of the PDSA Cycle.

Knowledge is built by an iterative process of developing a theory, making predictions based on the theory, testing the predictions with data, improving the theory based on the results, making predictions based on the revised theory, and so forth. Tests of change are designed to answer questions that come from a combination of theory about the subject matter and conclusions from analysis of data from past studies. When designing studies for testing a change, the planned tests should match this sequential nature of building knowledge.

Each PDSA Cycle is designed to answer specific questions related to the team's aim. Each cycle should build on the current knowledge about the changes being considered and answer specific questions required to implement the change into standard practice. Numerous small-scale cycles accumulate into large effects through synergy. Figure 1.3 illustrates this process.

In a typical improvement effort, most PDSA Cycles are designed to test and adapt changes. Developing a good plan is critical for an effective, successful test cycle. The plan

---

[6]Deming, W. E., *Out of the Crisis*, Cambridge, MA: MIT Press, 1986, 88.

FIGURE 1.2   The PDSA Cycle

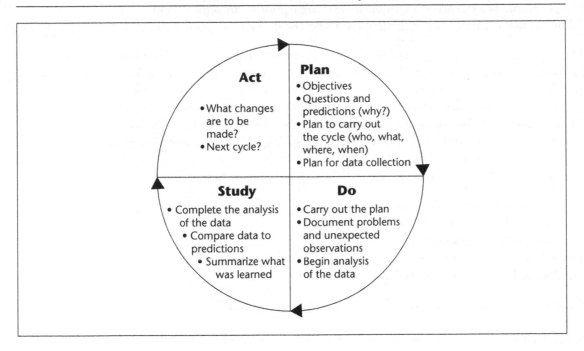

FIGURE 1.3   Sequential PDSA Cycles for Learning and Improvement

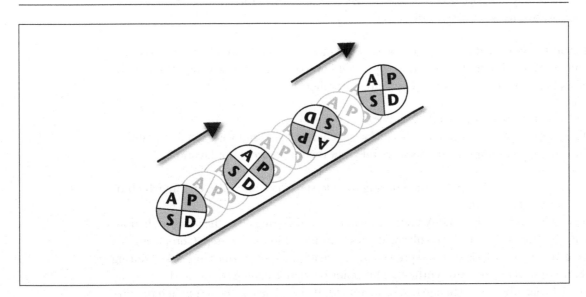

begins with a statement of the specific objective of the cycle. **Cycles to test a change** will have varying objectives depending on the current degree of belief about the change. Some typical objectives of a PDSA test are:

- Increasing degree of belief that the change will result in an improvement
- Deciding which of several proposed specific changes will lead to the desired improvement
- Evaluating how much improvement we can expect if we make the change
- Deciding how to adapt the proposed change to the actual environment of interest

- Evaluating cost implications and possible side effects of the change
- Giving individuals a chance to experience the change prior to implementation
- Deciding which combinations of changes will have the desired effects on the measures

The objective of the cycle described at the beginning of the plan step will clarify the specific focus of testing the change. After agreeing on the objective, the team should state the specific questions to be answered in the cycle. These questions provide the format for describing the team's predictions about the change(s) that will be tested in the cycle. The predictions should be worded in such a way that the results of the tests conducted in the cycle can be compared to the predictions. Thus, stating the predictions will have an impact on the data collection plan of the cycle.

Next, the team develops a plan for the test. The plan should include:

- Who will schedule and conduct the test?
- Exactly what changes will be made?
- Where will the test be conducted?
- When will the test be done?
- What data will be collected to answer the questions in the cycle?

Some hints for planning useful cycles for testing changes include:

- Think a couple of cycles ahead of the initial test (future tests, implementation).
- Scale down the size and decrease the time required for the initial test.
- Do not try to achieve buy-in or consensus for the test; recruit volunteers for the test.
- Use temporary supports to make the change feasible during the test.
- Be innovative to make the test feasible.

In the Do step of the cycle, the test is performed and the data collected is analyzed. The information obtained during this step should prepare for the Study step. What if the test of a change is not successful? There are a number of possible reasons:

1. The change was not properly executed.
2. The support processes required to make the change successful were not adequate.
3. The change was implemented successfully but the results were not favorable.

Information should be obtained during the Do step to clearly differentiate which of these situations occurred.

The third step of the PDSA Cycle for testing, Study, brings together the predictions made in the Plan step and the results of the test conducted in the Do step. Comparing the results of the data analysis with the predictions made for the specific questions asked during the planning step creates this synthesis. This point is where learning occurs and where the degree of belief about the change can be increased. If the results of the test match the predictions, our degree of belief about our knowledge is increased. If the predictions do not match the data, we have an opportunity to advance our knowledge through understanding why the prediction was not accurate.

In the Act step of the PDSA Cycle for testing a change, the project team must decide on the next course of action:

- Is further testing needed to increase our degree of belief about the change?
- Do alternative changes need to be tested?
- Do we need to learn about other implications (such as costs) of the change?

- Are we ready to implement the change on a full-scale basis?
- Do we need to modify the proposed change or develop an alternative change?
- Should we drop consideration of the proposed change?

The decision on course of action will lead to developing the next PDSA Cycle. The use of multiple cycles allows knowledge to increase as we progress from testing to implementing a change, thus minimizing risk and consequences of any failures. As degree of belief that the change will be successful is increased, the scale of the test can be increased. Based on the results of a test, a change or some part of the change could be implemented as is, the change could be modified and retested, or it could be abandoned.

Cycles for implementing a change differ from test cycles in a number of ways:

- Support processes need to be developed to support the change as it is implemented.
- Failures are not expected when the change is implemented.
- Increased resistance to the change can be expected as it affects more people.
- Cycles for implementing a change take longer than test cycles.

Figure 1.4 summarizes the use of the PDSA Cycle to test and implement changes.

Tools and Methods to Support the Model for Improvement[7]

The Model for Improvement with its cycle for learning and improvement provides the structure and road map for accomplishing improvement of health care processes. In many improvement efforts, that is all that is required. Other times, teams get stuck looking for an idea or trying to understand the problems in the current process. Over the past fifty years, the quality improvement profession has developed methods and tools to assist with the improvement process, which are described in Table 1.1. Many of the tools commonly used in improvement projects are shown in Table 1.2.

FIGURE 1.4   PDSA Cycles from Testing to Implementation

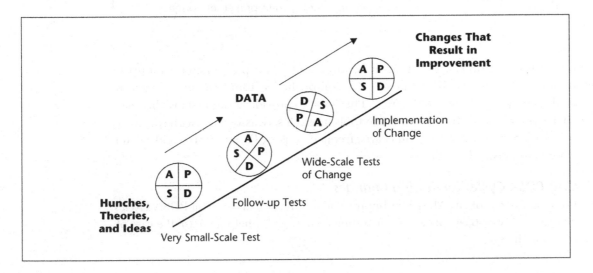

---

[7]Langley et al., *The Improvement Guide*, Appendix C.

Table 1.1   Overview of Methods for Improvement

Category	Method	Typical Use of Method
Viewing Systems and Processes	Dynamic Programming	Map relationships with mathematical equations and then simulate performance.
Gathering Information	Surveys	Obtain information from people.
	Benchmarking	Obtain information on performance and approaches from other organizations.
	Creativity Methods	Develop new ideas and fresh thinking.
Organizing Information	Quality Function Deployment (QFD)	Communicate customer needs and requirements through the design and production processes.
	Failure Mode and Effects Analysis (FMEA)	Used by process and product designers to identify and address potential failures.
	Problem Solving	A collection of concepts and tools (is/is not, five why's, stratification) to address the special case of improvement where a problem has been identified.
Understanding Variation	Statistical Process Control	A philosophy and a set of methods for improvement with its foundation in the theory of variation. SPC incorporates the concepts of an analytic study, process thinking, prevention, stratification, stability, capability, and prediction.
	Measurement System Analysis	Procedures to understand the impact of bias and precision of the measurement process on variation in data.
	Statistical Methods	Graphical and numerical procedures to help understand and quantify patterns of variation in data.
Understanding Relationships	Planned Experimentation	Design studies to evaluate cause-and-effect relationships and test changes.
Project Management	PDSA Cycle	Method for organizing learning, testing, and implementing during an improvement project.

When thinking about these tools, it is important to keep a perspective on the improvement initiative. If the aim can be accomplished without the use of any of the tools, then they do not need to be used. They exist to provide additional insight when solutions are not obvious. In this book, the tools most closely associated with statistical process control (Shewhart charts, run charts, frequency plots, Pareto charts, and scatter plots) will be emphasized.

Designing PDSA Cycles for Testing Changes

The art of effective use of the Model for Improvement is the design of useful PDSA Cycles to test changes.[8] Three basic principles of testing a change will help increase the rate of learning about changes:

---

[8]Langley, J. et al., *The Improvement Guide.*

Table 1.2   Overview of Tools for Improvement

Category	Tool	Typical Use of Tool
Viewing Systems and Processes	Flow Diagram	Develop a picture of a process. Communicate and standardize processes.
	Linkage of Processes	Develop a picture of a system composed of processes linked together.
	Causal Loop Diagrams	Identify reinforcing and balancing processes.
Gathering Information	Form for Collecting Data	Plan and organize a data collection effort.
	Operational Definitions	Provide communicable meaning to a concept by specifying how the concept will be applied within a particular set of circumstances.
Organizing Information	Affinity Diagram	Organize and summarize qualitative information.
	Force Field Analysis	Summarize forces supporting and hindering change.
	Cause and Effect Diagram	Collect and organize current knowledge about potential causes of problems or variation.
	Matrix Diagram	Arrange information to understand relationships and make decisions.
	Tree Diagram	Visualize the structure of a problem, plan, or any other opportunity of interest.
	Interrelationship Diagram	Identify and communicate logical and sequential connections between components of a problem.
	Radar Chart	Evaluate alternatives or compare against targets with three or more variables or characteristics.
	Driver Diagram	Display the theory for improvement in an improvement project.
Understanding Variation	Run Chart	Study variation in data over time; understand the impact of changes on measures.
	Pareto Chart	Focus on areas of improvement with greatest impact.
	Frequency Plot	Understand location, spread, shape, and patterns of data.
	Shewhart Chart	Distinguish between special and common causes of variation.
Understanding Relationships	Two-Way Table	Understand cause-and-effect for qualitative variables
	Scatter Plot	Analyze the associations or relationship between two variables; test for possible cause-and-effect.
Project Management	Gantt Chart	Organize the project tasks over time with key milestones identified.
	PERT Chart	Display the sequential relationships of the project tasks and determine the critical path.
	Work Breakdown Structure	Develop a hierarchical relationship between the tasks on a project.

- Initially test on a small scale and build knowledge sequentially.
- Collect data over time.
- Include a wide range of conditions in tests in latter cycles.

Following these principles will result in conducting tests where the effects observed can be clearly tied to the change of interest. Often, the simplest way to design a PDSA Cycle is to make the change and study run charts of the global measures and specific measures relevant to the cycle before and after the change. But even with run charts over a long period of time, it is always possible that some other cause that occurred near the same time that the change of interest was made could be responsible for the observed effects. Some other ways to increase the rigor of the test include:[9]

- Remove the change and see if the process returns to its initial levels. This can be repeated as many times as necessary (make the change, observe results over time, remove the change) until an adequate degree of belief is obtained.
- Adding some type of comparison group or control group to the study. The same measures would be made for the comparison group as for the environment where the change is made. A run chart for the control group can then be compared to the environment undergoing the change.
- Use the methods of planned experimentation to separate effects of changes of interest and background variables.

Planned experimentation[10] is a collection of approaches and methods to help increase the rate of learning about improvements to systems, processes, and products. An experiment is a change to a process or product and an observation of the effect of that change on one or more measures of interest. The methods of planned experimentation are appropriate for understanding the important causes of variation in a process and evaluating multiple changes to the process. Using these methods, it is possible to design a single PDSA Cycle to evaluate multiple changes. Planned experimentation allows the determination of the individual (main effects) and combined effects (interactions) for the changes being evaluated.

The theory of applying planned experimentation to improvement activities was described by Deming.[11] He differentiated studies designed to understand a fixed population (enumerative studies) from studies designed where the population of interest was in the future (analytic studies). Whereas enumerative studies are used to develop estimates of the population, the ability to predict future results is the focus of analytic studies. The approaches and methods in this book have their foundation in Deming's analytic studies framework. Chapter Two provides further discussion of analytic studies.

---

[9]Speroff, T., and O'Connor, G., "Study Designs for PDSA Quality Improvement Research," *Quality Management in Health Care*, Jan-Mar 2004, *13*, 17–32.

[10]Moen, R., Nolan, T., and Provost, L., *Quality Improvement Through Planned Experiment*, 2nd ed., New York: McGraw-Hill, 1999.

[11]Deming, W. E., "On Probability as a Basis for Action," *The American Statistician*, November 1975, *29*(4).

Planning one large PDSA Cycle in a study to attempt to get all of the answers should almost always be avoided. Testing the change during full-scale implementation should be considered only when:

- The team has a high degree of belief that the change will result in improvement.
- The risk is small (losses from a failed test are not significant).
- The team cannot find a way to test the change on a small scale.

During the design of studies to test a change, those responsible for developing the change should continually be asking themselves how they could reduce the risks of the test and still gain some knowledge. The following are some ways to design a test on a small scale:

- Simulate the change (physical or computer simulation).
- Have others in the organization with knowledge of the change review and comment on it.
- Have members of the project team test the change before introducing it to others.
- Incorporate redundancy in the test; make the change side-by-side with the existing process.
- Conduct the test in one facility in the organization, or with one group of patients.
- Conduct the test over a short time period (one hour or one day).
- Test the change with a small group of volunteers.

One of the most common designs for a test of change is the "before and after test" (or pretest/posttest design). In this design for a test, a change is made and the circumstances after the change are compared to the circumstances before the change. The collection of data before the change provides the historical experience that is the basis of the comparison. When considering the design of a PDSA test, a run chart that includes multiple measurements before and after the change is made provides minimal complexity and excellent protection from misinterpreting the results of the test.

Figure 1.5 shows the results of such a before-and-after test. Data was collected on week 4, the change was made during week 7, and then data was collected again on week 11. The reduction in delay time from 8 hours to 3 hours was considered very significant for the process of interest. The bar chart in Figure 1.5 shows a summary of the test data.

Summarized in this way, does this test provide an adequate degree of belief that the change, when implemented, will lead to an improvement? Are there other feasible explanations of the reduction in delay time after the change was introduced?

The run chart at the bottom of Figure 1.5 (Case 1) shows one possible scenario that *could have* yielded the results observed in the test. The delay on week 4 is 8 hours and the delay on week 11 is 3 hours as described by the before-and-after bar chart. The run chart shows results for delay times for weeks 1 to 14 (three weeks before the change was made until three weeks after the second test observation was made) is shown. The run chart in Case 1 confirms the conclusion that the change did result in a meaningful improvement.

FIGURE 1.5 Results of a Before-and-After Test: Case 1

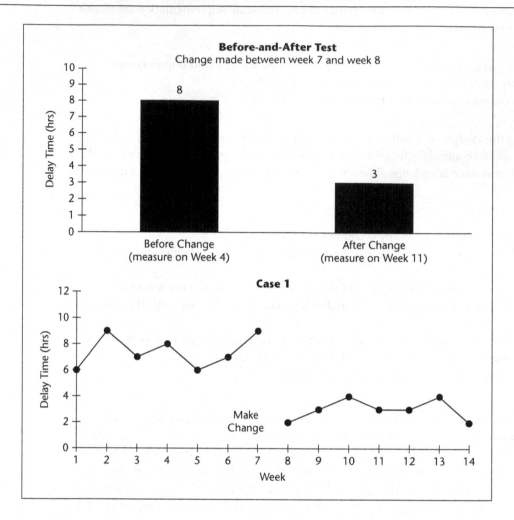

Figure 1.6 shows run charts for five other possible scenarios that offer alternative explanations of the test results. In each case a run chart of delay time for weeks 1 to 14 is shown. The test results for week 4 (delay time of 8) and week 11 (delay time of 3) are the same for all cases.

In Case 2 there is no obvious improvement after the change is made. The measures made during the test are typical results from a process that has a lot of week-to-week variation. The conclusion from study of the run chart is that the change did not have any obvious impact on the delay time.

In Case 3 it appears that the process has been steadily improving over the 14-week period. The rate of improvement did not change when the change was introduced. Although the delay time for the process has certainly improved, there is no evidence to show that the change made any contribution to the steady improvement in the process over the 14 weeks.

In Case 4 an initial improvement is observed after the change is made, but in the last three weeks the process seems to have returned to its prechange level of delay time. The results may be due to a "Hawthorne effect," which is named after some tests on productivity conducted at the Western Electric Hawthorne plant in the 1920s. Whenever changes were made in the work environment, initial improvements were observed. But performance quickly returned to normal levels after workers became accustomed to the change. This effect is similar to a "placebo effect." Because the workers are focused on

FIGURE 1.6   Other Possible Run Charts Associated with Before-and-After Graph

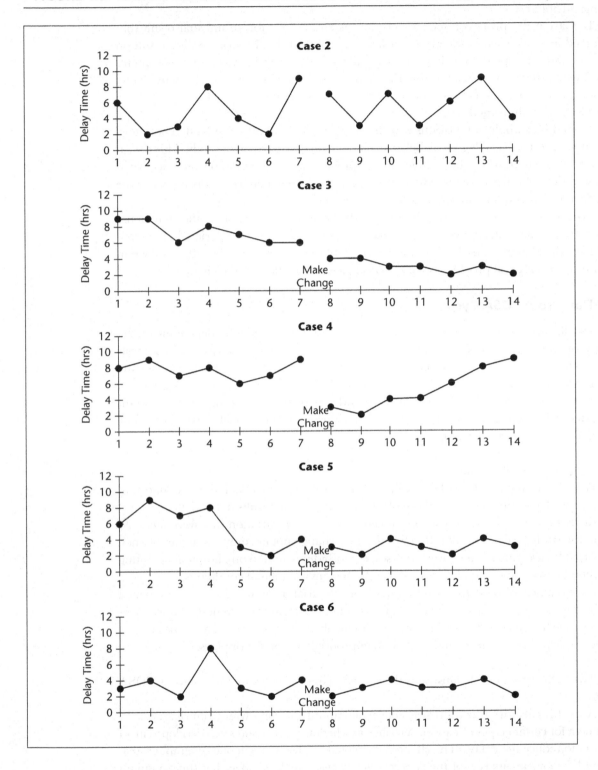

the process and paying particular attention to the measures of interest, observers see an initial improvement. Later, when focus on the change is lessened, the delay times revert to the original process levels.

In Case 5, an improvement in the process delay times has occurred, but it appears that the improvement occurred in week 5 before the change was made after week 7.

The improvement in delay time should be attributed to some other phenomenon, not the change of interest.

In Case 6 the process appears to be consistent, except for an unusual result that occurred in week 4 when the pretest results were obtained. The strange high result on week 4 made it appear that the more typical result on week 11 was an improvement. Once again, there is no evidence that the change contributed to any improvement. (Note: a visual analysis was used to interpret these run charts. Chapter Three will introduce some more formal analysis methods.)

From this example, it is obvious why the simple before-and-after test is often not rigorous enough to increase degree of belief about a change in an analytic study. This design should only be used when the change has had previous testing and has proven effective in a wide variety of environments. Then the test is being done to confirm performance in the specific environment of interest or to measure side effects of the change.

What can be done to increase the rigor of the before-and-after test in other situations? Often, the simplest alternative is to conduct the test over a longer time period, both before and after the change is made. Plotting the test results on a run charts like those shown in Figure 1.6 usually will provide convincing evidence of the effect of the change.

Analysis of Data from PDSA Cycles

The specific approach to analysis of data from a PDSA Cycle will differ depending on the design of the study that is conducted. Classical statistical methods based on hypothesis tests, confidence intervals, or probability analysis usually are not applicable because of the nature of the analytic studies in improvement work (described earlier in this chapter and discussed in more detail in Chapter Two). Knowledge of the subject matter is important in studying the results of tests of a change. The following elements will usually be part of the analysis of all tests of change:

1. Initially show all the data.
2. Plot the raw data in the order in which the tests were conducted. This is an important means of identifying the presence of trends and unusual results in the data.
3. Rearrange this plot to study other potential sources of variation that were included in the study design, but not directly related to change under study. Examples of such variables are patient categories (age, sex, comorbidities, and so on), hospital, operating room, clinic, physician, laboratories, and other environmental conditions.
4. Use graphical displays to assess how much of the variation in the data can be explained by the change(s) of interest. These displays might include using different symbols to identify the change or ordering the test results to highlight data before and after the change.
5. Summarize the results of the study with appropriate graphical displays.

The following example illustrates these approaches to analyzing the results of PDSA Cycles.

A health care organization was concerned about the long wait from diagnosis to treatment for certain types of cancer. A change in scheduling procedures was developed in an attempt to reduce the delays. The change was piloted for five weeks in one geographic area. Figure 1.7 shows an analysis of the data collected to evaluate the change. The three hospitals in the area reported the average wait time to treatment for cancer patients over an 11-week period. The change in scheduling was introduced after week 6 in each of the hospitals.

The first run chart (see Chapter Three for details on run charts) in Figure 1.7 shows the data from each hospital in time order. No unusual results or unexpected changes are obvious. There appeared to be a slight downward trend in the data after week 6.

FIGURE 1.7   Analysis of Data from a PDSA Cycle

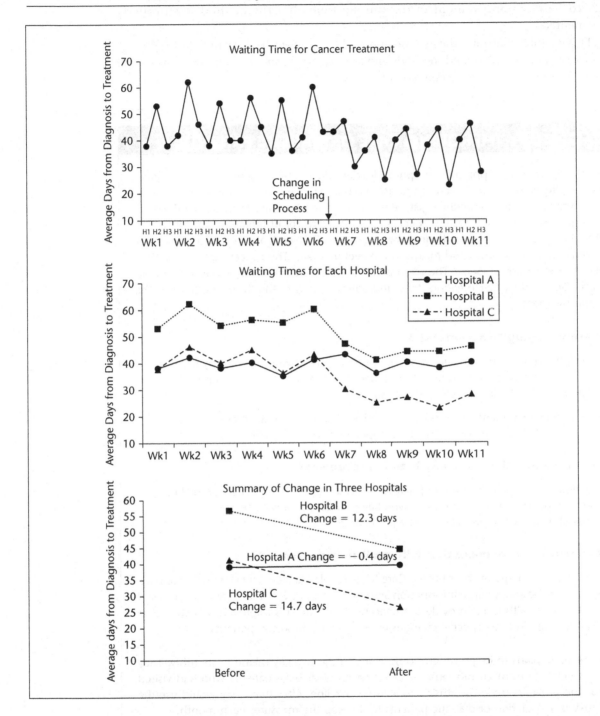

The second run chart separates the data for each hospital. There are obvious differences in average waiting times from the three hospitals. From this graph, it appears that there was no change in Hospital A. After investigation, it was found that the new scheduling procedure was not properly implemented in Hospital A. But both Hospitals B and C had properly implemented the change.

The third graph in Figure 1.7 summarized the effects of the scheduling change in the three hospitals. Based on these results, the health care organization spread the implementation of the scheduling change to the rest of their system, expecting about a 12- to 15-day improvement in the waiting time after the method was properly implemented.

This example illustrates the general approach to analyzing data from PDSA Cycles. A number of more sophisticated methods and tools for analyzing the data from Cycles will be described in the remaining chapters of this book.

CASE STUDY: IMPROVING CARE OF DIABETIC PATIENTS

This case study illustrates the approach and principles described in this chapter to use the Model for Improvement to guide an improvement project in a primary care health care clinic.

A team composed of an endocrinologist, two primary care physicians from the south clinic, a nurse manager, an information system specialist, and the director of the clinic was formed to redesign the office system of care for their diabetic patients. This work also served as a pilot for the care of other chronic diseases and for general preventive care. The concept design for their work was the Chronic Care Model.[12] The team used the Model for Improvement as a road map for their work. During their first meeting, they attempted to answer the three questions of the Model for Improvement:

What are we trying to accomplish?

During the next 10 months, improve the care of patients with diabetes by redesigning the office practice using the Chronic Care Model. Pilot the system in the South Clinic with a population of about 200 diabetic patients so that:

- >80% of diabetic patients have set collaborative goals (self-management).
- The average HbA1c level for the diabetic population will be <8.0%.

How will we know that a change is an improvement?

1. The average HbA1c of the pilot population using a registry of patients with diabetes
2. Percentage of patients in the registry who have set collaborative goals
3. Additional measures of progress on the key changes

What changes can we make that will result in improvement?

The six components of the Chronic Care Model (Self-Management, Decision Support, Delivery System Design, Clinical Information System, Community Resources and Policies, and Organization of Health Care) provide the concept design for this improvement effort. The team will develop and test specific changes under each of these components.

The team made plans to begin reporting the data on the two key measures monthly. They decided to collect data from 20 randomly selected charts of diabetic patients who had visited the clinic for the previous three months to establish a baseline. After that, they would use the current registry of population of diabetic patients to develop the measures each month.

They then begin planning their first series of PDSA Cycles to test and implement the concept design. Table 1.3 describes their initial 14 cycles planned in four of the Chronic Care Model components.

---

[12]Wagner, Edward H. et al., "Quality Improvement in Chronic Illness Care: A Collaborative Approach," *Journal of Quality Improvement*, *27*(2), February 2001, 63–80.

Table 1.3   Initial Team Plan for PDSA Cycles

Concept	PDSA Cycle #	Description of PDSA Cycle	Responsibility
A: Clinical Information System	A.1	Develop simple database in Access for diabetic patients. Download list of patients based on system codes for diabetics. Begin completing records during initial chart review.	Jones
	A.2	Develop method to put laboratory and visit data directly into the database.	Jones
	A.3	Test visit sheet printed from database with two physicians on the team.	Jones
B: Self-Management	B.1	Dr. Smith trial self-management goal setting process with five patients during next week.	Smith
	B.2	Test incorporating the self-management process into the diabetic visit flow sheet.	Smith
	B.3	Distribute information to diabetic patients on self-management.	Marshall
	B.4	Develop 2-hour session to educate staff and prepare for broader rollout of collaborative goal setting.	Marshall
	B.5	Schedule a documented encounter at least annually to promote patient identification of their appropriate self-management opportunities.	Rogers
C: Decision Support	C.1	Develop electronic prompts to communicate evidenced-based standards based on ADA guidelines.	Allen
	C.2	Recently established monthly QA review as part of the faculty meeting.	Allen
D: Delivery System Design	D.1	Test with two patients a letter to inform diabetics of the redesign of the diabetic care system. Requested them to schedule an appointment if they have not visited in the last six months.	Rogers
	D.2	Established a protocol for routine HbA1c measurements.	James
	D.3	Test a system for blood pressure documentation and tracking with protocols for identification and drug management.	James
	D.4	Develop an intervention program that advocates regular foot exams for all diabetics and protective foot care behaviors for diabetics with high-risk feet.	James

Exhibit 1.1 shows example of the documentation for one of the first PDSA Cycles completed. The team met over lunch every Friday during the next two months to work on the plan and study of the PDSA Cycles.

(continued)

EXHIBIT 1.1 DOCUMENTATION FOR INITIAL SELF-MANAGEMENT PDSA CYCLE

PDSA Cycle B.1 Self-management

Objective: Begin to understand the issues involved in implementing self-management practices with all diabetic patients.

Plan

Question: Can the providers incorporate self-management methods into the visit of a diabetic patient? Will patients accept self-management?

Predictions: There will be some initial problems with overrunning appointments, but visit can be adjusted to accommodate. Most patients will be receptive to collaborative goal setting.

Plan for test: Develop interviewing tool. Dr. Smith will trial self-management goal setting process with five patients during next week.

Data collection: Ms. Rogers reviews Dr. Smith's notes from visit. Receptionist interviews patients on their reaction to offer of self-management. Dr. Smith summarizes his perceptions of the process after completing with five patients.

Do: Dr. Smith offered collaborative goal setting with five patients during a two-day period. One patient was not interested in participating. Script was modified after visit with second patient.

FIGURE 1.8 Run Charts of Key Measures for Diabetes Improvement Project

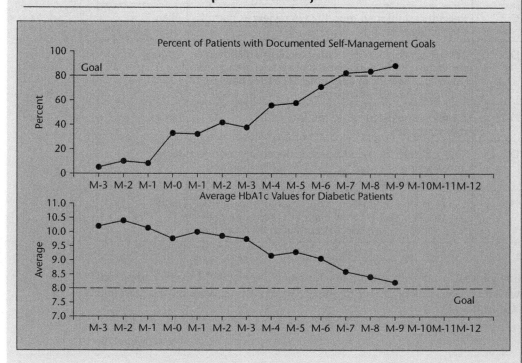

Study: Three of the five patients left the visit with an agreed goal to be accomplished during the next month. Four of the five patients were appreciative of the opportunity and one patient was delighted with his involvement in setting a goal. Dr. Smith has some other ideas to modify the interviewing tool and for better incorporating the methods into the visit by modifying the visit flow sheet.

Act: Dr. Smith will continue to use the revised interviewing tool with all diabetic patients. Dr. James will try with one patient next week.

The team had an offsite meeting two months later to review progress on the project and make additional plans. They reviewed their aim and the run charts (Figure 1.8) of their two global measures related to the aim. They reviewed their progress on each of the components of the care model. For the next three months, they decided to concentrate on delivery system design and patient self-management. Table 1.4 shows some of the PDSA Cycles planned for continued testing and implementation of the changes.

Table 1.4   Some Additional Plans for PDSA Cycles

Concept	PDSA Cycle #	Description of PDSA Cycle	Responsibility
A: Clinical Information System	A.5	Test use of registry for follow-up phone calls by office staff, office initiated scheduling of visits with diabetics needing routine screening, and a reminder system for office-initiated patient notification of annual foot exams.	Jones
B: Self-Management	B.11	Update patient education material for use in clinic. Monitor patient satisfaction with education material and improved where appropriate.	Smith
	B.12	Worked with HMOs to make it possible for all patients to receive education regardless of health plan coverage.	Marshall
	B.13	Develop the concept of a clinical educator to lead self-management with providers, staff, and patients for all chronic diseases.	Marshall
C: Decision Support	C.8	Develop a set of decision support information (ASA, general guidelines to specialists, diabetes medication information and dietary recommendations) and made available in every examination room.	Allen
	C.9	Begin offering smoking cessation courses and document patient response to the offer.	Allen
	C.10	Test an annual meeting for the entire care team to assess their working relationships and make the appropriate improvements to maximize cooperation and the application of the best clinical expertise.	Allen
D: Delivery System Design	D.7	Develop prewritten prescriptions for glucometers and medical shoes to aid in the wording requirements for Medicare reimbursement.	James

(continued)

The team continued testing, adapting, and then implementing specific ideas for each of the components of the Chronic Care Model. They reviewed their progress with the organization's senior leaders in the fifth month of the project. Their measures (Figure 1.8) confirmed the progress of the team. The senior leaders offered to get involved in the *Community Resources and Policies* and the *Organization of Health Care* components of the care model.

The team held a second meeting with their senior leaders after the ninth month of the project. They had accomplished their self-management goal and predicted accomplishment of the clinical outcome measure with the next two months. Plans were begun to spread this work with diabetic patients to other chronic diseases.

SUMMARY

This chapter introduced the Model for Improvement as a road map for execution of an improvement project. The important connection of the use of data with the model was emphasized:

1. To answer: How do we know that a change is an improvement?
2. To provide for learning in PDSA cycles.

The rest of the book will assume the Model for Improvement as the backdrop for the tools and methods used to learn from data. A listing of the methods and tools used in improvement work was included in Tables 1.1 and 1.2.

The case studies in Chapter Thirteen illustrate the use of the Model for Improvement as a framework for the improvement project. Most of the case studies are focused on a portion of the project that emphasizes the use of data for learning on the project. Case Study F on readmissions presents the three questions of the model and describes three PDSA cycles on the project.

KEY TERMS

Aim statement

Implement changes

Model for Improvement

Plan, Do, Study, Act Cycle (PDSA)

Run chart

Shewhart charts

Test and adapt changes

## CHAPTER 2

USING DATA FOR IMPROVEMENT

This book is about using data for improvement; thus, this chapter provides the foundation for the entire book. In this chapter, as we focus on working with data for improvement, we will also make connections to other major ways in which data are traditionally used in health care to include accountability and research.

Improvement projects are about testing, adapting, implementing, and spreading changes. Data and measurement play important, but supportive, roles. Some of the important uses of data and measurement include: using key measures to assess progress toward the project's aim; using specific measures for learning during PDSA cycles; using balancing measures to assess whether the system as a whole is being improved; and using data from the system to focus improvement and refine changes.

In support of the use of data for improvement this chapter will aid the reader in: identifying the role and characteristics of data as it is used for improvement, for accountability or for research; identifying basic types of data; identifying outcome, process and balancing measures for improvement projects; developing operational definitions; sampling data for improvement projects; distinguishing between the use of data in enumerative and analytic studies and analysis and presentation of data for improvement.

Throughout this book we will use the term *measure* where others may mean the same thing using such terms such as *indicator, metric, key process variable (KPV), key quality characteristic (KQC)*, or *critical to quality (CTQ)*.[1]

WHAT DOES THE CONCEPT OF DATA MEAN?

Data are documented observations or the results of performing a measurement process. The concept of data refers to strings or patterns of characters (for example computer bits) that describe some aspect of the world. The availability of data offers opportunities to obtain information and knowledge through inquiry, analysis, or summarization of these strings or characters. Data can be obtained by perception (for example, observation) or by performing a measurement process.

Observations come from our unique perceptions using our senses of sight, taste, smell, hearing, and touch. As Figure 2.1 shows, observations are a valuable source of data, but there are some weaknesses with relying only on observations when learning or testing changes for improvement:

---

[1]Lloyd, R., *Quality Health Care: A Guide to Developing and Using Indicators*, Boston: Jones and Bartlett, 2004.

FIGURE 2.1   Sources of Data

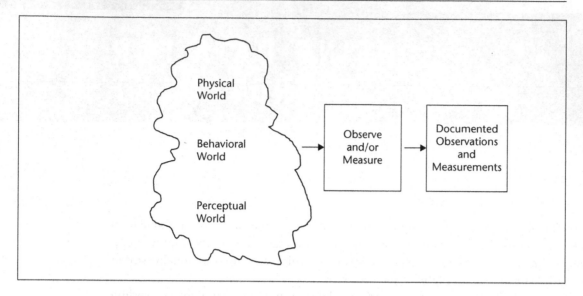

1. Recent observations tend to be more heavily weighted in our minds than observations from the more distant past.
2. New observations depend on previous observations. If we are used to a temperature of 30 degrees, a temperature of 60 degrees feels warm. But if we are used to a temperature of 95 degrees, 60 degrees feels cool.
3. Our minds automatically filter perceptions. Sometimes we observe what we want or expect to observe.

Because of the first three issues, improvement teams learn better from data based on measurements than on observations. Measuring a patient's temperature may help us learn more and faster than the patient's perception of whether or not she has a fever.

This doesn't mean that data from observation isn't useful; sometimes it's very important to learning and improvement. Recording data from patients' perceptions of their pain levels, for instance, could be a valuable aid to learning about and improving patient pain levels. And many times, no measurement process is available. Combining observation and measurement data is a useful approach to obtaining data for improvement. For example: measurement on cycle time for admitting patients can be combined with patient and staff observations related to their experience of the process.

How Are Data Used?

The focus of this book is on using data for improvement. Improving health care processes is difficult to do without some type of feedback to help figure out where to focus, or to tell whether changes actually improved the system of interest. Unfortunately, getting data for improvement can be a challenge. Solberg, Mosser, and McDonald suggest that getting data for improvement is made more difficult by confusion between data for improvement, judgment, and research.[2] Table 2.1 summarizes some key differences between data designed to be used these three ways.

---

[2]Solberg, L. I., Mosser G., and McDonald S., "The Three Faces of Performance Measurement: Improvement, Accountability, and Research." *Journal on Quality Improvement*, 1987, *23*(3), 135–147.

Table 2.1   Data for Improvement, Accountability, Research

Aspect	Improvement	Judgment or Accountability	Clinical Research
Aim	Improvement of care process, system, and outcomes	Judgment, choice, reassurance, spur for change	New generalizable knowledge
Methods			
Test observability	Test observable	No test, evaluate current performance	Test blinded
Bias	Accept consistent bias	Measure and adjust to reduce bias	Design to eliminate bias
Sample size	"Just enough" data, small sequential samples	Obtain 100% of available and relevant data	"Just in case" data
Flexibility of hypothesis	Hypothesis flexible; changes as learning takes place	No hypothesis	Fixed hypothesis
Testing strategy	Sequential tests	No tests	One large test
Determining if change is improvement	Run charts or Shewhart charts	No focus on change	Hypothesis tests (T-tests, F-tests, Chi-square), p-value
Confidentiality of data	Data used only by those involved in the improvement	Data available for public consumption	Research subjects' identities protected

Data used for improvement are typically collected by those working within the health care system to observe process performance, obtain ideas for improvement, test changes to see if they are improvements, and to see whether improvements are maintained. When we are collecting and using data for improvement we are observing the changes we are testing. This enables us to adjust our changes and also adjust our hypothesis as we work incrementally toward improvement by small sequential tests of the change. When in the improvement mode various types of bias can exist in our data. We attempt to design our data collection so that the bias is stable. Thus, if bias exists in our process, we can assume it is there all the time. If changes tested yield improvement, then they have done so in the face of these biases. When collecting data for improvement we are aware that we are doing so while also providing ongoing care to our patients and our community. Therefore, when using data for improvement, we try to develop measures from data that are already available or to develop a few new measures that are relatively easy to obtain. In improvement, small samples are used, as the strategy is to obtain just enough data to plan the next small sequential test of a change. Run or Shewhart charts are used to determine if changes yield improvement.

Often concerns about reliability and validity surface when dealing with data. A useful reference related to reliability and validity for accountability and research data is Judd, Smith, and Kidder.[3] When using data for improvement unknown biases may exist. We collect and display samples over time as a means of dealing with bias rather than performing

---

[3]Judd, C., Smith, E., and Kidder, L., *Research Methods in Social Relations*, 6th ed., Chapter 3, "Measurement: From Abstract Concepts to Concrete Representations," New York: Holt, Rinehart and Winston, 1991.

Table 2.2 Useful Aspects of Measurement for Improvement

Measure Aspect	Definition
High priority for maximizing the health of populations	Measure addresses a process or outcome that is strategically important to maximize the public's health. Medical condition defined by high prevalence, incidence, mortality, morbidity, or disability.
Demonstrated variation in care and gap between what is known through science and done in health care	Measure addresses an aspect of health care for which there is a known gap in what is evidenced-based care and current care and quantifies the potential for improvement. Demonstrates progress in quality of care that closes the gap identified in the Charter.
Based on established clinical recommendations	Process Measures: Evidence that process measure improves health outcomes. Outcome Measures: Evidence that there are improvements (change concepts) that health care organizations can make to improve the outcome.
Meaningful and interpretable to multiple users	Can the health care organization use the information generated to improve quality of care? Progress on the measures is reportable in a manner interpretable and meaningful to health center staff, consumer-led governing boards, DHHS/HRSA.
Well-defined specifications	Measure is operationally defined: numerator, denominator, data sources, and collection methodology, method of measurement.
Useful variation in data	Data on the measure are not all 0s or 100%. Variation in data is useful for learning.
Feasibility	Data required for the measure available through electronic registry system with reasonable effort. Cost of data collection and reporting is justified by the potential improvements in care and outcomes that result from the act of measurement.
Acceptable to the patient population	Measure is acceptable and meaningful to diverse populations.

the tests for reliability and validity necessary for accountability and research data. When using data for improvement, concerns about reliability and validity are translated into practical terms. Some of the more useful attributes to think about when developing data for improvement are summarized and defined in Table 2.2.[4] These attributes include developing measures that are: of high priority when working to improve patient care; actionable; meaningful for multiple users; acceptable to patients; respect confidentiality; are feasible to obtain; use established clinical recommendations; reflect known gaps between current practice and science; follow established clinical recommendations; and use well-defined specifications or current industry standards.

Data for judgment or accountability are collected first and foremost for the purpose of evaluating or judging the performance of a provider, medical group, or organization, rather than for improving a process. These data are often collected for an external customer, such as a payer or regulator. When using data for accountability a hypothesis is not being tested; rather, performance is being evaluated. When collecting data for accountability one typically tries to use 100% of the relevant available data rather than rely upon small samples. Substantial resources, understandably, are invested to measure and account for factors, such as severity or risk, that may bias the data. Risk or severity adjusting usually takes time, and adds complexity and cost to the data collection process and is not

---

[4]Adapted from Center for Medicare and Medicaid Services, *Doctors' Office Quality Project and Performance Measurement Coordinating Council*, 2006.

FIGURE 2.2   Measurement for Judgment Versus Improvement

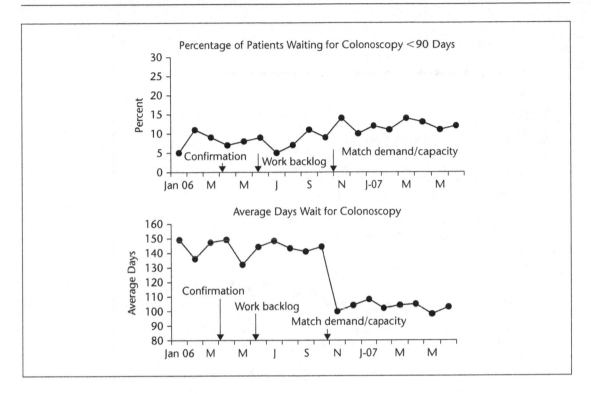

without controversy[5] (see later discussion on case-mix adjustment in this chapter). All of this means that data collected for accountability are typically more difficult to obtain than data for improvement purposes. In addition, data collected for accountability are designed to evaluate, compare, or judge and therefore may not always be useful for improvement purposes. Although it may be useful in terms of accountability to know that only 62% of patients needing a colonoscopy waited less than 90 days, that data may not be very helpful to the improvement team that is testing changes to reduce waiting time. Tracking actual waiting time as the team tests changes will be more helpful than solely tracking the percentage meeting the waiting time standard. Figure 2.2 illustrates this principle.

Measurement for judgment may result in data that are often recorded as 100% or 0. These data are not useful for teams trying to learn from the measure. In the example in Figure 2.3 it is evident that patients were counseled regarding smoking cessation 100% of the time each month, a requirement in the organization. The team wanting to help people to stop smoking will not find these data useful as they work to improve smoking cessation. They need to see variation in data in order to tell whether their changes are improvements. They selected a different measure, one of more benefit to patients and more use to the team as they test changes. Using the new measure, the percentage of patients who have not smoked in two months, they had a strong degree of belief that their changes yielded improvement. If they had used the percentage of patients counseled it would have been impossible to learn whether their changes were improvements.

Another common practice with data for judgment is the use of percentile ranking. Though useful for understanding how the organization compares to others, percentile rankings are less helpful in improvement. Percentiles are influenced not only by the

---

[5]Nicholl, J., "Case Mix Adjustment in Non-Randomized Observational Studies: The Constant Risk Fallacy," *The Journal of Epidemiology and Community Health*, 2007, *61*, 1010–1013.

FIGURE 2.3 Moving from Judgment to Improvement Measures

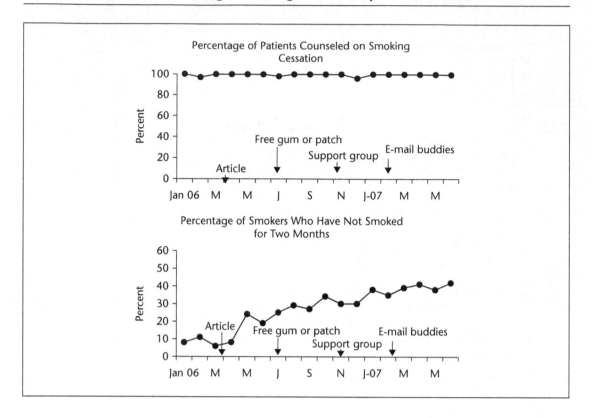

performance of one organization, but by all that are included in the comparison. Thus, it is possible to see an increase in an organization's percentile ranking, not because that organization improved, but because another organization's performance degraded. This becomes a confusing situation for improvement teams as they test changes. Did the improvement in their organization's percentile ranking occur because of the changes the team tried or because of the poor performance of others in the comparison pool? In the following example, Figure 2.4, the team found it much more helpful while testing changes to track the actual average patient satisfaction in their organization rather than the percentile ranking.

Some tip-offs that one is working with data for judgment rather than data for improvement include: data not viewed over time, the use of percentiles, case-mix adjustment, and a measure that yields nearly all 0s or all 100%. The difference between measurement for judgment and improvement is important to consider when developing operational definitions for measures (described later in this chapter).

The use of data is very important for clinical research. When collecting and using data for research every effort is made to identify and control for important forms of bias. Issues about the validity and precision of measures are an important part of the research. When collecting and using data for research we aren't able to observe the impact of the change and learn from it while we are testing because the test is typically blinded to reduce potential biases. Research can be a challenge to develop and fund. Researchers may have only one shot at the research project they've worked so hard to develop. When asked whether or not they should also collect research participants' weight, even if they can think of no reason for doing so, they're likely to collect the data "just in case."

FIGURE 2.4   Using Percentile Rankings

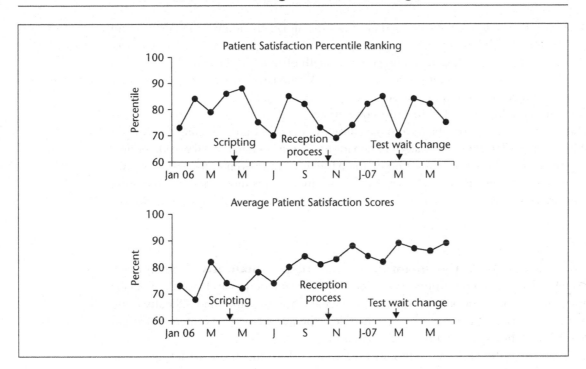

Experience in health care with accountability data and research studies can prove both an advantage and a challenge when it comes to using data for improvement.[6] Some of these challenges include:

1. Many clinicians will not want to collect data when working to improve a process because they assume that they must use the rigorous, expensive, time-consuming data collection methods necessary for research.

2. Other clinicians may discount or dismiss data others have collected to improve a health care process because it is not of "research-level quality." This attitude dampens enthusiasm for learning and improvement.

3. Some clinicians are very committed to collecting data for learning and improvement but believe that "research-level quality" data collection is necessary for improvement. The cost and time involved in using research-level data collection constructs in an improvement project makes improvement so slow it can effectively halt vital improvement work.

4. Most of the data collected to help improve medical processes will be far too crude and specific to meet a payer's or regulator's need for data for accountability. Mixing a system designed to collect data for improvement and a system reporting to external sources for accountability creates chaos with neither purpose satisfied. If clinicians suspect data being collected for improvement will really be used for accountability, data may be difficult to obtain.

5. Collecting data for accountability is an important social responsibility, but these data are rarely specific or timely enough to be useful for process improvement. Sometimes the data may point out that performance in a particular clinical area is undesirable, but the data doesn't help to determine what to change about the current process to yield improvement. Accountability data can eventually be used to track the results of an improvement effort or a series of improvement efforts.

[6]Randolph, G., Provost, L. et al., "Model for Improvement—Part Two: Measurement and Feedback for Quality Improvement Efforts," *Pediatric Quality*, August, 2009, *56*(4), 779–798.

Some guidelines for collecting data for improvement include:

- Be sure to have a few key measures that clarify the aim of the improvement effort and make it tangible. These should be regularly reported throughout the life of the project (daily, weekly, or monthly, depending on the length of time for the project).
- Be careful about overdoing process measures. A balance of outcome, process, and balancing measures is important (see discussion in next section).
- Plot data visually on the key measures over time.
- Make use of existing databases and data already collected for developing measures.
- Whenever feasible, integrate data collection for measurement into the daily work routine.
- Be aware that the second question of the Model for Improvement—"How will we know that a change is an improvement?"—usually requires more than one measure. A balanced set of three to eight measures will ensure that this question can be answered.

Types of Data

The two basic types of data are **quantitative** (numeric) and **qualitative** (nonnumeric). Most qualitative data comes from observations, but measurements can be qualitative (for example, blood type). Examples of qualitative data are "the customer had difficulty using the form," "the appointment was not on schedule," "people seemed very interested in the health fair," or "the assessment tool was not completed."

Though quantitative data are usually preferred for learning, there are a number of reasons to use qualitative data:

- Quantitative data can be difficult or expensive to obtain.
- The information of interest is so dramatic that qualitative data are sufficient to meet all needs.
- Observations of people best describe the phenomena of interest.

Rating scales can be used to obtain data on personal experience. Figure 2.5 contains three such rating scales. Following the figure are some examples of questions and statements that could be used with the scales.[7] It should be noted that the response can be put

FIGURE 2.5   Simple Scales for Turning Personal Experience into Data

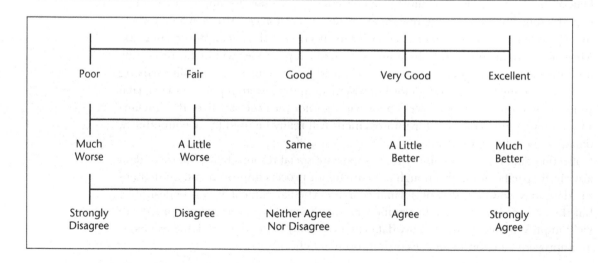

[7]Langley, G., Moen, R., Nolan, K., Nolan, T., Norman, C., and Provost, L., *The Improvement Guide*, 2nd ed., San Francisco: Jossey-Bass, 2009, Appendix B, 422–423.

anywhere on the scale; it need not be limited to the five discrete labels. The scales are provided to establish a basic level of measurement for almost any application. Recent research has dispelled some of the myths in using these scales and shown their usefulness, even with traditional statistical analysis.[8] These qualitative scales can be converted to quantitative data by establishing a point scale that corresponds to the word scale (for example, 1–5). These scales, along with common measurements such as time and cost, will allow those improving quality in service or administrative applications to use quantitative data as readily as their manufacturing counterparts.

Examples of Questions Used with the Poor–Excellent Scale

- How would you rate your health in the last four weeks?
- How would you rate the relationship you have with your therapist?
- How would you rate the courtesy shown to you during your visit at this clinic?
- How would you rate the cleanliness of your room during your hospital stay?

Examples of Questions Used with the Worse–Better Scale

- How would you rate your overall health now compared to four weeks ago?
- As a resident of this senior living community, how would you rate your social life now compared to three months ago?
- How would you rate the ease of use of scheduling process A compared to scheduling process B?
- How would you rate the new medication ordering process compared to the old one?

Examples of Statements Used with the Agree–Disagree Scale

- Our providers welcome questions from patients and family.
- It is easy to find your way around our facility.
- Your health care team members always knew what one another were doing.
- Our pharmacy always has your medication ready when we say we will.

Traditionally in the science of improvement, there are three types of data: **classification**, **count**, and **continuous**. Classification and count data are often grouped together as attribute data to distinguish them from continuous data, and continuous data are often referred to as variables data. For *classification* data, attributes are recorded in one of two categories or classes. Examples of these classes are conforming units/nonconforming units, go/no-go, complete/incomplete, pass/fail, or good/bad. *Count* data focuses on attributes that occur that are unusual or undesirable: number of mistakes, number of accidents, or number of no-shows. At times data are counted with a different intent. Data are counted to obtain the volume or amount of a particular entity, typically workload or productivity, such as a hospital census, the number of visits to a clinic, or the volume of lab tests completed. These counts are treated as *continuous* data because of their intent. Table 2.3 outlines the relationship between qualitative and quantitative data and the three types of data used in improvement.

Table 2.3   Relationship of Nature of Data to Improvement Terms

Nature of Data	Continuous	Attribute
Quantitative	Continuous	Count
Qualitative		Classification

[8]Carifio, J., and Perla, R., "Ten Common Misunderstandings, Misconceptions, Persistent Myths and Urban Legends about Likert Scales and Likert Response Formats and Their Antidotes," *Journal of Social Sciences*, 2007, *3*, 106–116.

Traditional measurement theory categorizes data as nominal, ordinal, interval, and ratio. Table 2.4 briefly describes these terms.

Figure 2.6 shows the relationship of data that come from observation or measurement to these traditional categorizations of data.

Table 2.5 compares the traditional measurement scale typology (nominal, ordinal, interval, and ratio) to types of data as treated in improvement and then to the type of recommended Shewhart chart. (These charts are described in Chapter Five). Velleman

Table 2.4   Traditional Data Typologies

Traditional Categories of Data	Description	Health Care Examples
Nominal	Data are non-numeric and placed in distinct and totally separate categories. These data are in categories that have no order.	Smokers/Nonsmokers Gender, Ethnicity (such as African American, Asian, Caucasian)
Ordinal	The data suggest a certain order. These data are categorized and may be ranked in some numerically meaningful way on a scale. With ordinal data the order matters but not the difference between values (e.g., a patient satisfaction rating of 4 does not mean the patient is twice as satisfied as a patient rating satisfaction at a 2).	Some patient satisfaction scales Rankings
Interval	Data are measured along a scale in which each position is an equal distance from the next on the scale. With interval data the difference between two values is meaningful (e.g., the difference between a weight of 120 and 110 is the same difference as between 90 and 70 pounds.).	Some patient satisfaction scales Temperature Personal experience scales
Ratio	In a ratio scale, numbers can be compared as multiples of one another. In addition, the number zero has meaning. (10 grams is twice as much as 5 grams. We can have 0 grams.)	Height, weight, blood sugar Waiting time in days

FIGURE 2.6   Relationship Between Nature of Data and Data Typology

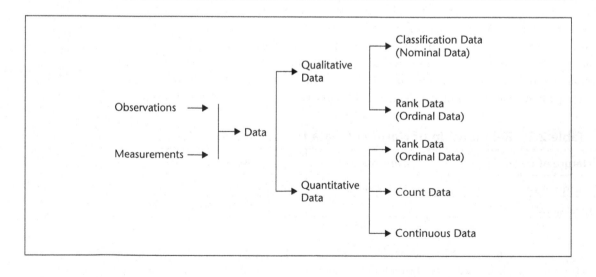

Table 2.5 Comparison of Traditional Data Categories with Science of Improvement Categories

Traditional Categories of Data	Science of Improvement Data Groupings		
	Continuous (Variable) Data	Attribute Data	
		Count	Classification
Nominal			P Chart
Ordinal	X Chart, Median Chart		P Chart
Interval	$\bar{X}$, S Chart, X Chart		
Ratio	$\bar{X}$, S Chart, X Chart	U or C Chart	

and Wilkinson address traditional measurement scales and conclude that additional flexibility in measurement typology is needed in order to more effectively learn from data.[9]

For continuous data, a measured numerical value is recorded: a dimension, physical attribute, or calculated number. Some type of measurement device or scale is required to obtain the data. Continuous data include measurements of time, money, physical properties, scaled data, and throughput (workload).

When a choice exists, continuous data will be more useful for learning about the impact of changes tested than will count or classification data. For example, a team working to reduce colonoscopy waiting time tested a number of changes (see Figure 2.2). The percentage of patients who waited 90 days or less showed no improvement month after month. The team was discouraged. One of the team members noted that staff working in the clinic reported that waiting time seemed better and that patients complained less about waiting time. The team decided to look at another measure, the average monthly waiting time per patient. They learned that although the percentage of patients waiting 90 days or longer had not dropped, the average waiting time per patient had dropped from a median of 144 days to 104 days; a substantial improvement. Their changes were resulting in improvement. The team could better see this improvement using continuous data than they could by using classification data. For an additional example, see Figure 2.23 near the end of this chapter.

We also commonly use the terms **global project measure** and **PDSA measure** when using data in improvement work. Global measures focus at the project level and are maintained throughout the life of the improvement project. For example, the percentage of patients experiencing perioperative harm may be an appropriate global measure for a project improving perioperative safety. Other measures are done on an as needed basis as part of PDSA Cycles for diagnosis and for assessment of the changes tested. For example, in a perioperative safety project, the percentage of patients assessed for bleeding risk preoperatively might be a PDSA Cycle measure.

A perioperative safety team used the following as global measures for their improvement efforts:

[9]Velleman, P., and Wilkinson, L., "Nominal, Ordinal, Interval and Ratio Typologies Are Misleading," *The American Statistician*, 1993, *47*(1), 65–72.

- Percentage of patients harmed
- Percentage of unplanned returns to the operating room
- Percentage of unplanned surgical readmission
- Percentage of patients with on-time prophylactic antibiotic administration
- Percentage of patients with appropriate DVT prophylaxis
- Percentage of patients with appropriate Beta Blocker use

In an improvement project it is useful to include measures of the three types mentioned in the last section: **outcome**, **process**, and **balancing measures**. The perioperative safety project's measures were organized as follows in Table 2.6: Table 2.7 provides some of the dimensions of system performance a team could consider to develop a good balancing measure(s). The concept of a family of outcome, process, and balancing measures for an improvement project is discussed in more detail at the end of this chapter.

Table 2.6   Outcome, Process, and Balancing Measures

Type of Measure	Description	Perioperative Example
Outcome	<ul><li>The voice of the customer or patient.</li><li>How is the system performing?</li><li>What is the result?</li></ul>	<ul><li>Percentage of patients harmed</li><li>Percentage unplanned returns to the operating room</li><li>Percentage unplanned surgical readmission</li></ul>
Process	<ul><li>The voice of the workings of the process.</li><li>Logically linked to obtaining the outcomes.</li><li>Address how key parts or steps of the system are performing.</li></ul>	<ul><li>Percentage of patients with on-time antibiotic administration</li><li>Percentage of patients with appropriate DVT prophylaxis</li><li>Percentage of patients with appropriate Beta Blocker use</li></ul>
Balancing	<ul><li>Look at a system from different directions or dimensions.</li><li>What happened to the system as we improved the outcome and process measures?</li><li>Could relate to unintended consequences or competing explanations for project success.</li></ul>	<ul><li>Volume of surgical workload</li><li>Percentage of prophylactic antibiotics appropriately discontinued</li></ul>

Table 2.7   Dimensions of System Performance

Dimensions of System Performance
Outcome (quality, timeliness)
Transaction (volume, number of patients)
Productivity (cycle time, efficiency, utilization, flow, capacity, demand)
Cost (charges, staff hours, materials)
Appropriateness (validity, usefulness)
Patient satisfaction (surveys, complaints)
Staff satisfaction (surveys, absenteeism, turnover)

THE IMPORTANCE OF OPERATIONAL DEFINITIONS

If you are going to obtain data useful for improving a health care process, that data needs to be of use in learning when changes tested are an improvement. Earlier in this chapter we addressed the importance of ensuring that measures be useful for improvement. Many measures start as accountability measures and, though useful for judgment, they are of limited usefulness for improvement. (See the section "How Are Data Used?" in this chapter for further discussion.) If the data are collected differently by different people, or differently each time the data are collected, it makes it hard to know whether changes in the data are due to the changes tested or from inconsistencies in data collection. To learn from data, you need an agreement as to how the data will be collected in order to maintain data collection consistency.

An **operational definition** is the term used for such an agreement. An operational definition is one that gives communicable meaning to a concept (such as error, waiting time, and appropriate care) by specifying how the concept is applied within a particular set of circumstances. An important component of an operational definition is the statement of the measurement process used. The physicist Percy Bridgeman was one of the first to point out that a concept has no communicable meaning until it is known how it will be used in a particular application or operation. He noted: "The true meaning of a term is to be found by observing what a man does with it, not what he says about it."[10]

Similarly, Walter Shewhart wrote: "Being free from grease is not rigorously definite; to some people it means clean enough to eat on; to the experimental physicist it may in some instances mean baked out at a high temperature under vacuum."[11]

Operational definitions are used in collecting health care data.[12] Often an operational definition is converted into a checklist or form that delineates what is meant by "appropriate" or "complete" and helps multiple data collectors to remain consistent in their use of the operational definition. One hospital wanted to track and improve appropriate pain assessment and used the definition in Table 2.8.

Developing an operational definition requires agreement on two things:[13]

1. A method of measurement or test
2. A set of criteria for judgment

Table 2.8 Operational Definition Appropriate Pain Assessment

Pain is appropriately assessed and documented if defined as:	Source of data:
A. Documentation using 0–10 pain scale upon admission **B.** Documented reassessment within 4–12 hours if admission level 3 or less **C.** Documented reassessment within 2 hours while awake if admission level >3, and/or receiving active pain/nausea Rx **D.** Documented intervention to initiate Rx for level >5 on any two consecutive assessments	Daily Patient Care Flow Record and Notes, physician orders, MAR
Documented reassessment appropriate for the given intervention	

[10]Bridgeman, P. W., *The Logic of Modern Physics*, New York: MacMillan, 1927, 7.

[11]Shewhart, W. A., *Statistical Method from the Viewpoint of Quality Control*, Washington, D.C.: The Graduate School of the Dept. of Agriculture, 1939.

[12]Lloyd, *Quality Health Care*, 71–75.

[13]Deming, W. E., *Out of the Crisis*, Cambridge, MA: Massachusetts Institute of Technology, 1986, Chapter 3.

Measurements could be for physical characteristics, like pulmonary capacity and make use of a measurement device. The operational definition then needs to bring clarity to which device(s) will be used, how they will be used, how the users will know the devices' precision (calibration and statistical stability) and to what degree of discretion the data will be collected (that is, whole number or one or more decimal place?)

A set of criteria for judgment may be necessary in some situations. What constitutes an error, a fall, or a delay? Sometimes a measurement is taken and converted to an attribute that was either possessed or not possessed when the measurement was obtained. For example, to operationally define "late" time is measured in an agreed-upon fashion. Some criteria are still needed to judge at what point "late" is declared. What are the agreed-upon criteria for deciding something is "late" or "appropriate"? Agreed-upon criteria for judging such concepts are crucial in order to learn whether or not a change tested was an improvement. An organization wanting to track progress in improving the severity of symptoms for people with asthma formatted their operational definition as a checklist as seen at Table 2.9.

Operational definitions abound in health care.[14] An example of an operational definition of providing aspirin at arrival from the National Hospital Quality Measures (Centers for Medicare & Medicaid Services and the Joint Commission) follows in Exhibit 2.1.[15] This example illustrates some of the detailed complexity that must be addressed to have a clear operational definition of many concepts and measures in health care systems.

The example shown in Exhibit 2.2 provides a starting point for developing measures for an improvement project.

Table 2.9   Asthma Severity Operational Definition

Asthma Severity Diagnosis					
Rate symptoms/signs in each category; Severity Code corresponds with highest cell checked.					
Daytime cough, wheeze, SOB, or chest tightness	Nighttime cough, wheeze, SOB, or chest tightness	B2-Agonist Use	Impact on activity	FEV1 / PEF	Code Severity
☐ All the time	☐ Frequent	☐ 1–2x/wk	☐ Interferes with any activity	☐ <60%	**☐ 4 Severe Persistent**
☐ Daily	☐ >5x/month	☐ 3–6x/wk	☐ Interferes with moderate activity	☐ 60–80%	**☐ 3 Moderate Persistent**
☐ 3–6x/week	☐ 3–4x/month	☐ 7x/wk	☐ Only with a lot of activity	☐ >80%	**☐ 2 Mild Persistent**
☐ < 2x/week	☐ <2x/month	☐ 7x/wk	☐ Not at all unless an attack	☐ >80%	**☐ 1 Mild Intermittent**

---

[14]Lloyd, *Quality Health Care*, 71–75.

[15]The Joint Commission and Centers for Medicare and Medicaid Services, Specifications Manual for National Hospital Quality Measures. Version 3.2c, October 2010. This manual is periodically updated by The Joint Commission. Users of the Specifications Manual for Joint Commission National Quality Core Measures must update their software and associated documentation based on the published manual production time lines.

EXHIBIT 2.1 OPERATIONAL DEFINITION ASPIRIN AT ARRIVAL

Performance Measure Name: Aspirin at Arrival

Description: Acute myocardial infarction (AMI) patients who received aspirin within 24 hours before or after hospital arrival

Rationale: The early use of aspirin in patients with acute myocardial infarction results in a significant reduction in adverse events and subsequent mortality. The benefits of aspirin therapy on mortality are comparable to fibrinolytic therapy. The combination of aspirin and fibrinolytics provides additive benefits for patients with ST-elevation myocardial infarction (ISIS-2, 1988). Aspirin is also effective in patients with non-ST-elevation myocardial infarction (Theroux, 1988; RISC Group, 1990). National guidelines strongly recommend early aspirin for patients hospitalized with AMI (Antman, 2004; Anderson, 2007).

Type of Measure: Process

Improvement Noted As: An increase in the rate

Numerator Statement: AMI patients who received aspirin within 24 hours before or after hospital arrival

Included Populations: Not Applicable

Excluded Populations: None

Data Elements: Aspirin Received Within 24 Hours Before or After Hospital Arrival

Denominator Statement: AMI patients

Included Populations:

Discharges with an *ICD-9-CM Principal Diagnosis Code* for AMI as defined in Appendix A, Table 1.1 Specifications Manual for National Hospital Inpatient Quality Measures Discharges 10-0-10 (4Q10) through 03-31-11 (1Q11) AMI-1-1

Excluded Populations:

- Patients less than 18 years of age
- Patients who have a Length of Stay greater than 120 days
- Patients with *Comfort Measures Only* documented on day of or day after arrival
- Patients enrolled in clinical trials
- Patients discharged on day of arrival
- Patients discharged or transferred to another hospital for inpatient care on day of or day after arrival
- Patients who left against medical advice or discontinued care on day of or day after arrival
- Patients who expired on day of or day after arrival
- Patients discharged or transferred to a federal health care facility on day of or day after arrival
- Patients with a documented *Reason for No Aspirin on Arrival*

Data Elements:

Admission Date; Arrival Date; Birthdate; Clinical Trial; Comfort Measures Only; Discharge Date

Discharge Status; ICD-9-CM Principal Diagnosis Code; Reason for No Aspirin on Arrival

Risk Adjustment: No

Data Collection Approach: Retrospective data sources for required data elements include administrative data and medical records.

Data Accuracy: Variation may exist in the assignment of ICD-9-CM codes; therefore, coding practices may require evaluation to ensure consistency.

Measure Analysis Suggestions: None

Sampling: Yes, please refer to the measure to set specific sampling requirements; for additional information see the Population and Sampling Specifications section.

Data Reported As: Aggregate rate generated from count data reported as a proportion

EXHIBIT 2.2   EXAMPLE OF FORM FOR DEVELOPING IMPROVEMENT PROJECT MEASURES

Form for Developing Improvement Project Measures

1. Basic Information

   Improvement project name:

   Name of this measure:

   Objective of this measure:

   What is the numerical target or goal for this measure?

   Is this an outcome, process or balancing measure for this improvement project?

2. Operational Definition of the Measure

   What actual data elements need to be collected? Define both numerator and denominator if appropriate. Is this definition different from standard definitions used in other places? List inclusions or exclusions to the data you will collect. What identifying information you will capture with the data (for example, coding, location)?

   Will you sample to obtain the data? If so, describe your sampling plan.

   For each data element, define the measurement unit and degree of precision (for example, is length of stay in days, hours, or minutes? Is pain scale captured in whole numbers or is it possible to record a 3.5?). Will you round the data?

   If your data involve making a judgment such as "late" or "inappropriate," list the criteria you will be using to make that judgment.

3. Administration

   Where are the data located (for example, encounter form, chart, data base, specific computer system, file)?

   How frequently will you measure? When? (for example, daily, weekly, monthly)

   Who will collect the data?

   How will you display this data, that is, which graph(s) will you use?

   Who will make the graph(s)?

   Who will review the graphs and in what setting? How often?

4. Additional Information

   Do you have baseline data for this measure? If yes, what is it and what time frame is it from? Was it collected exactly the same way that you will be collecting the data for this measure now? If not, how was it defined?

   Improvement projects require more than a single measure. What other measures will complement this measure as part of your measurement set?

Data for Different Types of Studies

Before discussing sampling and analysis of data in improvement work, it is useful to review an important distinction on the types of studies (introduced in Chapter One). W. E. Deming classified studies into two types depending on the intent for action that will be taken based on the study.[16] It turns out that understanding the two types of studies is crucial as we approach sampling, displaying, and analyzing data for improvement.

An **enumerative study** is one in which action will be taken directly on the population from which the data were obtained. The population in an enumerative study is static or fixed, much like the water in a pond. Sampling of the population is done randomly so that probability theory can be used in analysis. If one wanted to determine the water quality of the pond they would sample randomly to reduce potential bias (for example, not all samples from spots easy to reach). Data in an enumerative study is often collected, analyzed, and displayed as an aggregate measure(s) before the study intervention and again after the intervention is made. Data are analyzed using classic statistical methods such as a T-test or confidence interval. The result of the study would be knowledge about *the* population from which the samples were taken or measurements were made. For an enumerative study, one has the ability to make estimates for the population sampled. Using the analogy of a pond, such as that in Figure 2.7, one would be able to estimate the water quality in *that* pond. Action based on an enumerative study is taken *only on the population in that study*. What was learned from this population, this pond in our analogy, could not be used to predict the water quality in another pond, nor even the water quality in this pond in the future.

An analytic study is one in which action taken will be on an underlying causal system with the intent of improving performance of a product, process, or system in the future. An analytic study is conducted in a dynamic, rather than static, population. Our analogy is that of a stream or river, such as that in Figure 2.8, rather than a pond. Data are obtained from an active process or system. An example might be all people with diabetes seen in the clinic each month. Data in an analytic study are collected at regular ongoing intervals

FIGURE 2.7   Image Reflective of an Enumerative Study

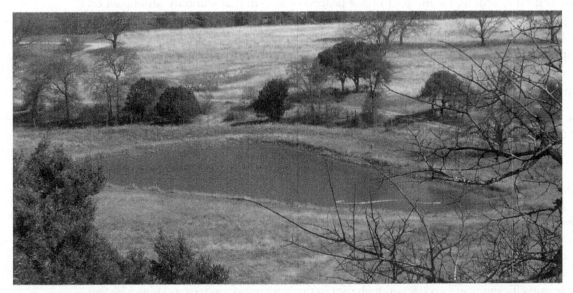

[16]Deming, W. E., *Some Theory of Sampling*, Wiley, New York, 1950. (Reprinted by Doer, 1960); Deming, W. E., "On Probability as a Basis for Action," *The American Statistician*, 1975, *29*(4), 146–152.

Provost, L. P., "Analytical Studies: A Framework for Quality Improvement Design and Analysis," *BMJ Quality and Safety*, 2011, 20 (Supplement 1), 92–96.

FIGURE 2.8   Image Reflective of an Analytic Study

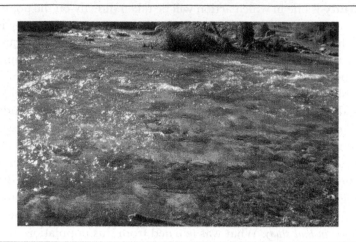

(such as daily, weekly, or monthly) rather than solely before and after a change. Using our stream analogy, one would dip into the stream at intervals to obtain data on an ongoing basis. Sampling in an analytic study usually makes use of judgment sampling rather than random sampling. If sampling water quality in a stream, would it be important to know that a manufacturing plant upstream empties its waste at 11 PM each night? Would one want to obtain samples from both fast- and slow-moving portions of the stream? This kind of sampling involves the judgment of subject matter experts. In an analytic study, data are analyzed by graphical means (for example, run or Shewhart charts). The results of an analytic study are used for prediction of future performance of the process of interest. One can predict the water quality tomorrow in our stream. Knowledge from an analytic study is used to redesign some part of the process or system that will have an impact on the performance of the system in the future.

Since most quality improvement (QI) studies have analytic intents, the discussion of sampling and data analysis in the remainder of this chapter are focused on analytic studies.

Use of Sampling

The purpose of measurement for improvement is to speed learning and improvement, not to slow it down. It is easy for improvement teams to get trapped in measurement and put off making changes until they have collected all of the data they believe they require. Measurement is not the aim; improvement is the aim. In order to move forward to the next step, a team needs just enough data to make a sensible judgment as to next steps.

Sampling involves deciding how much and which data are going to be collected in order to aid the improvement effort. Sometimes the number of patients or other volume of work available is small enough that it makes sense to obtain all of the data in the set (for example, we only have seven people with newly diagnosed diabetes each month so we obtain data from all of them). But when working with a great deal of data, sampling can be a simple and efficient way to collect enough data so that a team can understand how a system is performing. Sampling can save time and resources while accurately tracking performance.

One organization learned this lesson when an improvement team sought some baseline data regarding the age distribution of people with diabetes in their population with HbA1c levels greater than 8. They requested the information from their Information Systems (IS) department. They waited, and waited, and waited. Impatient that the request was taking too long, one team member decided not to wait for the IS department but to obtain a smaller amount of data himself. He went through the charts for all people with diabetes with an HbAlc of >8 for a three-month period (89 people with diabetes), and noted the age of each.

The team felt confident enough in these data that it decided to proceed with its improvement agenda. When the IS department eventually delivered the report months later, it confirmed the team's decision not to wait on the IS data. Figure 2.9 illustrates the pattern of the data based on the team's small sample size compared to that of the much larger sample. The results were nearly identical. This team would have learned nothing additional by waiting for more data. They saved valuable time by sampling and depending on their own sound judgment to know when enough data was enough.

We can think of sampling in relation to cooking. If we add salt to a pot of soup we *could* collect all of the data, eat all of the soup, to tell if adding salt was an improvement. Obviously, we know that we can use much smaller samples to tell if we've added enough salt to the soup. The same principle applies to health care data. We can often use sampling strategies other than collection of all of the available data to learn more efficiently from our data.

There are number of different sampling strategies; three are discussed here:

- Simple random sampling
- Systematic random sampling
- Judgment sampling

Random sampling is a sampling strategy with which many are familiar. A **simple random sample** is the selection of data from a frame by use of a random process such as a mechanical device or random numbers. The random numbers can be obtained from a computer or from a published list such as a random number table.

A team working to improve the care of patients with diabetes by using the Chronic Care Model used a simple random sample for their two key measures:

- The percentage of people with diabetes who had established self management goals
- The average HbAlc level for the population of people with diabetes

They collected data from 20 randomly selected charts from the frame of people with diabetes who had visited the clinic for the previous three months to establish a baseline. These charts were already tracked by the use of a six-digit patient chart identification

FIGURE 2.9   Large Sample Compared to Small Sample

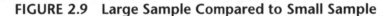

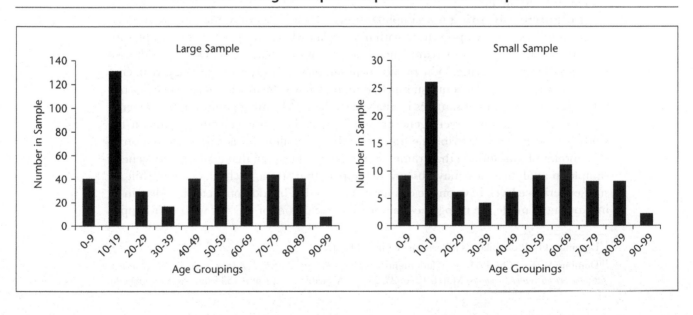

number that had been assigned when that patient entered the group's practice. The team used the following process in obtaining a random sample for their baseline:

- Ran a computer search and created a list of each of the patient chart identification numbers for those patients with diabetes seen at the clinic for the previous three months; 207 were identified.
- Numbered this list sequentially from one to 207.
- Used a random number table to generate a list of 20 numbers between 1 and 207.
- Obtained the patient records whose line number on the computer listing corresponded to the 20 random numbers between 1 and 207 they had previously generated.

After establishing this baseline, the team would develop the measures each month using all of the data from the documented population of people with diabetes being entered into the registry.

A **systematic random sample** is created by choosing a random starting point from a frame and then selecting data at specified intervals. For example, suppose the frame consisted of 1,000 medical records and a team wanted to select 100 medical records for review. Because one out of every ten records is to be selected, a random number between 1 and 10, for example 8, is obtained. The eighth record on the list is selected as well as the eighteenth, twenty-eighth, and so on. The systematic sample is vulnerable to bias occurring from repeating patterns in the frame. In practice this is unusual and the systematic sample is often a convenient way to produce a useful random sample.

In one example of a systematic sample taken over time, a hospital was interested in improving post–knee replacement outcomes. Post-discharge self-care was seen as problematic. Patients reported that they had had a difficult time following the self-care regime. The improvement team wanted to determine the effect of a patient video they had just begun using on patients' ability to follow the prescribed self-care regime. They developed a plan to select every fifth eligible patient and ask them about their ability to follow the self-care regime. They used a random number table to determine that the second patient the next day would be selected and then every fifth patient after that. The patients were contacted one week after discharge. One of the questions asked the patients to rate the amount of difficulty they had following the home care regime on a scale of 1–5. Their responses were plotted on a run chart as they were obtained. In addition to evaluating the efficacy of the change, the comment section of the survey provided some ideas for further improvement.

Judgment sampling is a sampling strategy useful in improvement work. In judgment sampling we rely upon those with process knowledge to select useful samples for learning about process performance and the impact of our changes. Dr. Deming addressed judgment sampling saying, "Use of judgment samples is hardly ever necessary in an enumerative problem. . . . In contrast; much of man's knowledge in science has been learned through use of judgment samples in analytic studies."[17] Deming points out that an enumerative study requires a very general sample, spread out over the entire frame, if the study is to accurately describe the frame and therefore allow for accurate estimation of the amount of variation in that frame. Deming notes, however, that taking a very general sample in analytic study may obscure the impact that strata, such as location, shift, or staff experience level, have on the change being tested.[18] In addition, in testing ideas in an improvement mode, we recognize that the exact conditions of our test will never happen

---

[17]Deming, "On Probability as a Basis for Action," 146–152.

[18]Deming, W. E., "On the Use of Judgment-Samples," *Reports on Statistical Applications, JUSE (Union of Japanese Scientists and Engineers)* March 1976, *23,* 25–31. Available as reprint # 153 from www.deming.edu.

again (same staffing, same patients, same level of acuity, and so on). So, judgment is used to select samples over a range of conditions such that, by seeing how the change performs under each of these circumstances, the degree of belief that this change will or will not work in the future is raised. Deming also pointed out that in improvement work (analytic studies) the learner typically benefits from using judgment to obtain samples that constitute a convenient starting place ("Which clinic, unit, provider, and so on will be most willing to test this change with us?"). Such a convenience sample is, by its very nature, a judgment sample. Selecting judgment samples requires input from subject matter experts and is crucial to improvement work. Some examples of judgment samples are:

- Select specific times of day to collect STAT lab turnaround times
- Select the first 10 patients that arrive after 2:00.
- Select the charts from only patients with three or more comorbidities
- Interview the next person with diabetes that comes in the office for care.

A team working in the Emergency Department (ED) wanted to learn about variation in ED patient waiting time and be able tell if the changes they were going to test to reduce waiting time were improvements. The team wanted to use a sampling strategy to reduce the amount of data they would need to collect. The team discussed using random sampling until a member noted that it would help them learn more effectively if waiting time data was collected at particular times of the day. Random sampling or systematic random sampling would be less effective in helping them learn about their system than would data they decided to collect based on their process knowledge. They collected samples and plotted the data for waiting times at 1000, 1900, 2200, and 0200 each day. This allowed them to learn about the impact of time of day on their process performance. They also plotted the weekly average waiting time (average of 140 waiting times per week) on a run chart to tell over time if their changes were improvements.

A team working in a primary care clinic wanted to learn about their ability to see clinic patients at the time promised (on-time service). The team decided that if a physician was going to be behind in seeing patients he or she would be behind by 11 AM. If they could not catch up in the afternoon it would be evident by 2 PM. Some team members were concerned that "on-time" performance varied by day of the week and by physician with some days and some physicians having more impact on "on-time" performance than others. After considering all these factors, the team developed the sampling strategy in Table 2.10.

Using this sampling strategy, the team could learn about variation between days of the week by plotting the average of each day's delay time (all physicians' delay times for Tuesday added and then averaged, repeat for Wednesday, and so forth) They could also choose to learn about the difference between physicians by plotting Physician One's average delay each day, then Physician Two's average delay each day, and so on. They could learn if the clinic was making an improvement in "on-time" performance by plotting the average delay at 11 AM each day and plotting the average delay at 2 PM each day.

What About Sample Size?

Those who have worked with research studies will be familiar with classic methods used to determine the sample size required to obtain a desired level of confidence in the results (such as power calculations[19]). In research the sample size decision will depend on the

[19]Jones, S. R., Carley, S., and Harrison, M., "An Introduction to Power and Sample Size Estimation," *Emergency Medicine Journal*, Sep 2003, *20*(5), 453–458.

Table 2.10   Judgment Sampling Data Collection Strategy

Sampling Strategy for Measuring Delays in an Outpatient Clinic									
Year	**Delays in Minutes 11 AM/2 PM**								
Date	**Day**	**Phy 1**	**Phy 2**	**Phy 3**	**Phy 4**	**Phy 5**	**Phy 6**	**Phy 7**	**Phy 8**
1/2	Tues	/	/	/	/	/	/	/	/
1/10	Wed	/	/	/	/	/	/	/	/
1/18	Thur	/	/	/	/	/	/	/	/
1/26	Fri	/	/	/	/	/	/	/	/
1/29	Mon	/	/	/	/	/	/	/	/
2/6	Tues	/	/	/	/	/	/	/	/
2/14	Wed	/	/	/	/	/	/	/	/
2/22	Thur	/	/	/	/	/	/	/	/
3/1	Fri	/	/	/	/	/	/	/	/
3/4	Mon	/	/	/	/	/	/	/	/
3/12	Tues	/	/	/	/	/	/	/	/
3/20	Wed	/	/	/	/	/	/	/	/
3/28	Thur	/	/	/	/	/	/	/	/

type of data (attribute versus continuous) that will be collected, the variability associated with continuous data or the rate associated with attribute data, the magnitude of the difference we hope to detect in the study, and our degree of belief or desired confidence in the result. In improvement projects, the sample size is a less well-defined issue because data are usually collected over time. As we use data for improvement, however, there are a number of different issues raised related to size of the sample or the amount of data collected. Different approaches are used to address these sample size issues with data for improvement than are used with data for research. Some of the elements of an improvement project that affect the sample size decision include:

1. The specific objective of the data collection (getting ideas, making comparisons, testing a change, and so on).
2. The type of data (attribute, where larger sample sizes are required or continuous).
3. The expected rate of the attribute of interest. The smaller the rate, the larger the sample size required to detect changes in process performance. Rare events data may require very large sample sizes to detect changes (Note: Chapters Three, Four, Five, and Seven will cover this issue in detail).
4. The availability of data or resources to obtain data.
5. The importance or expected visibility of the objective. Do the results need to be used to influence others or just the team members?

For data used as part of an improvement effort, getting data across a wide range of conditions (locations, days of the week, shift, and so forth) may be more important than the amount of data collected under a specific condition. In general, more data (larger sample sizes) lead to more information and better precision of results. Unless the data are already collected and reported, larger sample sizes also involve more effort and cost.

In Figure 2.10 we see average clinic waiting time plotted over the life of the project. An important improvement (a 30% reduction) in the average waiting time has been made by the team around after period 12. The five run charts show a sample of one patient's waiting time per week, and the average of a sample of five patients' waiting times per week, 10, 20, and 50 patients' waiting times per week.

FIGURE 2.10   Sample Size and Ability to Detect Change

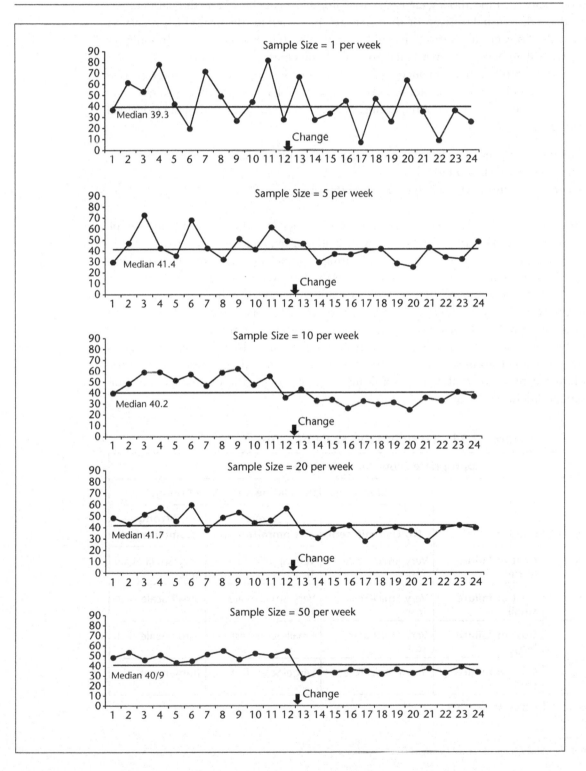

Is it obvious that a change in the measure has occurred looking at the data plotted with a sample size of one per week? What about sample sizes of 5, 10, 20, and 50? The picture is not as evident with the smaller sample sizes. For the sample size of 1, the run chart does not provide convincing visual evidence that an improvement has been accomplished. The information gained with a sample size of 5 and 10 begins to provide convincing visual evidence that the change resulted in improvement. A sample size of 50 per week is probably overkill. Sample size issues in improvement efforts are a balance between resources (time, money, energy, slowing improvement efforts) and the clarity of the results desired. A visual preview of the run charts predicted for the project key measures provides the "power calculation" usually done in research projects. (Note: In Chapter Three, we will go beyond simple visual analysis of run charts.)

The risks with failure and concept of "degree of belief" or confidence in the success of the change being made can act as aids in helping us plan our sampling strategy. The scope or scale (amount of sampling, testing, or time required) of a test should be decided according to:

1. The team's degree of belief that the change will result in improvement
2. The risks from a failed test
3. Readiness of those who will have to make the change

As shown in Table 2.11, very small-scale tests are needed when the consequences of failure are large and degree of belief is low, even if staff are eager for the change.

For example, a team is testing a new admitting approach designed to reduce time and improve billing accuracy. Negative consequences for their system could be considerable if the new system doesn't work. If they don't have a high degree of belief that their change is going to work they would be wise to plan very small-scale tests. Their initial sample size might be very small and consist of trying the change with one admission.

If the consequences of a failed test are major but the team's degree of belief in success is high, then small- to medium-scale tests should be considered. The test of the use of high-flow oxygen immediately post surgically on a pilot population to reduce infection rates might fall into this category.

Table 2.11   Deciding the Scale of a Test[20]

Appropriate Scope for a PDSA Cycle				
Current Situation		Staff/Physician Readiness to Make Change		
		No Commitment	Some Commitment	Strong Commitment
Low Belief that change idea will lead to Improvement	**Cost of failure large**	Very Small-Scale Test	Very Small-Scale Test	Very Small-Scale Test
	Cost of failure small	Very Small-Scale Test	Very Small-Scale Test	Small-Scale Test
High Belief that change idea will lead to Improvement	**Cost of failure large**	Very Small-Scale Test	Small-Scale Test	Large-Scale Test
	Cost of failure small	Small-Scale Test	Large-Scale Test	**Implement**

Source: Adapted from Langley, et al., 2009.

---

[20]Langley et al., *The Improvement Guide*, 146.

Table 2.12 Sample Strategy Guide for Planning a Run Chart[21]

Situation	Data Points Required
Expensive tests, expensive prototypes, or long periods between available data points, large effects anticipated.	Fewer than 10
Desire to discern patterns indicating improvements that are moderate or large.	11–50
The effect of the change is expected to be small relative to the variation in the system.	51–100

Once the appropriate sample size for a measure is selected, another issue is the number of times the measure needs to be plotted to understand the impact of changes tested. A helpful aid in planning sampling strategy is to consider the time required to increase the degree of belief that the improvement has occurred and that it will persist. The importance of viewing the impact of the change on the system over time sets a context for determining sample size for the test. The sample size needs to be adequate to detect patterns that indicate improvement. Some guidelines for determining the number of plotted points necessary to detect patterns on a run chart are shown in Table 2.12.

As discussed in Chapter One, improvement efforts rely on small repeated Plan-Do-Study-Act (PDSA) cycles to build a body of data over time. The Best Emergency Department wanted to test a number of changes aimed at reducing ED waiting time. They expected the effect of their changes to be small relative to the variation already existing in their system. They thought it was going to take awhile to see evidence of improvement and to be convinced that the improvement was being maintained. The team decided to collect data from 20 patients each day. The ED improvement team may have only collected waiting time data from a relatively small fraction of their patients but by the time the team completed their improvement project they had data from 38 weeks, or a sample of 5,320 patients.

Stratification of Data

When using data for improvement, people often intend to learn from the data to get ideas to test. Could the data be separated or grouped by some of the factors that might aid learning from the data? In other words, could the data be stratified? **Stratification** is the separation and classification of data according to selected variables or factors. The object is to find patterns that help in understanding the causal mechanisms at work. Stratification is used to gain clues as to the causes of variation in the process under study. Data may be stratified by time periods; organization or unit; by demographics such as age, sex, socioeconomic group, ethnic group; or by treatment location treatment method, and provider—the list is almost endless. Figure 2.11 illustrates the concept of stratification.

When using data for improvement the goal is learning, not judgment. This can be important to emphasize when stratifying data in ways that allow us to identify units or individuals. Sometimes stratified data are coded to protect privacy while still allowing people to learn about the variation between organizations or providers.

Stratification may be used when plotting data over time. Figure 2.12 shows monthly Post–Coronary Artery Bypass Graft (CABG) complication data, which are then stratified by protocol A and protocol B (shown in Figure 2.13). By stratifying the data the team begins to get some insight to the possible causes of variation in post-CABG infection rates

---

[21]Ibid., 159.

FIGURE 2.11   Stratification Involves Separation and Classification

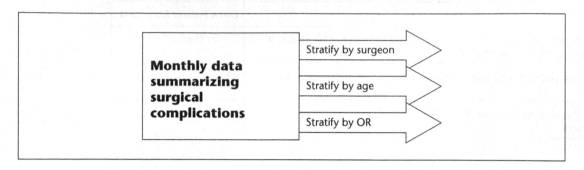

FIGURE 2.12   Run Chart of Post-CABG Complication Rate
Without Stratification

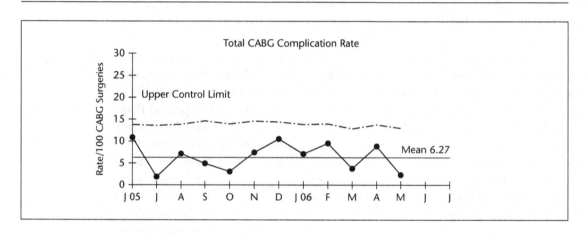

FIGURE 2.13   Post-CABG Complication Rate Stratified by Protocol

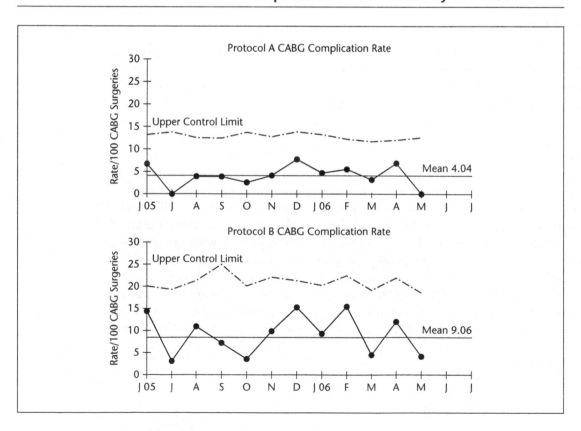

in their system. Protocol B is clearly exhibiting a higher rate of post CABG complications than is protocol A. Maybe the team can learn something useful for improvement here. Chapter Four has more examples of using stratification with run charts and other graphical methods to learn from variation.

What About Risk or Case-Mix Adjustment?

Risk, severity, or **case-mix adjusting** is the process of trying to account for differing levels of complexity or illness between groups of patients.[22] In general, risk adjusting is performed to make comparisons of outcomes across different providers or organizations. This is important when data are being used for judgment or accountability and it can be important in some research projects.[23] Some improvement projects would also benefit from taking into account differences in severity among subjects when studying practice patterns or the effect of changes made to clinical processes. Our ability in health care to risk/severity adjust our data is evolving as we continue to understand the factors that affect various health outcomes. Risk adjustment of data is not without its challenges.[24] Computer programs are available to do risk/severity adjustment for many measures using complex models. Logistic regression analysis based on data from patient records is one of the most common approaches to these programs. Examples of factors included in the adjustment models are age, race, gender, body size, and comorbidities. If your organization is able to risk adjust the data you are using for an improvement project without slowing down your improvement efforts then use the risk-adjusted data. Our ability to learn from unadjusted data increases if we can appropriately stratify or otherwise rationally group the data. Chapter Four further addresses stratification and rational subgrouping techniques.

Because data used for improvement are not used to judge people but to learn, the unadjusted data may still be very useful for learning and improvement. A team working to improve hip replacement complications wanted to learn from variation in current clinical practice that might be revealed by their current data. The team knew they could readily obtain both the raw data and the risk-adjusted data. Figure 2.14 shows both unadjusted

FIGURE 2.14   Little Difference Between Risk-Adjusted and Non-Risk-Adjusted Data

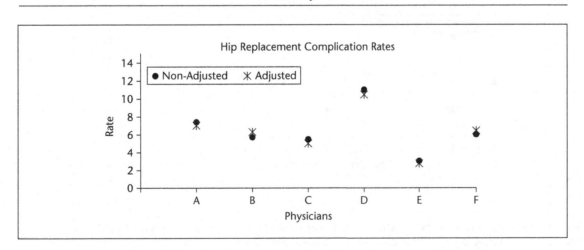

[22]Kuttner, R., "The Risk-Adjustment Debate," *New England Journal of Medicine*, 1998, *339*, 1952–1956.

[23]Tekkis et al., "Mortality Control Charts for Comparing Performance of Surgical Units: Validation Study Using Hospital Mortality Data," *British Medical Journal*, *326*(7293), April 2003.

[24]Nicholl, J., "Case Mix Adjustment in Non-randomized Observational Studies: the Constant Risk Fallacy," *The Journal of Epidemiology and Community Health*, 2007, *61*, 1010–1013.

and risk-adjusted data for each provider. Risk adjusting resulted in some additional accuracy and some change in complication rates for the providers in this system. However, they could have learned just as much from the more readily obtainable unadjusted data. Provider D had a much higher complication rate and provider E a much lower complication rate than the rest of the peer group. Risk adjusting their data resulted in some minor changes in their complication rates, but did not lead to a different conclusion. An opportunity for learning about their system was as evident to the team in the raw data as it was in the risk-adjusted. This team didn't have to slow down their progress to obtain the data. If, however, they had had to wait an additional two or three months to obtain the data in a risk-adjusted format they may have lost team focus and forward momentum.

In some instances risk-adjusted data are readily available and may lead to important opportunities to learn and improve. This post-CABG mortality data in Figure 2.15 reveals that physician B, who appears to have a high mortality rate, has a low rate when risk adjustment is considered. The opposite is the case for physician E.

A number of authors have studied the need for case-mix adjustment with control charts. In their study of mortality rates, Marshall and Mohammed concluded: "There is moderate-good agreement between signals of special cause variation between observed and risk-adjusted mortality."[25] Here, "observed" refers to raw or crude mortality (unadjusted data). The references below contain examples of using various risk-adjustment strategies in data analysis for improvement.[26]

Transforming Data

Sometimes it is useful to transform the basic data from the original scale in which it was recorded. Although it is usually best for data for improvement to remain in the scale in which it was recorded, there are a number of situations where a transformation can

FIGURE 2.15   Large Differences Between Risk-Adjusted and Non-Risk-Adjusted Data

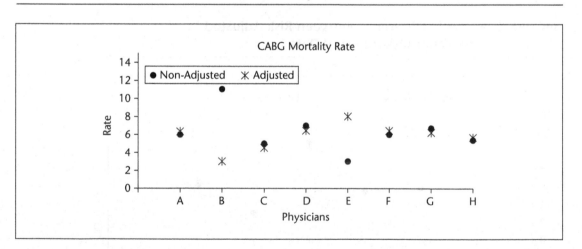

[25]Marshall, T., and Mohammed, M., "Case-Mix and the Use of Control Charts in Monitoring Mortality Rates after Coronary Artery Bypass," *BMC Health Services Research*, 2007, *7*, 63.

[26]Steiner S., and Cook, R., "Monitoring Surgical Performance Using Risk-Adjusted Cumulative Sum Charts," *Biostatistics*, 2000, *1*(4), 241–452.

Eisenstein, E., and Bethea, C., "The Use of Patient Mix-Adjusted Control Charts to Compare in-Hospital Costs of Care," *Health Care Management Science*, 1999, *2*, 193–198.

Webb, A., and Fink, A., "Surgical Quality of Care," *Hospital Physician*, Feb 2008, 29–37.

improve the ability to learn from the data. For example, an organization was certain that its problem with patient falls was worsening. They based this conclusion by looking at the number of patient falls each month (see Table 2.13 and Figure 2.16).

When presenting the data someone mentioned that the last several months had been extremely busy and wondered if they should consider this when thinking about the fall data. That led the group to collect data regarding the number of occupied bed days each month and transform their data from the raw data of the number of falls to a fall rate per occupied bed day. See Table 2.14 and Figure 2.17 for the display of their data and graphs.

Failing to consider both a numerator (the key measure) and a denominator (some appropriate unit of production or volume) is a common practice. One of the fundamental

Table 2.13   Number of Falls

Month	M-07	A	M	J	J	A	S	O	N	D	J-08	F	M	A	M	J	J	A	S	O	N
# Falls	6	5	7	3	4	6	2	5	4	2	4	3	7	4	5	7	6	8	10	7	9

FIGURE 2.16   Run Chart of Number of Falls

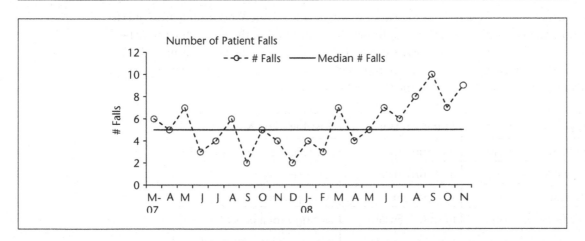

Table 2.14   Data for Rate of Falls

Month	Number of Falls	Number of Occupied Bed Days	Falls Rate	Month	Number of Falls	Number of Occupied Bed Days	Falls Rate
M-07	6	612	0.980	J-08	4	549	0.729
A	5	719	0.695	F	3	412	0.728
M	7	655	1.069	M	7	632	1.108
J	3	497	0.604	A	4	589	0.679
J	4	553	0.723	M	5	508	0.984
A	6	649	0.924	J	7	679	1.031
S	2	502	0.398	J	6	982	0.611
O	5	514	0.973	A	8	802	0.998
N	4	507	0.789	S	10	978	1.022
D	2	443	0.451	O	7	812	0.862
				N	9	917	0.981

FIGURE 2.17   Graphs of Fall Rate and Number of Falls

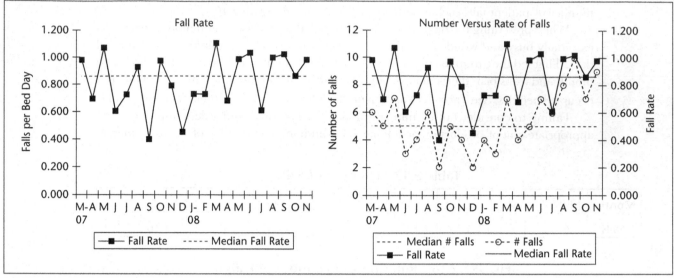

ways in which we transform data in order that we may learn more accurately from it is to use ratios. Using a ratio minimizes confusion from variation in the data which may be a result of changes in volume of workload rather than changes in the key measure. Moving from raw data to the use of ratios is an important step in transforming the data we use in improving health care. Some examples of useful ratios follow:

Key Measure	Standard Unit	Possible Ratio Measure
# of late surgeries	# of surgeries	late surgeries / total surgeries
Total OR costs	# of surgeries	cost / surgery
ED costs	# of patients	cost / patient
# patients waiting	hospital census	waiting / total patient
# patients leaving	total ED arrivals	# leaving / total # arrived

There are two types of ratios using a denominator: percentage and rate, which often creates confusion:

Percentage = # events of interest/total population of interest (numerator *cannot* be larger than denominator)

Example: # people given ACEI / # people who should have ACEI

Example: # bills with an error / # patient bills

Rate = # events over a specified time/population at risk for that event over time (numerator *can* be larger than denominator)

Example: # infections / # patients

Example: # errors in bills / # patient bills inspected

Another situation in which transformation is useful is when data are highly skewed. Data are not always symmetrically distributed; that is, they don't always form the classic bell-shaped curve. The distribution may be quite uneven with data skewed (long-tail) in one direction or another. Highly skewed data can create some difficulty when learning from that data for improvement. How do we know we are working with skewed data and what do we do about it? Several tip-offs exist that indicate that we are dealing with skewed data.

- We have data that are measuring time of tasks and some times are near zero.
- The data ranges over multiple orders of magnitude (10, 100, 1,000, and so on).
- The shape of the distribution on a frequency plot of the data shows a long tail (to the left, negative skew; to the right, positive skew).

Data measuring time is bounded by 0 and often displayed without any transformation of the data. Examples include waiting time; time to complete a procedure, or length of stay. These data often result in a skewed distribution that is evident when viewed on a frequency plot (Chapter Four has more on construction and use of frequency plots). Figure 2.18 includes a distribution plot showing a symmetric distribution (distribution of data not skewed) versus a skewed distribution of data.

Figure 2.19 shows a run chart for the time required to complete a report after close of business at the end of each week. The system was originally designed to produce a report

FIGURE 2.18 Distributions of Data Without and with Skew

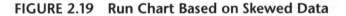

FIGURE 2.19 Run Chart Based on Skewed Data

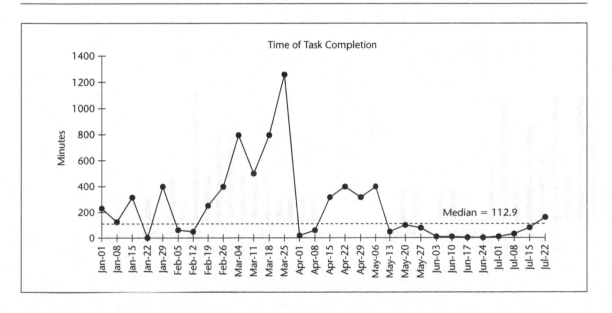

within 120 minutes of close of business. In March, some reports were not available until the following day. An investigation completed in July produced the data used to develop the chart. The chart shows high values in February and March, but a run of 10 points below the median in recent weeks.

Figure 2.20 shows the frequency plot for the data. The data are obviously skewed in to the left, toward taking little time to complete reports.

What do we do to improve our learning when our data are highly skewed? The square root and the logarithm function are both common transformations for skewed data that can be readily done on a spreadsheet. Figure 2.21 shows frequency plots of the time-to-completion data. The frequency plot using the square root transformation still shows some positive skewness (long right tail), whereas the logarithm transformation results in slight skewness to the left. We will return to the use of transformations in Chapter Eight discussing when they are useful for certain Shewhart charts.

FIGURE 2.20   Frequency Plot of Time to Complete Task

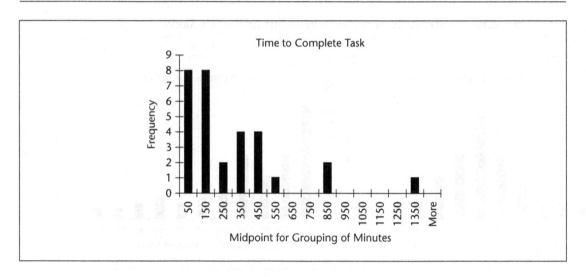

FIGURE 2.21   Frequency Plots of Time to Complete Task

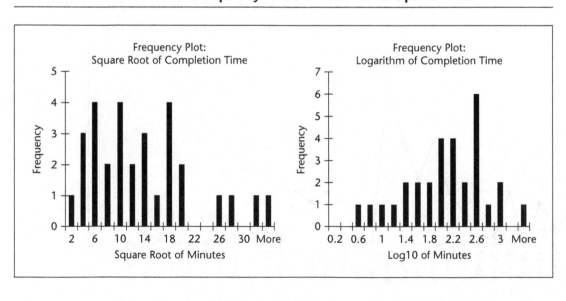

FIGURE 2.22   Monthly Incident Data and Transformed Data

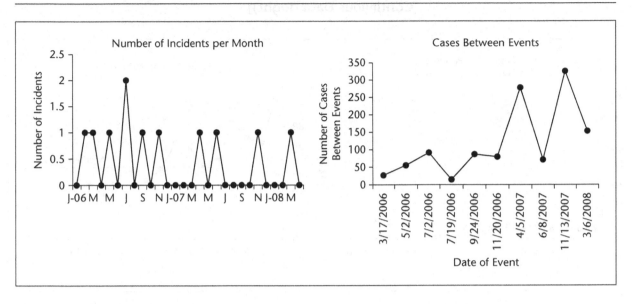

Another type of data transformation is useful when working with rare events data. The first graph at Figure 2.22 provides an example of a run chart for monthly data on incidents with many of the plotted values equal to zero. This is not unusual when dealing with relatively rare events such as infections or complications. More than 25% of the data points are zero, making it hard to tell whether changes are improvements. These data are counts of the number of incidents. Using an appropriate ratio would not help us here; we would still have too many months with zero. In this situation, transforming the data is useful in helping to learn whether the process is improving. The transformation is in the way the data are collected and displayed. Rather than collecting and graphing the number of incidents, the number of cases *between* incidents is collected and displayed. In other words, the graph displays the number of success between failures. Up is always good on this type of graph; increasing the number of cases between incidents is desirable (increasing successes between failures). Chapters Three and Seven include more information on this type of transformation.

One undesirable transformation often seen in health care measurement is to convert continuous data to attribute data. A team was working to improve waiting time in the clinic. Their goal was for 75% of patients to wait 30 minutes or less. The outcome measure they were using for their project was Percentage of Patients Waiting 30 Minutes or Less. The team worked diligently testing many changes. People working in the clinic said things were improving and patients seemed happier. In fact, patient satisfaction related to waiting time had improved, but the percentage of patients waiting 30 minutes or less had not. The left side of Figure 2.23 shows the graph they were using to evaluate their project. Someone on the team suggested that they look at the average waiting time each month (graph on the right). The result of their improvement work during the last year was clear on the run chart of the average wait time. As this example illustrates, if data are measured on a continuous scale they are best displayed with that continuous scale rather than being converted to an attribute measure.

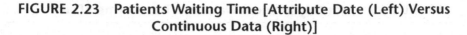

FIGURE 2.23   Patients Waiting Time [Attribute Date (Left) Versus Continuous Data (Right)]

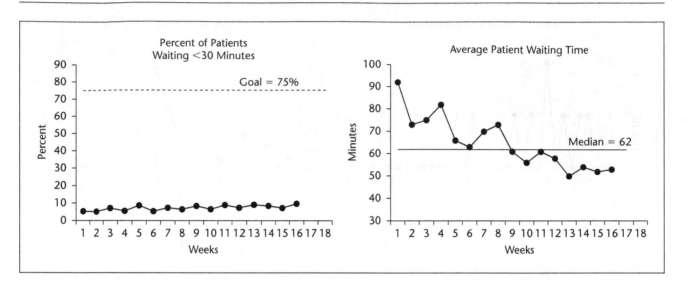

Analysis and Presentation of Data[27]

As mentioned earlier in this chapter, quality improvement projects are almost always analytic studies (rather than enumerative). The purpose of an analytic study is prediction. What is the degree of belief that the changes being tested will work under a wide range of conditions? In order to predict the impact of changes tested, the data are analyzed using principles and tools appropriate for analytic studies. Thus the methods for analysis of data from analytic studies do not use enumerative methods such as hypothesis tests and confidence intervals, which are appropriate when the objective is estimation.

Three basic principles underlie the methods of analysis for data collected in QI projects:

1. The analysis of data, the interpretation of the results, and the actions that are taken as a result of the study should be closely connected to the current knowledge of experts in the relevant subject matter.
2. The conditions of the study will be different from the conditions under which the results will be used. An assessment of the magnitude of this difference and its impact by experts in the subject matter should be an integral part of the interpretation of the results of the experiment.
3. Methods for the analysis of data should be almost exclusively graphical (always including a run order plot), with minimum aggregation of the data before the initial graphical display. The aim of the graphical display will be to visually partition the data among the sources of variation present in the study.

The first principle relates to the important role that knowledge of the subject matter plays in the analysis and interpretation of data from analytic studies. The PDSA cycle, as introduced in Chapter One, is used to build the knowledge necessary for improvement. The first step in the cycle is *Plan*. During the planning phase, predictions of how

---

[27]Moen, R., Nolan, T., and Provost, L., *Quality Improvement Through Planned Experimentation*, New York: McGraw-Hill, 2000, Chapter 3.

the results of the study will turn out are made by the team planning the cycle. This is a means of bringing their current knowledge into focus before the data are collected for the study.

In the *Do* step of the PDSA Cycle, the study is performed and the analysis of the data is begun. The third step, *Study*, ties together the current knowledge and the analysis of the study. This is done by comparing the results of the analysis of the data to the predictions made during the planning phase. The degree of belief that the study forms a basis for action is directly related to how well the predictions agree with the results of the study. This connection between knowledge of the subject matter and analysis of the data is essential for successful quality improvement work.

The second principle relates to the difference between the conditions under which a study is run and the conditions under which the results will be used. In some studies, the conditions are not too different. An example of a small difference is a study in which minor changes are made to a stable clinical or administrative process. Pilot studies or medical experiments on animals to develop drugs to eventually be used for humans are examples of substantial differences in conditions. Differences between the conditions of the study and the conditions of use can have substantial effects on the accuracy of the prediction. In most QI tests, some aspects of the product or the process are changed, and the effects of these changes are observed. Estimation of these effects is an important part of the analysis. However, it should not be assumed that the changes produce the same effects under all conditions. The changes made in the study may interact with one or more background conditions, such as hospital census, time of day, or type of clinician. This interaction can cause the effect of a change to differ substantially under different conditions. A wide range of conditions will allow the improvement team to assess the presence of such interactions and the implications for interpretation of results. Graphical methods of analysis will be used to determine the stability of effects over different conditions.

The third principle relates to the synthesis of theory and the data presented with the aid of graphical methods. In quality improvement projects, it is essential to:

- Include knowledge of the subject matter in the analysis
- Include those who have process knowledge: physicians, nurses, technicians, researchers, clerical personnel, microbiologists, and managers
- Apply this subject matter knowledge creatively to uncover new insights about the relationship between variables in the process

The following elements should be a part of the data analysis during QI projects:

1. Show all of the basic data with minimal aggregation.
2. Plot the data in the order in which the tests were conducted. In QI projects (analytic studies) plotting the data in time order is pivotal. This is an important means of identifying the presence of signals of unusual variation in the data. In an analytic study these signals are superb opportunities to learn. We don't want to miss detecting them. We want to discover what happened to create the signal and then use what we learned to strengthen our improvement. In an enumerative study data that are unusual, termed "outlier" data, are often removed from the study. In an analytic study these data are not removed. We learn from all of the data. In fact, signals of unusual variation may be key to learning for improvement. An example in Chapter One illustrated the importance of viewing data over time by comparing a before-and-after bar chart to data plotted in time order on a run chart.

3. Rearrange the data graphed in time order to study other sources of variation that were included in the study design but not directly related to the aim of the study. Examples of such variables are work shift, patient diagnosis, data collectors, and environmental conditions.
4. Use graphical displays to assess how much of the variation in the data can be explained by the changes that were deliberately made in the study. These displays will differ depending on the type of study that was run.
5. Summarize the results of the study with both appropriate graphical displays and essential text.

How a graph is constructed can make a great deal of difference in the ease and accuracy of learning for improvement.[28] A good graph is a well-designed presentation of interesting and relevant data.

Good graphics will tend to have the following characteristics:[29]

1. Complex ideas are communicated with clarity, precision, and efficiency.
2. A lot of information is provided with the least amount of ink in the smallest space.
3. Multivariate information (information about multiple characteristics) is presented on the same graph.
4. Graphical integrity (does not mislead the reader; when the data changes, the graph changes).

Key principles for useful data display include:

- Show all the data.
- Label axis and other elements to allow for self-interpretation.
- Be simple enough for the appropriate people to learn from quickly.
- Focus the reader on learning from the graph, not on the graph itself.
- Separate different sources of variation.
- Emphasize comparisons and relationships (use stratification).
- Make it possible to learn form a large amount of data.
- Minimize text, markings, colors, and so on that are not directly related to the data.
- Use annotations to facilitate understanding the graphical display.

Graphs that are useful for learning and communication should **not**:

- Distort what the data have to say.
- Mask important changes in the data.
- Change (scale or symbols, and so forth) in the middle of the graph.
- Use three-dimensional displays (unless the data are three-dimensional!).
- Use fancy art or borders to embellish the graphic.

These design principles of good graphical display owe a great deal to the work of Edward Tufte. An overriding principle is summarized in his words: "It is better to violate any design principle than to put graceless or inelegant marks on paper."[30] We have attempted to consistently use Tufte's principles throughout this book and apologize if we have failed in any instance.

[28]Carifio, J., and Perla, R. J., "A Critique of the Theoretical and Empirical Literature of the Use of Diagrams, Graphs, and Other Visual Aids in the Learning of Scientific-Technical Content from Expository Texts and Instruction," *Interchange*, 2009, *40*(4), 403–436.

[29]Associates in Process Improvement, *The Improvement Handbook*, Austin, TX: API, 2008.

[30]Tufte, E., *The Visual Display of Quantitative Information*, Cheshire, CT: Graphics Press, 1998.

When analyzing quality improvement studies involving multiple organization units (for example, collaborative QI projects"[31]), the data should be reviewed in several ways:

1. First show the key data for each participating site. This is best done as "small multiples"[32] of each of the participating sites for both outcome and process measures.
2. Based on the consistency of the individual sites, Show the aggregate outcome data over time ("intent to treat" analysis).
3. Similarly, show the aggregate process measures over time.
4. Show the aggregate outcome data for the participants that were successful in implementing the intervention ("per protocol analysis" or "on treatment analysis").

Chapters Three and Four have more information on the importance of using graphics to learn from health care data. Chapter Six includes additional information related to principles of good graphical display.

USING A FAMILY OF MEASURES

Health care systems are very complex. Any single measure used as the sole means of determining improvement to a particular system is inadequate. When working to improve a system, multiple measures are usually necessary to better evaluate the impact of our changes on the many facets of the system. For example, a team working to reduce the percentage of cases that exceed the length of stay (LOS) guidelines is excited about their progress. Figure 2.24 shows the percentage of cases exceeding LOS guidelines decreasing as they have tested, implemented, and spread a new protocol. But is it necessarily time to rejoice yet? What if the team checked their unplanned readmission data for this DRG and saw the percentage of unplanned readmissions increasing as shown in Figure 2.25? If both measures had been visible at the same time, maybe even on the same graph, the unintended impact of the protocol to reduce LOS on unplanned readmissions would have been readily evident. An example of placing both of these measures on the same graph is shown in Figure 2.26.

FIGURE 2.24   Percentage DRG Exceeding LOS Guidelines Indicating Improvement

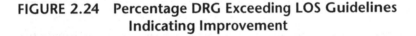

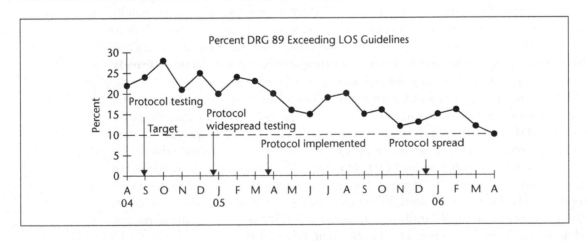

---

[31]Institute for Healthcare Improvement, *The Breakthrough Series: IHI's Collaborative Model for Achieving Breakthrough Improvement*, 2003, available from www.ihi.org/IHI/Results/WhitePapers/.

[32]Tufte, E., *The Visual Display of Quantitative Information*, Cheshire, CT: Graphics Press, 1998.

FIGURE 2.25   Percentage Unplanned Readmissions Worsening

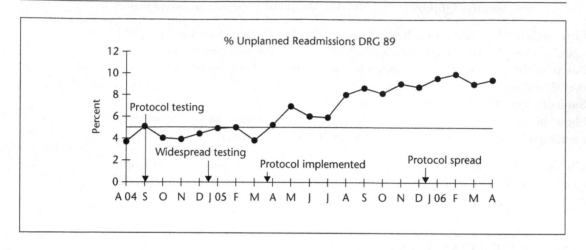

FIGURE 2.26   Multiple Measures on a Single Graph

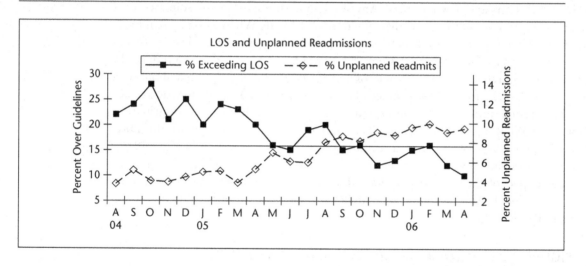

Health care processes are so interrelated that a single measure is not adequate to evaluate the impact of our changes on the system. A single measure simply cannot usefully represent the dynamic complexity between parts of our system. Typically a set of three to eight balanced measures are recommended for improvement projects. Frameworks such as the *Clinical Values Compass* are used in health care to help us develop a useful small **family of measures** (FOM) to better understand the impact of our changes.[33]

Thinking about measurement for improvement in terms of outcome, process, and balancing measures (introduced earlier in this chapter) provides a robust framework for designing a FOM to learn about the impact of changes on the system. Displaying the data on graphs over time allows us to see the impact of our changes on an individual measure and on the system represented by the FOM. This helps us avoid a local improvement that turns out to be a detriment to the larger system, such as a reduction in costs that increased waiting time and reduced satisfaction. The team working to reduce surgical site infections used this concept to develop a family of measures they would use to view the impact of their changes on the system. Their FOM is shown in Table 2.15.

---

[33]Nelson, E., Batalden, P., and Ryer, J., *Clinical Improvement Action Guide,* Chicago: Joint Commission on Accreditation of Healthcare Organizations, 1998.

Table 2.15 Family of Measures Including Outcome, Process, and Balancing Measures

Type of Measure	Description	The Surgical Infection Prevention FOM
Outcome	The voice of the customer or patient. How is the system performing? What is the result?	Surgical Site Infection Rate
Process	The voice of the workings of the system. Are the parts or steps in the system performing as planned?	Percentage of appropriate prophylactic antibiotic selection Percentage of on-time administration of prophylactic antibiotics Percentage of staff with a safety culture climate score greater than 4
Balancing	Looking at a system from different directions or dimensions. What happened to the system as we improved the outcome and process measures?	Patient satisfaction Cost per case

The Family of Measures aids us in answering question two of the Model for Improvement ("How will we know a change is an improvement?"). At least one **outcome measure**(s) is essential. If the surgical infection prevention team achieved improvement in all of their process measures, the percentage of appropriate prophylactic antibiotic selection, the percentage of on-time administration of prophylactic antibiotics, and the percentage of the staff with a safety culture climate assessment score greater than four, their colleagues would still want to know if the rate of surgical site infections had improved. Almost all improvement activities should include one or more outcome measures.

Process measures are useful because they are logically connected to the outcome measure(s) and typically show improvement before the outcome measure does. They are early indicators of whether or not our changes are improvements and therefore are very valuable as we test changes. It is easy to overdo measurement, particularly process measures. Vigilance is necessary here to ensure that we are using "just enough" measures to tell whether our changes are improvements. Improvement requires change. Collecting data for too many measures can reduce the time people have to devote to testing changes.

Balancing measures aid us in detecting unintended consequences. A team may have reduced STAT lab turnaround time but what was the impact on cost and accuracy? A balancing measure may also aid us in tracking events that would provide a rival explanation for the improvement. If we are working to reduce waiting time it may be useful to measure volume of workload to see if it, rather than our changes, explains any improvement in the waiting time.

The Institute of Medicine (IOM) report "Crossing the Quality Chasm"[34] suggests six dimensions of care to consider in developing a balanced set of measures. These are shown in Table 2.16 and may be useful as the team develops the FOM for the project.

The usefulness of the Family of Measures is increased when they are viewed as a time series and presented all on one page. Figure 2.27 is the surgical site infection prevention team's FOM displayed graphically and on one page. This display allows the team to view

[34]Institute of Medicine, *Crossing the Quality Chasm: A New Health System for the 21st Century*, Washington, D.C.: National Academy Press, 2001.

Table 2.16   Institute of Medicine's Six Dimensions of Care

Dimension	Description
Safety	As safe in health care as in our homes
Effectiveness	Matching care to science: avoiding overuse of ineffective care and under use of effective care
Patient-centeredness	Honoring the individual and respecting choice
Timeliness	Less waiting for patients and for those who give care
Efficiency	Reducing waste
Equity	Closing racial and ethnic gaps in health status

FIGURE 2.27   Surgical Safety Family of Measures

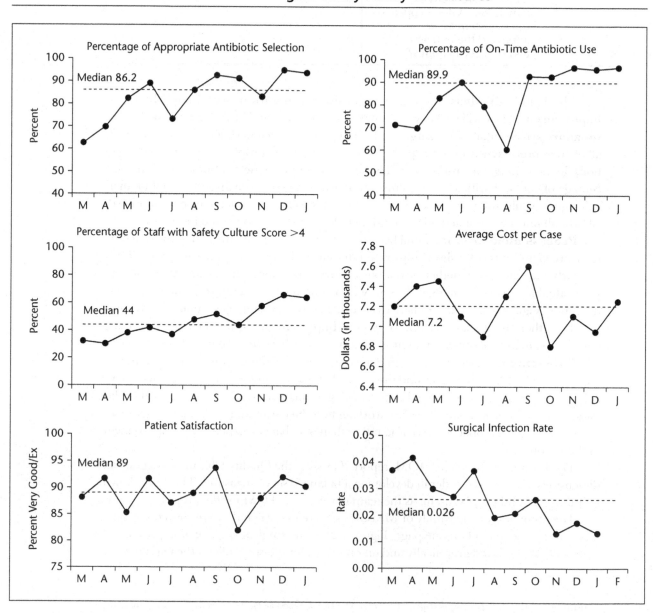

FIGURE 2.28   Tools to Learn from Variation in Data

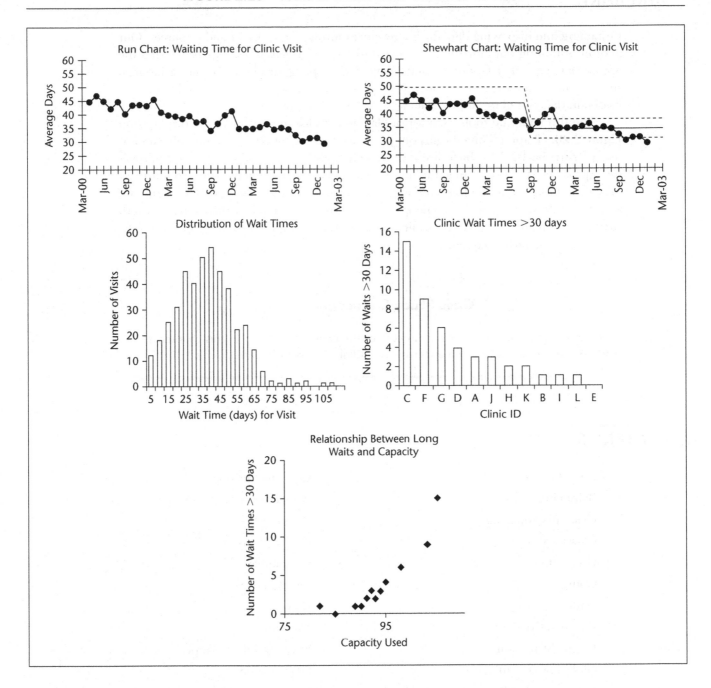

the impact their changes are having on the system, rather than on just a single measure. The surgical infection prevention team's FOM shows improvement in antibiotic use and safety culture and ultimately in the rate of surgical site infections. They have accomplished this without detriment to patient satisfaction or cost.

We've learned that any single measure is probably inadequate to support a system improvement. But when the measures are taken together, as a small family, they are powerful and useful. Chapter Thirteen contains more information on an organization's family of measures.

SUMMARY

Obtaining and displaying data for improvement involves some effort and resources. Our goal in obtaining data for improvement is to aim for *usefulness, not perfection*. Using the appropriate type of data, operational definitions, sampling, stratification, and including a small family of measures for improvement projects, are all key concepts aimed at helping us obtain data useful for improvement.

The fundamental tools used for displaying data for improvement are displayed in Figure 2.28. Chapter Three begins our journey into these tools with a thorough exploration of run charts. Run charts are a versatile tool and tremendously useful in improvement projects. We view them as the universal tool for improvement projects. They are not math-intensive, are useful for detecting early signals of improvement, easy to maintain, and straightforward to explain to people. We believe increased use of these tools in health care would greatly enhance the ability to learn from data and improve health care processes, systems, and outcomes.

Case Study Connection

To learn more about the application of a number of the concepts detailed in this chapter, **see Case Study A**, Improving Access to a Specialty Care Clinic, in Chapter Thirteen.

KEY TERMS

Analytic study	Outcome measure
Balancing measure	PDSA measure
Case-mix adjusting	Percentage
Classification	Process measure
Continuous	Qualitative
Count	Quantitative
Data	Rate
Enumerative study	Sampling
Family of measures	Simple random sample
Global project measure	Stratification
Judgment sample	Systematic random sample
Operational definition	

## CHAPTER 3

UNDERSTANDING VARIATION USING RUN CHARTS

INTRODUCTION

The run chart is a "universal tool" for virtually every improvement project. Run charts are easy to construct and interpret, yet so versatile that health care can make widespread use of them. This chapter introduces the many functions of this valuable tool. From this reading you will gain insights into: what a run chart is; how to make a great run chart; when to start a run chart; how to interpret a run chart; the many effective ways to display data with a run chart including the Family of Measures (FOM) multichart, displaying rare events data and more; and cautions and special uses for run charts.

WHAT IS A RUN CHART?

A **run chart** is a graphical display of data plotted in some type of order. The run chart has also been called a trend chart or a time series chart. Figure 3.1 shows a simple example of a typical run chart.

In this example, some Emergency Department (ED) staff thought that the percent of timely reperfusion (getting the blood flowing) after a heart attack had improved over the past two years. Other staff disagreed with this conclusion. The run chart was a useful

FIGURE 3.1   Run Chart Example

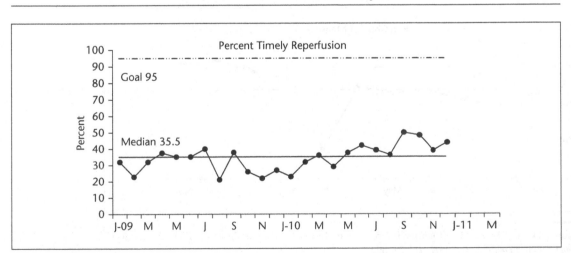

starting point with which to display their data in time order to see changes in the percentage of timely reperfusion in the ED over the past two years.

A run chart is easy to construct and simple to interpret. This simplicity makes it an attractive method for communicating and understanding variation. The run chart is a visual tool that encourages users to ask good questions based on the data they are viewing and thus learn about the process or system that the measure represents. Important uses of the run chart in improvement activities include:

- Displaying data to make process performance visible
- Determining whether a change resulted in improvement
- Determining whether gains made through the improvement effort are being sustained

Making variation visible is a constant theme throughout this book. Table 3.1 shows data presented at a meeting where, although comments were made about the organization having recently reached their goal of 90% for this measure, no other comments or questions were raised by participants. The run chart for these data is shown in Figure 3.2. This visual presentation of the data immediately opened up new discussions about the data, especially about the July data point.

The run chart allows us to learn a great deal about the performance of a process with minimal mathematical complexity.[1] Displaying data on a run chart can also be the first step in developing a Shewhart control chart (discussed in Chapter Four). This chapter describes the construction, interpretation, and use of run charts.

USE OF A RUN CHART

The primary use of run charts in this book is to answer the second question in the Model for Improvement "How will we know that a change is an improvement?" There

Table 3.1   Run Chart Data

Month	Jan	Feb	Mar	Apr	May	Jun	Jul	Aug	Sep	Oct	Nov
Measure	83	80	81	84	83	85	68	87	89	92	91

FIGURE 3.2   Run Chart Leading to Questions

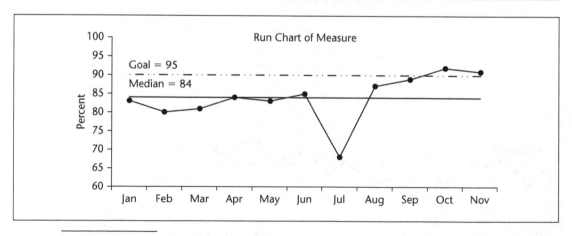

[1]Neuhauser, D., and Diaz, M., "Quality Improvement Research: Are Randomised Trials Necessary?" *Quality and Safety in Health Care*, 2007, *16*, 77–80.

are both practical and statistical answers to this question. A change in the data may be practically important, but may not provide any "signal," or probability-based statistical indication, of change. Or a change may indicate a statistical signal, but not be of practical importance. A change in the data could be both practically important and also exhibit evidence of a statistical signal. The following three scenarios illustrate these possibilities.

Scenario 1: The team was excited after the first week of testing when the percentage of patients agreeing to develop self-management goals jumped from 30 to 40%. But for the next three weeks, the reported percentages were 23%, 35%, and 27%. The team realized that there was a lot of random variation in their weekly percentages, and they needed to be careful in declaring that they had an improvement of practical importance. The initial jump in their data appeared to be of practical importance but was not a signal of real improvement.

Scenario 2: The team's goal was to increase the use of self-management methods from the current 30% of patients to greater than 70% of patients in their practice. Over six months of hard work, the percentage increased from 30 to 35%. One of the team members did an analysis and concluded that this increase was a statistical signal. But this was of little interest to the team who knew they still had a lot more work to do in order to meet their goal of 70% use of self-management methods. A rate of 5% improvement in five months, even if a significant statistical signal, was not of great value to their patients.

Scenario 3: The team was interested in testing whether use of a visit script developed by another organization could increase patients' interest in learning self-management methods. There was a lot of controversy about the approach, so they wanted to see, as soon as possible, if the percentage of patients adopting self-management methods had improved. After five weeks, they were able to show that an increase of 11% had occurred and that this increase was also a statistical signal. This provided encouragement to continue to develop the method for broader use in the practice.

The emphasis in this book is on describing how to design run charts that will make practical significance readily apparent. In addition, rules based on basic probability theory will be provided that can be used to detect nonrandom evidence of change (signals). These signals could indicate improvement or degradation of the process. Although there are other uses for run charts (for example, awareness of process performance level) most of the guidance in this book has been developed to help detect nonrandom changes, or signals of change, in process performance using probability-based rules. The objective is to detect these signals as rapidly as possible without an unreasonable risk of overreacting to random variation in the data series.

CONSTRUCTING A RUN CHART

There are seven steps to constructing a run chart. Exhibit 3.1 summarizes these steps.

The example in Exhibit 3.2 illustrates how these seven steps were used to develop the run chart (see Figures 3.3 and 3.4). When using software to develop a run chart, you will find that many of these steps are done by default. It is important, however, to ascertain that decisions made by the software program follow the guidelines given here.

EXHIBIT 3.1   CONSTRUCTING A RUN CHART

Seven Steps to Constructing a Run Chart

1. State the question that the run chart will answer and obtain data necessary to answer this question.
2. Develop the horizontal scale for the run chart. This will usually be a time scale, but other alternatives can be used. Appropriate time increments to develop the axis will typically be days, weeks, months, quarters, years, sequential patients, sequential procedures, and so on. A useful practice is to label several future time increments even though no data yet exist for that time frame. The scale should cover the time period of interest for the graph, not just the time when data are currently available.
3. Develop the vertical scale for the run chart. A good scale is one that is easy to plot, easy to read, and leaves ample room for future data that might be larger or smaller than the values used to create the initial run chart. Criteria for a good scale include:

   - Most of the data lies in about the middle half of the graph.
   - Labeled values on the axis should be round numbers and should be equally spaced.
   - Unlabeled tic marks should be easily plotted and read. They should be easy to work with and interpolate between.

   The completed chart should be sized with a 2:5 vertical to horizontal ratio. Estimate the range of the data points to be plotted on the vertical scale (the smallest value to the largest value). Then use this range to develop a vertical scale for the run chart. Be sure to construct your vertical scale so that it is high or low enough to encompass variation in future data and reference values such as your goal, a benchmark, or zero if it is meaningful to the chart.

4. Plot the data points. Make a dot (or another symbol). Connecting the dots with a line is optional, but the dots should always be distinguishable from the line. The data are communicated through the dots, not the line.
5. Label the graph completely with a useful title. Label the horizontal axis with the sequence of the data (for example, case 1, case 2, case 3, week 1, week 2, week 3, or Jan, Feb, Mar, and so forth). Label the vertical axis with the name of the measure or characteristic that you are studying.
6. Calculate and place a median of the data on the run chart. The **median** is the number in the middle of the data set when the data are reordered from the highest to the lowest value. If the number of observations is even, the median is the average of the two middle values. The median is required when applying some of the rules used to interpret a run chart. Placing the median on a run chart with a small number of data points or on a run chart with more than one series of data can add complexity to the interpretation of the run chart.
7. Add additional information to the chart. Add a goal or target line if appropriate. Annotate unusual events, changes tested, or other pertinent information on the run chart at an appropriate time location.

Examples of Run Charts for Improvement Projects

Analyzing a run chart always starts with simple visual analysis. The chart in Figure 3.5 is from a team working to improve lab turnaround times (for STAT tests). Simply looking at the run chart in Figure 3.5 allows us to conclude that the changes tested have not led to improvement.

No single measure is sufficient to gauge the progress of an improvement project. Improvement projects require tracking multiple measures. A team working to improve Chronic Heart Failure (CHF) treatment and outcomes in their organization tracked several

EXHIBIT 3.2   EMERGENCY DEPARTMENT REPERFUSION RUN CHART EXAMPLE

Step 1. State the question(s) the run chart will attempt to answer and obtain data necessary to answer this question. The question for the Emergency Department (ED) in this example was "Is the percentage of patients who obtain reperfusion in a timely manner improving?" Table 3.2 shows the monthly data of the percentage of reperfusions achieved in the prescribed time frame:

Table 3.2   Percentage Timely Reperfusion in the Emergency Department each Month

J 0 9	F	M	A	M	J	J	A	S	O	N	D	J 1 0	F	M	A	M	J	J	A	S	O	N	D
32	23	32	38	35	35	40	21	38	26	22	27	23	32	36	29	38	42	39	36	50	48	39	44

Note that any type of data or statistic calculated from data can be plotted on a run chart. This example plots a percentage based on multiple patients. Other examples might plot individual data values, averages, medians, counts, rates, etc.

Step 2. Develop the horizontal scale for the run chart. As shown in Figure 3.1, the ED staff used time increments of months on the horizontal axis. They extended the time period to March 2011 to prepare for future data. The horizontal scale will usually be time based, but other orderings are possible and illustrated later in this chapter.

Step 3. Develop the vertical scale for the run chart. A good vertical scale is one that is easy to plot, with easy-to-use increments and some room for future data.[2] The hospital group curious about the percentage of timely reperfusion in their ED noted that their data ranged from 21 to 50% each month and decided to scale their chart from 0 to 100%. This scale was a bit broad, but was necessary in order to encompass their goal of 95% timely reperfusion. Figure 3.3 shows how the ED team labeled their vertical axis in easy-to-use increments of 10%, making sure that labeled values on the vertical axis were whole numbers and were equally spaced.

Step 4. Plot the data points. The ED team plotted the data. They decided to connect the dots because their data were in time order. They made certain that the data line was relatively faint so that the dots were easy to distinguish from the data line.

FIGURE 3.3   Run Chart with Labels and Median

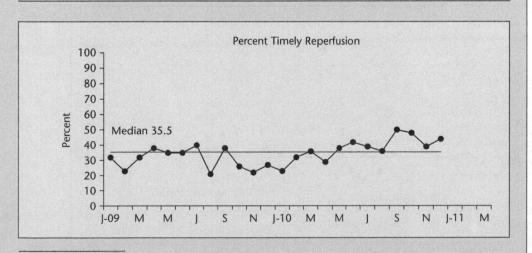

[2]Mowery, R., "Scaling Control Charts: What We Forgot to Tell You," *Quality Progress*, Nov 1991, 65–67.

(continued)

EXHIBIT 3.2 Continued

Step 5. Label the graph. Figure 3.3 shows the title and appropriate labels for the horizontal and vertical axes. Note that in this instance a label for the x-axis is not needed since the meaning of the units is obvious.

Step 6. Calculate and place a median of the data on the run chart. The **median** is the number in the middle of the data set when the data are reordered from the highest to the lowest value. Because the median is a positional value, it is physically in the middle of the data set and will have half the data above or equal to it and half below or equal to it. The median, rather than the mean, is generally the preferred center line for a run chart because probability-based rules used to interpret the run chart (introduced later in this chapter) rely on an equal chance of data points being above or below the center line. In addition, unlike the mean, the median won't be influenced by an unusually high or low value in the data set. There are a variety of useful methods for determining the median of a set of data:

Method 1: After plotting the data on the run chart in time order, reorder the data from high to low. Either count down the list of data to find the middle point, or physically cross off the highest value, then cross off the lowest value and continue until you locate the median. If the data set contains an odd number of data points a single point will represent the median. If the data set contains an even number of values, add the two middle data points and average them to calculate the median. See Table 3.3.

Method 2: Plot all of the data on the run chart. Slide a ruler or piece of paper down from the top of the graph counting the data points until you find the data point that represents the median. If the run chart contains 25 data points, the median data point is the 13th point down from the top of the graph (12 points are above it or equal to it, 12 below it or equal to it). If the run chart contains 24 data points, locate the spot halfway between point 12 and point 13 and label it the median. (Figure 3.3 will illustrate a run chart with the median.)

Table 3.3   Method 1: Run Chart Data Reordered and Median Determined

11 Largest Values											Two Middle Values		11 Smallest Values									
50	48	44	42	40	39	39	38	38	38	36	36	35	35	32	32	32	29	27	26	23	23	22	21

Median = (36 + 35) / 2 = 35.5

FIGURE 3.4   Run Chart with Goal Line and Tests of Change Annotated

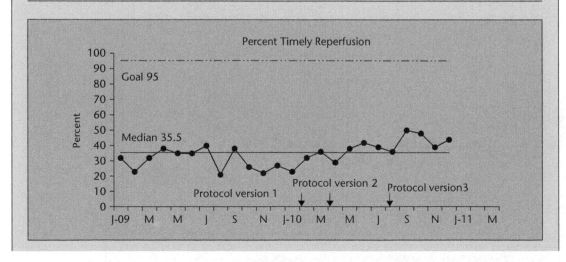

Step 7. Add additional information to the chart. The ED team made certain to include the goal line and to annotate key changes the team had tested on the run chart in Figure 3.4. Run charts lead to more effective learning when annotated in this way.

The visual display of a run chart, such as that in Figure 3.4, aids in the interpretation of a measure at any given time by placing variation in historical perspective. Studying a run chart can often reduce the risk of overinterpretation or tampering with the process. The run chart also offers a first look at a measure of a process before a Shewhart chart is developed. First, the chart should be assessed visually. Does the chart speak for itself? That is, does it show evidence of improvement that is obvious to all viewers? Sometimes such evidence is not obvious to all viewers. One may then choose to analyze a run chart using a set of rules useful for detecting nonrandom change, or signals, in the data. These rules are introduced later in this chapter. When using these rules, placing a median on the run chart is required.

FIGURE 3.5   Stat Lab Run Chart with No Evidence of Improvement

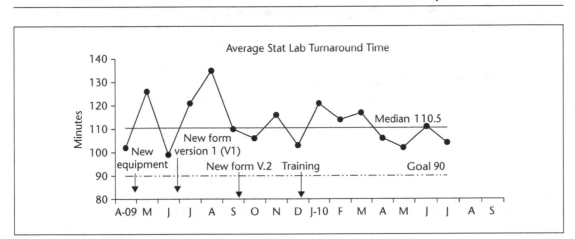

measures. Their run charts in Figure 3.6 readily reveal that the organization has improved the rate of patients who monitor their weight and the percentage of patients with Left Ventricle (LV) function documented. By annotating the major changes one can learn about the impact of these changes on key process measures. The outcome measure for this project, the number of admissions for heart failure, is also clearly declining. The fact that the related process measures are improving increases the degree of belief in the improvement noted in the outcome measure.

As mentioned earlier, multiple measures are usually required for an improvement effort. A single measure used to evaluate the impact of an improvement effort may miss key interactions in the system. Tracking cost while failing to track clinical outcome or patient satisfaction in an improvement effort is an obvious example. Looking at the CHF team's measures at the same time and all on one page made evaluating the impact of changes on the measures that represent the system easier and more effective.

Run charts can sometimes be displayed using the format called "small multiples."[3] Small multiples of run charts consist of a set of run charts. Each run chart is of the same measure but for a different location, segment of the organization or provider. All of these

---

[3]Tufte, E., *The Visual Display of Quantitative Information*, Cheshire, CT: Graphics Press, 1998.

FIGURE 3.6   Improvement Evident Using a Set of Run Charts Viewed on One Page

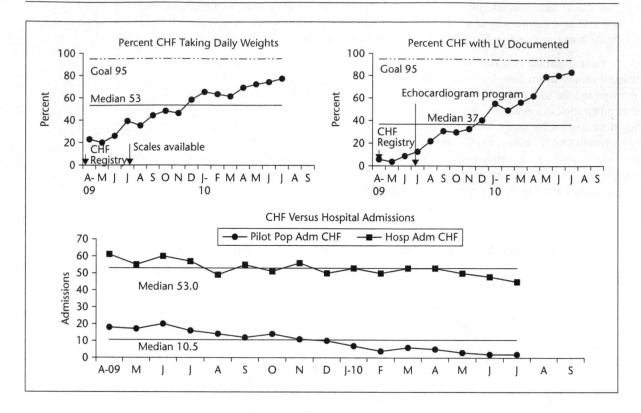

run charts are presented on the same "page" and with the same scale for rapid visual comparison. Figure 3.7 illustrates the concept of small multiples for a set of six patient satisfaction measures. Note that each run chart uses the same vertical and horizontal scales to aid in visual comparison.

Run charts may be used to display more than one measure on a chart. A single run chart may display multiple measures utilizing the same scale. Figure 3.8 provides an example of this. This run chart reveals that a great deal of improvement has been made and sustained related to the percent of people with diabetes who obtain foot exams and the percent of people with diabetes who obtain eye exams. The percent of people with diabetes who use self-management goals improved rapidly but then leveled off and remained in the 35% range.

The run chart may also display multiple measures which are quite dissimilar in scale by using two different vertical axes. Figure 3.9 displays the median wait time for the clinic in minutes and the volume of workload that week in number of visits. By using two vertical axes, these data can be displayed effectively. This chart reveals that the improvement in waiting time has not occurred because of any reduction in clinic workload. This type of run chart can be useful to display related or competing aspects of the system this way (for example, balancing measures).

Sometimes it is useful to display multiple statistics related to the same measure on the same run chart. Figure 3.10 shows a run chart used to display both the average HbA1c and the percent of the panel population with an HbA1c less than 7. While the average HbA1c has steadily decreased that might be skewed by a reduction in a relatively few patients with very high HbA1c values. Seeing the improvement in the percent of the population with a good HbA1c increases the degree of belief in the improvement.

FIGURE 3.7   Run Charts Used as Small Multiples

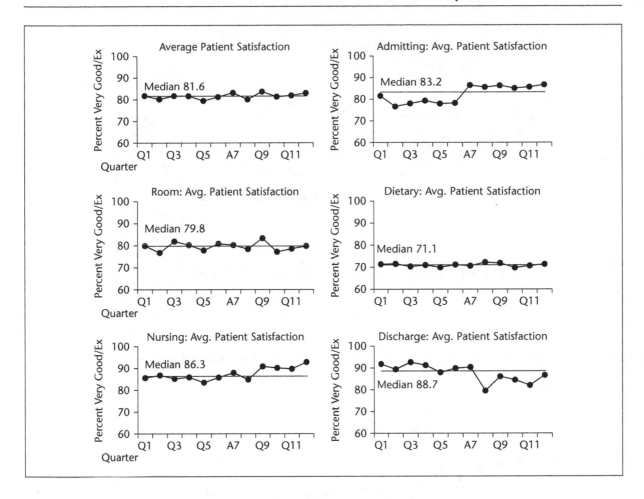

FIGURE 3.8   Run Chart Displaying Multiple Measures

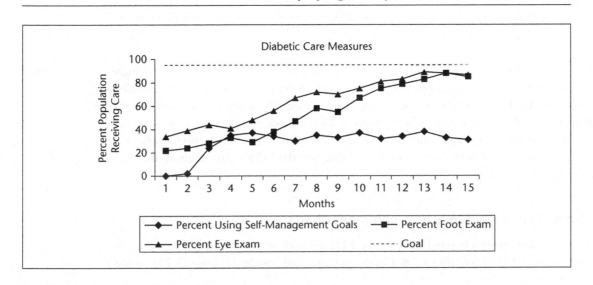

FIGURE 3.9   Run Chart Displaying a Different Measure for Each Axis

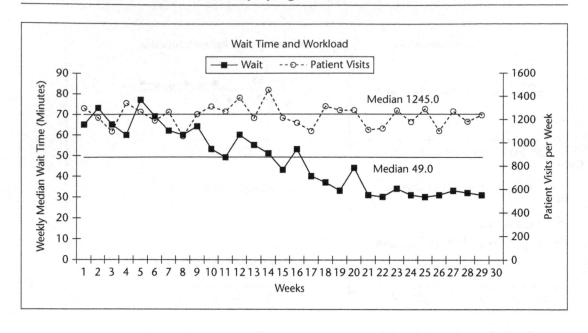

FIGURE 3.10   Run Chart Displaying Multiple Statistics for the Same Measure

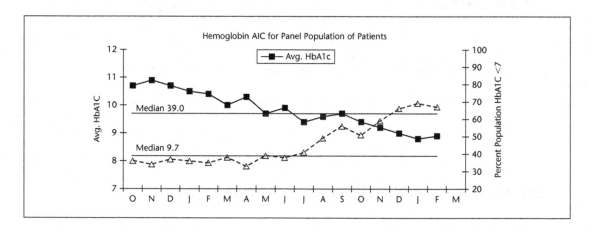

Some improvement projects are not rich in data, but the data may lead to a high degree of belief that the changes tested have led to improvement. When reporting results, it is important to characterize that improvement by sharing the median of the before data and the median of the after data rather than describe the process improvement by presenting just the first and last data points. The median minimizes the point-to-point variation and more accurately reflects the process performance than does any single point. See Figure 3.11 for an example.

Probability-Based Tests to Aid in Interpreting Run Charts

The team working on timely reperfusion in the ED had made some changes to their process but they were not sure whether or not improvement had resulted (Figure 3.12). What

FIGURE 3.11   Run Chart with Little Data

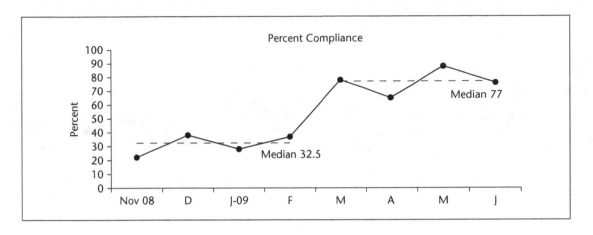

FIGURE 3.12   Run Chart with ED Team Uncertain About Improvement

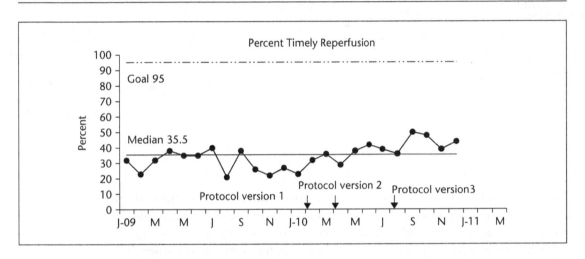

conclusions can be made by looking at the run chart? If improvement is not visually obvious on the run chart, probability-based rules may be of use to analyze the run chart for a *signal*, nonrandom evidence of change.

In addition to the overall visual analysis, four rules may be used to identify nonrandom signals of change in the data displayed on the run chart. These are:

- Rule One: A shift
- Rule Two: A trend
- Rule Three: Too many or too few runs
- Rule Four: An astronomical data point

There is evidence of a nonrandom signal in the run chart if one or more of the circumstances depicted by these four rules are seen when we analyze the run chart. Figure 3.13 illustrates the four rules. Rules One and Three are violations of random patterns and are based on a probability of less than 5% chance (or $p = 0.05$) of occurring just by chance when there is no real change.[4] Although there is nothing magical about

---

[4]Ott, E., *Process Quality Control*, New York: McGraw-Hill, 1975, 39–44.

FIGURE 3.13   Four Rules for Identifying Nonrandom Signals of Change

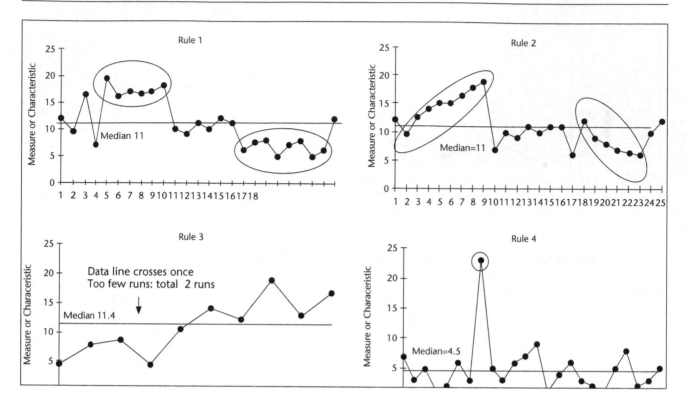

the 5% level of significance, it provides an objective threshold for whether the patterns on the chart represent a real nonrandom pattern and is consistent with typical practice in health care research. The threshold could be made more or less stringent based on the situation, but an agreed-upon approach is important so that the chart leads to action. The rules are appropriate for quality improvement projects where improvement is planned and predicted, and they have been shown to be effective in detecting signals in a wide range of health care applications.

The probability calculations for these rules assume that the data are continuous. Some problems can arise with these rules when the data are whole numbers when collected (discrete data) or when percentage data are bounded by 0 or 100%. Later in the chapter we address these issues. It is always fine to use a run chart with discrete data, but sometimes the rules should be interpreted with caution.

Rule One—Shift: *Six* or more consecutive points either all above or all below the median. Values that fall on the median do not add to nor break a shift. Skip values that fall on the median and continue counting. The decision rule of 6 comes from a simple probability calculation of an event with a 50% probability happening six times in a row ($P = 0.03$ for 6 points either above or below the median, which is less than $P = 0.05$).

Rule Two—Trend: *Five* or more consecutive points all going up or all going down. If the value of two or more successive points is the same, ignore the like points when counting; like values do not make or break a trend. The trend rule has been studied by others.[5] We have based our decision rule of 5 for a trend on our experience. Because most people are comfortable with the concept of a trend, it is important to define this value for consistent interpretation of a run chart.

Rule Three—Runs: A nonrandom pattern is signaled by too few or too many runs, or crossings of the median line. A run is a series of points in a row on one side of the median. Some points fall right on the median, which makes it hard to decide which run these points belong to. So, an easy way to determine the number of runs is to count the number of times the line connecting the data points crosses the median and add one (Figure 3.14). The data line must actually cross the median in order to signify that a new run has begun. Figure 3.14 provides an example of a data line that ends on the median rather than crossing it.

We still have only two runs because the line has crossed the median only once. After counting the number of runs we can determine whether we have a nonrandom signal of change due to too few or too many runs using the table in Table 3.4.[6]

The first step is to count the number of data points that do not fall on the median. In this example at Figure 3.14 there are 10 data points that do not fall on the median. Referring to Table 3.4, locate the row for 10 data points that do not fall on the median. Following that row across the page to the right, locate the column that lists the *minimum* number of runs the chart can have without indicating a nonrandom signal of change (for this example, 3). Continuing across the page to the right, the last column lists the *maximum* number of runs the chart can have without indicating a signal of change (for this example, 9). So, for this example, given 10 data points that don't fall on the median, the graph may have as few as 3 or as many as 9 runs without the number of runs indicating a signal. This example revealed only two runs. This is too few runs for the number of data points on the run chart and indicates a nonrandom pattern or signal of change.

FIGURE 3.14   Run Chart Evaluating Number of Runs

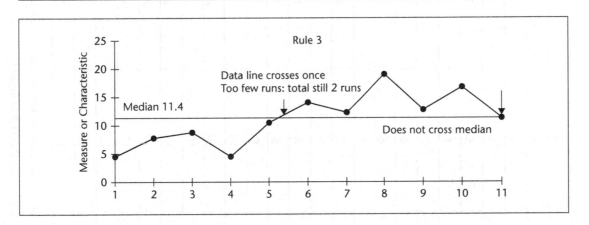

[5]Ott, *Process Quality Control*, p. 43; Olmstead, P., "Distribution of Sample Arrangements for Runs Up and Down," *Annals of Mathematical Statistics*, 1945, March, *17*, 24–33;

Davis, R., and Woodall, W., "Performance of the Control Chart Trend Rule Under Linear Shift," *Journal of Quality Technology*, 1988, *20*(4), 260–262.

[6]Swed, F. S., and Eisenhart, C., "Tables for Testing Randomness of Grouping in a Sequence of Alternatives," *Annals of Mathematical Statistics*, 1943, *Vol. XIV*, 66, 87, Tables II and III.

Table 3.4 Runs Rule Guidance—Table for Checking for Too Many or Too Few Runs on a Run Chart

Total number of data points on run chart not falling on median	Lower limit for number of runs (< than this is "too few")	Upper limit for number of runs (> than this is "too many")
10	3	9
11	3	10
12	3	11
13	4	11
14	4	12
15	5	12
16	5	13
17	5	13
18	6	14
19	6	15
20	6	16
21	7	16
22	7	17
23	7	17
24	8	18
25	8	18
26	9	19
27	10	19
28	10	20
29	10	20
30	11	21
31	11	22
32	11	23
33	12	23
34	12	24
35	12	24
36	13	25
37	13	25
38	14	26
39	14	26
40	15	27
41	15	27
42	16	28
43	16	28
44	17	29
45	17	30
46	17	31
47	18	31
48	18	32
49	19	32
50	19	33
51	20	33
52	20	34
53	21	34
54	21	35
55	22	35
56	22	36
57	23	36
58	23	37
59	24	38
60	24	38

Table is based on about a 5% risk of failing the run test for random patterns of data.

Source: Adapted from Frieda S. Swed and Churchill Eisenhart.[7]

[7]Ibid.

An example of too few runs providing a **signal of improvement** is illustrated in Figure 3.15. A team was testing changes to raise the percentage of patients who gave their organization the highest possible satisfaction rating (rated them in the "top box" on the survey). They noted too few runs on their graph with the most current data headed in the desired direction. This was a signal of improvement.

Figure 3.16 illustrates a run chart with too many runs. Given 20 data points that do not fall on the median, as few as 6 or as many as 16 runs are expected. This example contains 19 runs. This is too many runs for the number of data points on the run chart and is a signal of nonrandomness in the data. A pattern such as this most often represents data in need of stratification rather than data that truly reflect improvement. An example could be data displayed by alternating evening shift and day shift data on the graph. When plotting the results, evening shift might tend to be low, whereas the next point plotted, day shift, tends to be higher. Thus, every other point could be above or below the median. The fact that there are too many runs on this graph is a signal of nonrandom variation in the data. The signal, however, does not indicate improvement but rather indicates a need to separate the data from the two shifts and learn from each.

FIGURE 3.15   Measure with Too Few Runs

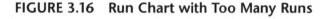

FIGURE 3.16   Run Chart with Too Many Runs

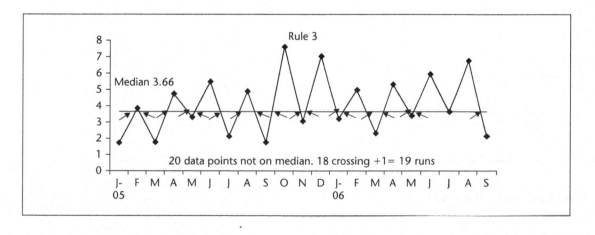

How do we arrive at the number of runs we expect to see on a run chart? The criterion for the number of runs for k data points as seen in Table 3.4 is based on the distribution of runs in random samples of continuous data. The parameters of this distribution are:

$$k_{bar} = \text{Mean} = (k + 2) / 2$$
$$S_k = \text{Standard deviation} = \sqrt{(k/2 * (k/2 - 1) / (k - 1)}$$

(Note: the minimum number of runs on a run chart with k points is 2 and the maximum number is k, so the mean is the average of 2 and k). These formulae and a probability of 5% are the basis for Table 3.4 on too few or too many runs. The values in the table can be approximated by using:

$$\text{Lower Limit} = k_{bar} - t_{k-1, .05} S_k$$
$$\text{Upper Limit} = k_{bar} + t_{k-1, .05} S_k$$

where k is the number points on the run chart (not on the median) and t is the tabled t-statistic.[8] Table 3.4 is applicable for 10 to 60 eligible points on a run chart. With more than 60 points, the equations above can be used. An approximate t value of 2.0 can be used in the equations with more than 60 data points.

Rule Four—Astronomical Point: This non-probability-based rule aids in detecting unusually large or small numbers. An astronomical data point is one that is:

⊛ An obviously, even blatantly, different value.

⊛ Anyone studying the chart would agree that it is highly unusual.

⊛ Caution: Every data set will have a high and a low data point. This does not mean the high or low are astronomical.

A team was working to reduce the daily average cycle time for patients in a clinic. Their initial data are at Figure 3.17 and shows their current state.

FIGURE 3.17   Early Run Chart of Clinic Daily Average Cycle Time

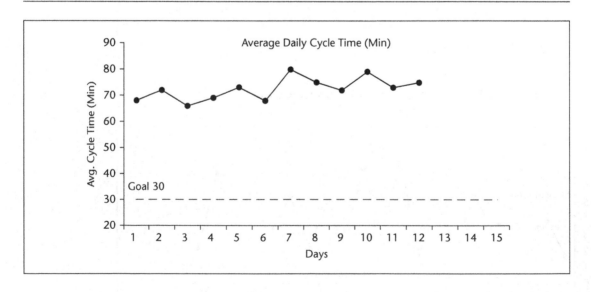

[8]Ott, *Process Quality Control*, Table A.15.

The team decided to test a smoothing technique starting on Day 13. Their results (see Figure 3.18) illustrate the astronomical rule for detecting a signal in their data. The team was excited by the reduction in average daily cycle time.

As they continued to track the data they became increasingly convinced that the smoothing technique was resulting in an improvement. See Figure 3.19.

Returning to the Emergency Department with data from Table 3.2 and the graph in Figure 3.20, the ED believed that the percent of timely reperfusion post–myocardial infarction had improved over the past two years. By applying each of the four rules, they could evaluate the graph for a signal of change. All four rules should be applied to each graph; however, it is not necessary to find evidence of change with each of the four rules

FIGURE 3.18   Clinic Daily Average Cycle Time with Astronomical Value

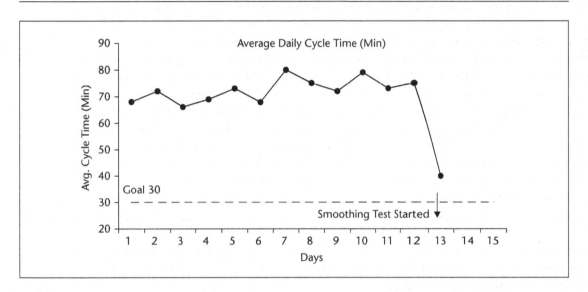

FIGURE 3.19   Clinic Daily Average Cycle Time with Continued Evidence of Improvement

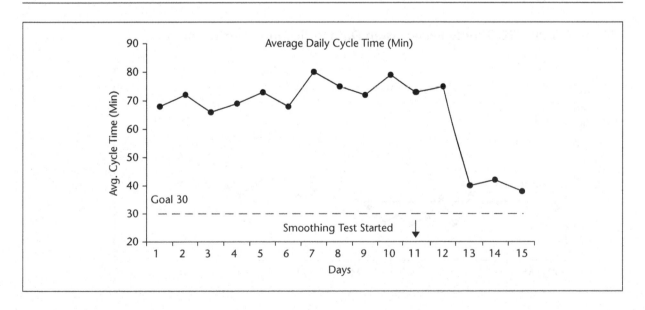

to determine that a signal has occurred. Any single rule occurring is sufficient evidence of a nonrandom signal of change.

- Rule 1, a shift of 6 or more consecutive points above the median, is present on the graph.
- Rule 2, trend, does not provide a signal of change.
- Rule 3, too many or too few runs, does not provide a signal of change. The run chart has 10 runs and 24 data points not falling on the median. Using Rule 3, the ED team should expect 8 to18 runs. The data are not outside of these parameters.
- Rule 4, an astronomical value, does not provide any additional signal of change.

Is the change in the percentage of timely infusion seen in Figure 3.20 an improvement? It is a signal of change in the desired direction, so in that sense it is a signal of improvement. However, it is important to ask if this change is an improvement in the *practical* sense, from the perspective of the team, the organization, and their patients. The goal of the ED was to reach 95% on-time reperfusion within a year. Given the patients' need this change is not yet of tremendous practical significance, even if it is a nonrandom pattern, or signal, of improvement. A small celebration may be appropriate, but much more work remains to be done.

Run charts play a pivotal role in improvement projects. They are used to answer the second question of the Model for Improvement (see Chapter One) "How will we know a change is an improvement?" The graphs in Figures 3.19 and 3.20 are examples of run charts used with improvement project measures. As improvement teams test changes they are waiting for the run chart to show a nonrandom pattern, a signal. The signal, evidenced by any of the four rules discussed here, provides evidence of improvement if it is in the desired direction. Of course, a signal does not have to indicate improvement. If the signal is in an undesirable direction it may indicate an unanticipated negative consequence or that some other factor is negatively influencing the measure. When a signal is noted, the team's job is to understand what happened to cause the signal and then use that information appropriately. If the signal was indicative of improvement the team will want to hold on to the gain, perhaps to replicate it elsewhere. If the signal was in an undesirable direction the team will want to learn from the signal in order to remedy the problem and to prevent it from happening in the future.

What if a team tests changes but sees no signal on their run charts? The changes tested did not yield evidence of improvement. Perhaps the tests of change were not carried

FIGURE 3.20   ED Timely Reperfusion Data Indicating Improvement

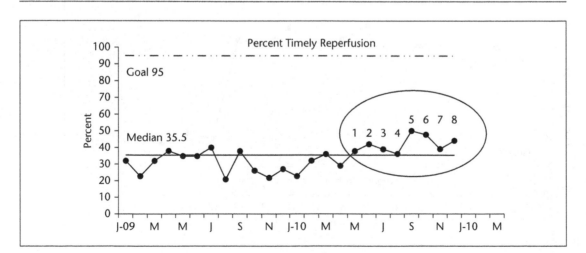

out as intended. Or the changes tested were not powerful enough to lead to improvement. The team may need more powerful ideas to tests. Or perhaps the ideas had potential but the tests of change were still quite small. As the tests increase in size or scope the team may logically expect to see improvement.

SPECIAL ISSUES IN USING RUN CHARTS

The previous sections have illustrated some of the uses of run charts to:

- Display data to make process performance visible
- Determine whether a change resulted in evidence of improvement
- Determine whether we are holding the gain made by our improvement

To summarize, Figure 3.21 illustrates these three important uses of the run chart:

Display data to make process performance visible (Graph A, Figure 3.21): The trauma center team was concerned about the length of time it was taking them to get a patient with an isolated femur fracture from their emergency department (ED) to the operating room (OR). They displayed their data on a run chart. On the y-axis they noted the time in minutes it took each patient to get from the ED to the OR. On the x-axis they listed sequential patients. The process showed no nonrandom signal as evidence of change during this time period, and it certainly was not performing at a level they wanted for their patients. It was time to test some of the changes to the process that they had recently been discussing.

Determine whether our change resulted in improvement (Graph B, Figure 3.21): The trauma team had learned of a protocol used by another organization with good results. They wanted to test it and adapt it to work in their organization. As they tested they were careful to annotate the run chart. After a few weeks of testing and adapting this protocol to their organization, the team saw evidence that their changes resulted in improvement in the form of a shift below the median. They decided to permanently implement the changes they had tested.

Determine whether we are holding the gain made by our improvement (Graph C, Figure 3.21): The trauma team continued to collect and plot data on the run chart to see if they were maintaining the improvement. Some improvements are maintained for a short time by extra effort or vigilance of those working in the system. The aim of improvement is to build improvement into the process of care. The run chart was a useful tool for both purposes, to tell if they had incorporated the change into the system and they were holding the gain.

The rest of this section describes a number of special issues that can arise when using run charts for these three situations. The following frequently asked questions are used to introduce the situations.

- When should the run chart be started?
- When should we apply a median? When should we extend the median?
- What do we do about run chart rules when the measure is not continuous data?
- Is there a useful run chart for plotting rare events data?
- Are there any cautions with percent or rate data on run charts?
- Do run charts always have to be in time order?
- What if the time intervals for the data are not equal?
- When should one consider using a trend line on a run chart?
- What about auto-correlated data?

FIGURE 3.21   Three Key Uses of Run Charts in Improvement Initiatives

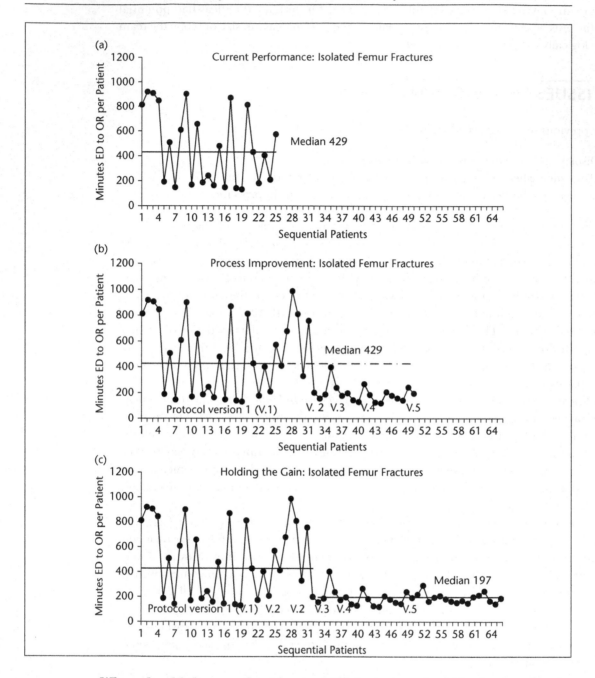

When should the run chart be started? A run chart should begin when data for the first point to be plotted is available. There is no downside to presenting these data on a run chart compared to presenting it solely in table form. This practice facilitates learning from the data as soon as possible. Beginning the run chart with a single data point also sets a clear expectation that data will be graphically displayed and allows important annotations to be captured in real time.

In Figure 3.22 the team learns about their baseline performance, and then learns that the three changes they are testing appear to be improvements. By the sixth week they detect evidence of improvement in the form of a trend. The rules for detecting signals of improvement can be applied to the run chart as soon as it becomes practical to do so.

FIGURE 3.22   Beginning a Run Chart as Soon as the First Data Are Available

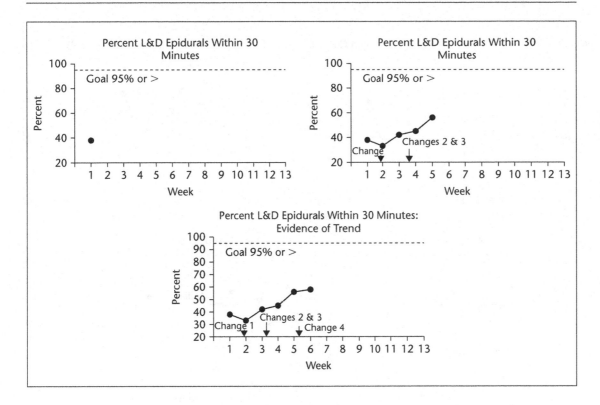

People often ask how much data is needed before each of the rules for detecting a signal on a run chart may be used. In this example, Rule Two, a trend was detected early in the improvement effort. This trend will remain a trend no matter the amount of additional data added to this graph. Rule One, a shift, and Rule Three (number of runs) require a minimum of 10 data points before becoming practical. We chose not to add the median to the run charts illustrated by Figure 3.23 because of the small number of data points on these run charts. Rule 4, because it is a visual analysis, can be applied at any time.

When should we apply and extend a median? The decision about when to create and extend a median will be based on the situation you face. A baseline median could be created from any number of data points. When we want to apply the probability-based rules for run chart analysis, however, the median should be created using 10 or more data points. When this is not possible the trend and run rules will not be applicable. If no baseline data exists, we suggest that the first few data points collected while the project is getting up and running may be used to create a baseline median. Chances are that the process hasn't been improved much during this start-up timeframe so this early data may provide the best information about baseline performance. This is crude, but can be useful in many cases. (See Figure 3.11 for an example of a run chart with little data which uses a median effectively for visual analysis.) Often historical data are available and may be used to create a baseline median. Of course, all the cautions with operational definitions related to the data (discussed in Chapter Two) should be considered in interpreting the data.

If a median is calculated from baseline data which exhibits no signals (shift, trend, runs, and astronomical data point), recommended practice is to extend this initial median into the future. By "freezing" and extending the baseline median, new data added to the chart do not influence the median. Any changes in the new data stand out against the baseline median more clearly, thus allowing better detection of signals of improvement.

FIGURE 3.23 Run Charts for Waiting Time Data

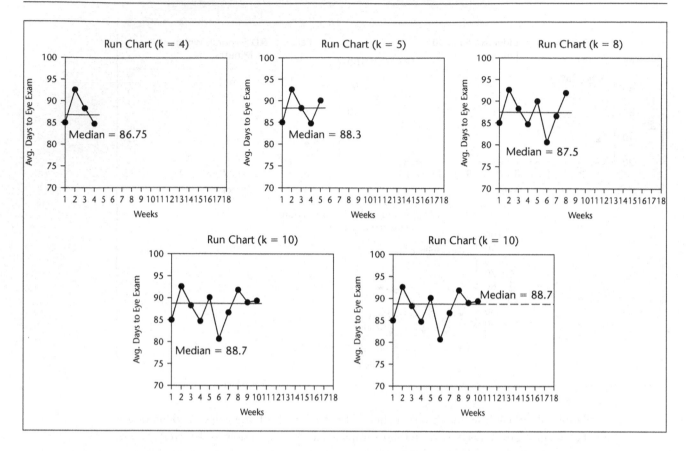

This is particularly important for understanding the impact of different changes to a system. The following charts at Figure 3.23 illustrate a group that chose to make a median with a small amount of data, updating it with each data point and then freezing and extending the median when reaching 10 data points. Ultimately, it is up to the user to decide when to calculate the median and when to apply the probability-based rules when starting the run chart. The rules are conditional on the median that is used, so any issues with this median will have an impact on the interpretation of the rules.

A signal in the new data being plotted on the run chart will be detected more accurately using proper technique for calculating the median. The team working to reduce waiting time for an eye exam continued to test changes and collect and plot their data. They knew by week 16 that they had a signal of improvement evidenced by a shift that began at week 11. If they had allowed all the data to be used in the determination of the median rather than solely the baseline data, the shift would not have been detected. Figure 3.24 contrasts proper and improper technique.

The rules for detecting a signal on a run chart are used for both data surrounding the original median and the extended median. Figure 3.25 displays a different pattern of data than the previous examples. In this instance a signal (shift) was detected that began in week 9. Part of this shift was detected using the baseline median, the other part using the extended median.

Sometimes it is appropriate to create a second median for new data added to the run chart. When changes made to the process result in a signal of improvement on the run chart it may be useful to create a new median for the new data representing improved performance. Some judgment is required to decide whether the improvement has been

FIGURE 3.24   Delay Detecting Signal with Improper Median Technique

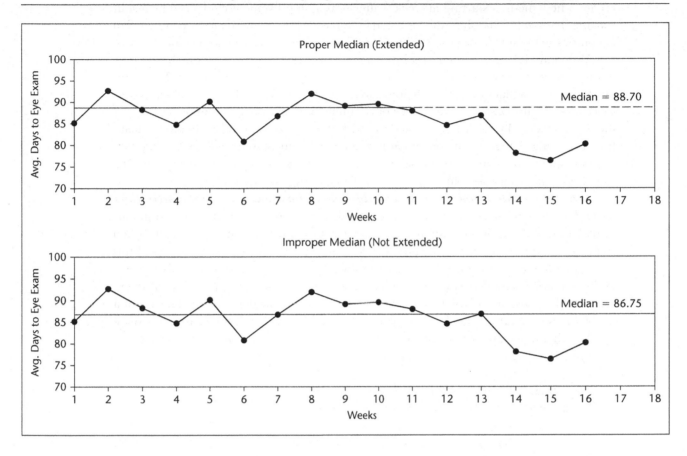

FIGURE 3.25   Detecting Signal with Proper Median Technique

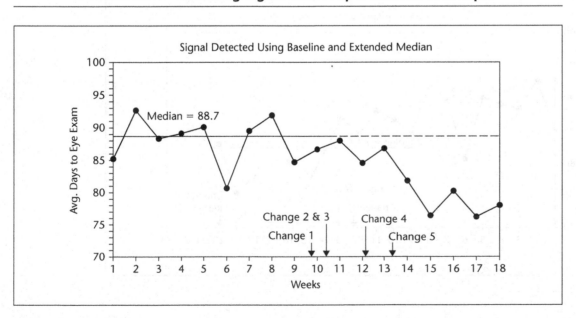

sustained long enough to warrant a new median. In this instance the team decided to create a new median starting at week 9 after noting improvement evidenced by a shift starting that week. That shift was sustained for quite a while. They created second median encompassing points 9 through 19. Figure 3.26 illustrates this chart with two medians.

When analyzing a run chart with two medians, the rules for detecting a signal of improvement must be applied separately to the data surrounding each median. For example, to detect a signal of a shift all 6 points would have to either be below or all above *their own median*. Figure 3.26 shows evidence of continued improvement. A shift below the new median is evident by week 19 (it started week 14). We can see on this graph that the team tried removing change 5 and noted their previous improvement went away. Next, they plan to put change 5 back in place and see if they get the same initial improvement. This is a useful strategy to increase our degree of belief in a change we are testing.

What do we do about run chart rules when the measure is not continuous data? Although the run chart rules are established based on a theoretical continuous distribution of data,[9] it is common to use run charts for attribute data and discrete (often rounded) continuous data (see Chapter Two for discussion of data types). Examples of this are count data, measures on a Likert scale, or time data rounded to days. This discreteness of the recorded data (for example, due to the scale that is used or to rounding of data), can actually cause more points than expected above or below the median. This is not a problem unless it affects the three probability-based rules used with run charts. When are the data that make up a run chart too discrete or repetitive to allow the run chart rules to be applied? There are two cases when problems occur:

1. More than half the data points fall on the median.
2. Too many data points fall on the extreme value.

More than one-half of data points fall on the median: When greater than 50% of the data points are on the median we can no longer use the probability-based run chart rules

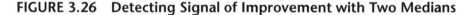

FIGURE 3.26   Detecting Signal of Improvement with Two Medians

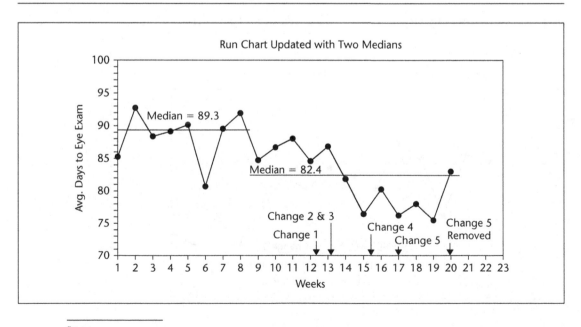

[9]Ibid.

because the symmetry around the center line breaks down significantly. If it is still desirable to have an estimate the of process central tendency, the mean should be used. Since data will usually not be symmetric around the mean, the shift and run rules (Rules 1 and 3) should still not be applied.

Too many points on the extreme value: If more than half the data on the run chart are at the extreme values on the scale (for example 0 or 100% on a percentage scale), the criteria for detecting a nonrandom statistical signal using the median cannot be applied. In these cases, the median will be the extreme absolute value itself (0 or 100%) and thus cannot be used to apply the rules. If it is desirable to have a measure of central tendency, one could use the mean of the data as described earlier. Figure 3.27 shows run charts that illustrate these two cases.

Another option in this case would be to display the time (for example, days) or workload (for example, number of cases) between the event on the run chart, plotting each time an event occurs (see next discussion)

Is there a useful run chart for plotting rare events data? Too many 0s can occur on a run chart if the measure involves undesirable events that are relatively rare, such as surgical site infections, employee needlesticks, falls, adverse drug events, or failure to follow protocol for a highly reliable system. Here, the data displayed on the run chart may result in time periods with too many zeros (more than half of the data points are zero). Figure 3.28 shows a run chart for a rare event incidence rate.

An alternative in this case is to use a run chart that displays time or workload *between* undesirable events.[10] (See earlier discussion in Chapter Two, Figure 2.20). More time or workload (such as cases) between undesirable events, such as a surgical site infection, is good and may be indicative of improvement. Figure 3.29 illustrates tracking cases between events. This method makes it easier to detect improvement than does Figure 3.28.

Creating a run chart displaying time or cases between a failure requires some finesse. Data are displayed on the graph each time the undesirable event occurs *after* an initial occurrence. For example, if the first undesirable event occurred on November 3rd and the next on November 8th, we would plot a single data point on November 8th, the number of cases between the November 3rd event and the undesirable event on November 8th. Figure 3.30, Chart A, shows that there were 38 cases between November 3rd and November 8th. If another event occurred on November 12th we would graph another data point, the

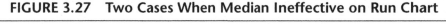

FIGURE 3.27   Two Cases When Median Ineffective on Run Chart

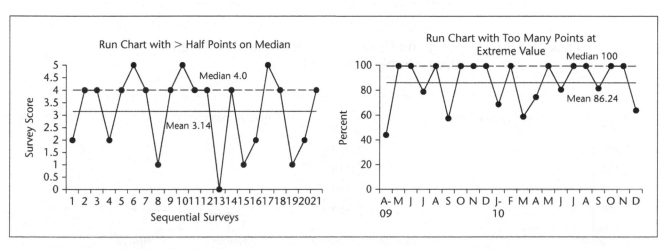

[10]Benneyan, J. C., Lloyd, R. C., and Plsek, P. E., "Statistical Process Control as a Tool for Research and Healthcare Improvement," *Quality and Safety in Health Care*, 2003, *12*, 458–464.

FIGURE 3.28   Run Chart Resulting in Too Many Zeros

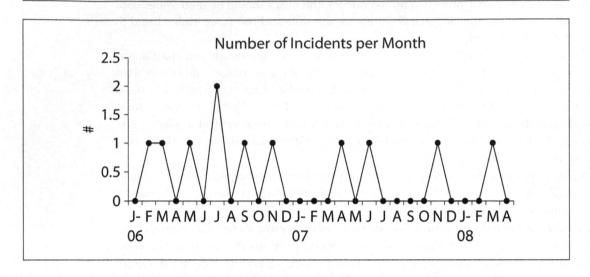

FIGURE 3.29   Run Chart of Cases Between Undesirable Events

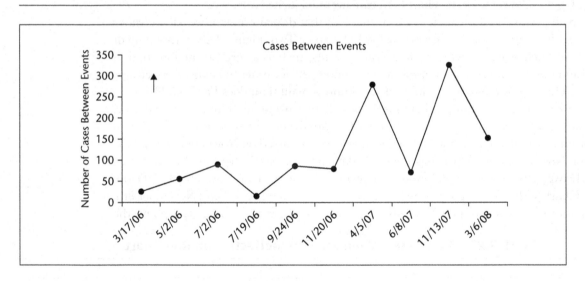

FIGURE 3.30   Starting and Updating Chart of Cases Between Undesirable Rare Events

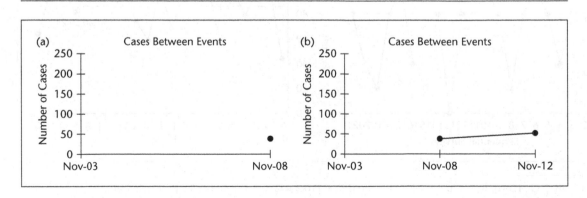

FIGURE 3.31   Plotting Monthly Data in the Absence of Events

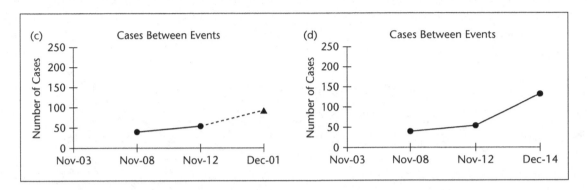

number of cases (53 in this example) between the event on November 8th and the event on November 12th. Figure 3.30, Chart B, illustrates updating the run chart.

It's common practice to enter data monthly (for a monthly report) even if no event occurred during that month. For example, if no event occurred between November 12th and December 1st, but reporting was required the first of each month, update the graph with the current count of cases between events as of 1 Dec. However, use a different symbol for this data point and connect it to the prior data point with a dashed line rather than a solid line (see Figure 3.31, Chart C). It is important to update the graph as soon as an undesirable event occurs. For example, if an event occurred on December 14th, determine the number of cases between November 12th and the event on December 14th. Then update the graph by changing the December 1st date to December 14th and entering the total number of cases between November 12th and the event on December 14th. See Figure 3.31, Chart D.

As these run charts mature with additional data added over time, patterns indicative of improvement may become evident. See Figure 3.32 for some examples of more mature run charts that track the number of cases between undesirable events and provide evidence of improvement. Both Cases 1 and 2 show evidence of a trend in a desirable direction. Case 3 reveals that the most recent data point is a huge improvement. Case 4 may at first glance be disconcerting to some who are thinking that the process has more variation in it now than at the beginning of the process and looks a bit chaotic. How can that run chart indicate improvement? Reflection reveals that the beginning of the process had few cases between each event. The median number of cases between events was 55.5. It appears smooth yet this really means that events are occurring frequently, which is undesirable. The later data appear to swing widely. These data reveal that there are now many cases between event occurrences. The median number of cases between events is 231.5. Even at its worst there are more cases between events than in any of the baseline time frame. In fact, the more recent data reveals a signal of improvement, a shift above the initial median of 55.5.

Are there any cautions with percent or rate data on run charts? One important caution is to be aware of the impact of unequal denominators when viewing data on a run chart. A team was plotting the percentage of patients who returned on an unplanned basis to the operating room (OR) each month. Their run chart is at Figure 3.33. When they saw the run chart they reacted strongly to the most recent data point, which revealed a percentage nearly double that of their usual performance.

Upon looking more closely at the data they noticed that the volume of surgeries performed that month was very different from the other months. When placing rate or

FIGURE 3.32   Mature Run Charts Tracking Cases Between Rare Events

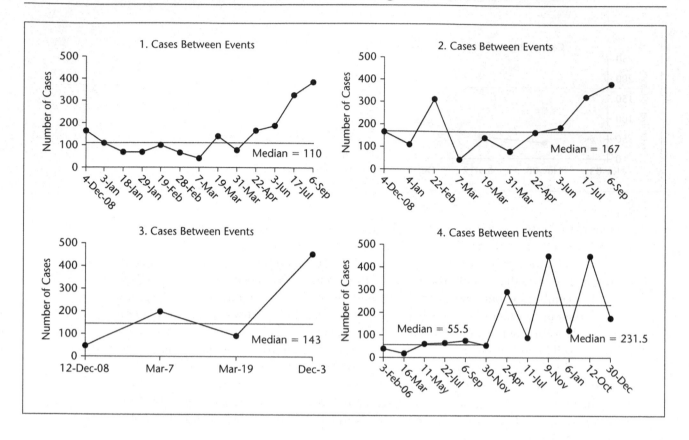

FIGURE 3.33   Run Chart with Percent Doubled in Most Recent Month

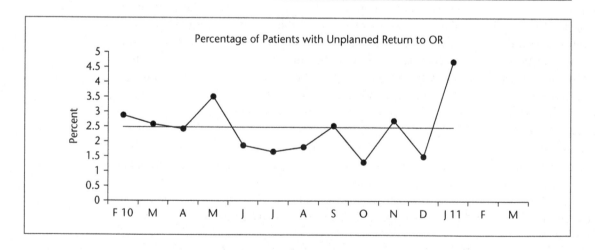

percent data on a run chart it is important that each data point has a roughly equal denominator, + or − 25% of the average denominator size. The average denominator size for the months up to the month in question was 488. Plus or minus 25% of the average yields a range of 366 to 610 surgeries. Each month, except the month in question, the denominator was within this range. If the team used a more sensitive chart, a Shewhart control chart (p chart, Chapter Five), they would discover that the month in question was probably not a signal but was more likely to have been caused by the small denominator size.

FIGURE 3.34   Shewhart Control Chart (P Chart) Adjusting Limits
Based on Denominator Size

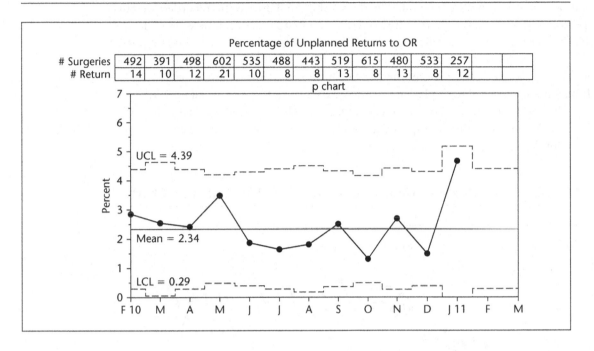

Percentage of Unplanned Returns to OR

# Surgeries	492	391	498	602	535	488	443	519	615	480	533	257		
# Return	14	10	12	21	10	8	8	13	8	13	8	12		

FIGURE 3.35   Use of Data Line on Run Chart

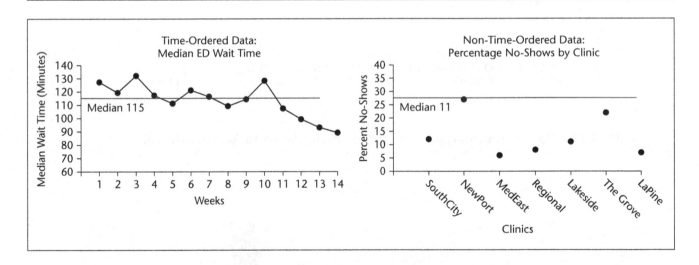

The Shewhart chart, Figure 3.34, reveals that the data point does not exceed the process limits and represents typical process variation. As a general rule, if the denominators of the points on the run chart are expected to vary more than a small amount, a Shewhart chart should be used instead of a run chart.

Do run charts always have to be in time order? Run charts commonly display data in time order. When data are displayed in time order, the data points may be connected by a data line to facilitate the visual interpretation of the data. Other orderings of data may by useful, such as location, patient, or provider order. When data are not in time order the data points should not be connected with a line. See Figure 3.35 for examples.

What if the time intervals for the data are not equal? When graphing time-ordered data, the run chart typically spaces the data points equally, implying that the interval between data points is equal. The data in Figure 3.36 are the recorded weights of a person with congestive heart failure (CHF). The first 20 data points were collected irregularly over three years, usually several months apart when the person visited his physician. The remainder of the data was collected much more frequently, nearly daily, as the patient entered an extended care setting and began recording his weight every day.

It may be more useful to display time- ordered data collected at unequal time intervals in a way that makes the impact of the unequal time periods more evident. Figure 3.37 displays the CHF data with the data spaced across the x-axis relative to the time that passed between obtaining the patient's weight.

FIGURE 3.36   Data from Unequal Time Intervals Displayed in Usual Run Chart

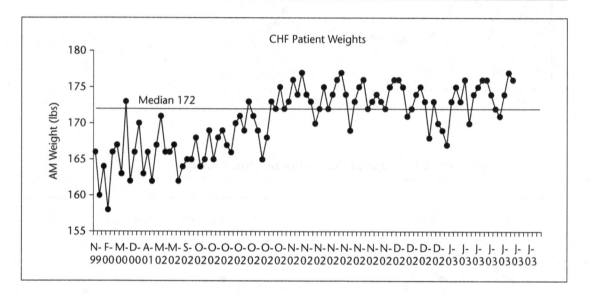

FIGURE 3.37   Data from Unequal Time Intervals Displayed to Reveal Intervals

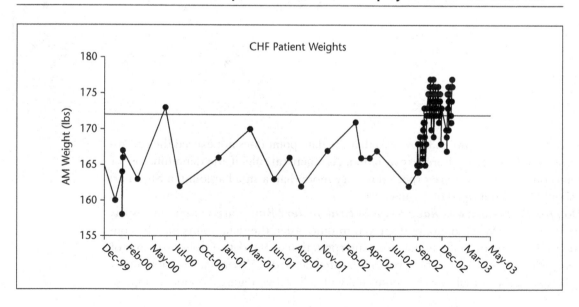

This patient's weight gain was not a slow creep, as implied by the first run chart with equal intervals. Rather it occurred rapidly from September to December 2002. His weight had actually been very consistent for quite some time; then he suddenly gained weight. This view of the data makes it more evident that the weight gain occurred in a short time span. A rapid gain in weight in a person with congestive heart failure can indicate fluid retention and have clinical significance. The rapidity of the change in some other clinical measures such as weight, blood sugar, hemoglobin, and hematocrits, blood pressure, and so forth may be an important piece of information influencing treatment. To produce a run chart with an un-equal x-axis develop a scatter plot with the time intervals (date) on the x-axis. Place the value being measured on the y-axis. Connect the data points with a data line and add the median. This is readily done using Excel™ or other software to create a scatter plot.

When should one consider using a trend line on a run chart? It can be misleading to place a trend line on a run chart if there is no signal of change using the four run chart rules. When there is no signal on a run chart, but a trend line is added, it may imply to someone studying the chart that there has been meaningful change. Best practice is to place a trend line on a run chart only if that chart provides a signal of change (such as a trend, shift, or too few runs, and so on) and the data appears to move in a consistent downward or upward direction on the run chart. In this case the trend line may effectively illustrate the magnitude of the change. Note: we will illustrate a linear trend here, but more complex trends (quadratic, cubic, exponential, and so forth) could also be added to the run chart.

Figure 3.38 illustrated a run chart for epidurals during labor and delivery. The improvement team was working on new protocols that encouraged cooperation between two departments that were critical to the process. They were working with the clinicians in small groups to train on the new protocols. After seven weeks, the team was encouraged by the improvement (they had a signal on the run chart from the trend rule). The team wanted to estimate when they would expect to meet their 95% goal (assuming their progress continued at the same rate). Using the data from the first seven weeks, they calculated a regression line[11] and extrapolated it into the future. They concluded that if they could maintain the same rate of improvement, the team should meet their goal by week 12.

FIGURE 3.38 Run Chart from Figure 3.22 with Seventh Week Added

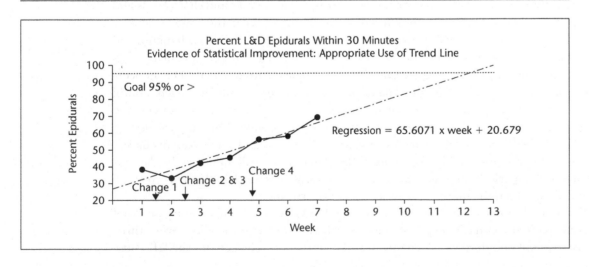

---

[11]Mosteller, F., and Tukey, J. *Data Analysis and Regression*, Reading, MA: Addison-Wesley, 1977.

FIGURE 3.39   Run Chart with Inappropriate Use of Trend Line

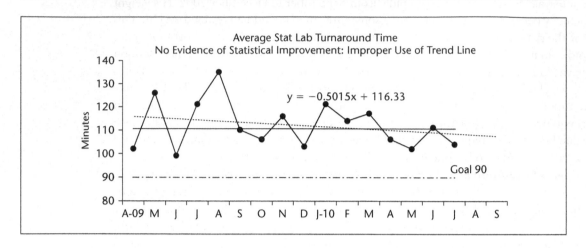

As a second example, the team working on STAT turnaround times wanted to quantify the results of their improvement work (see Figure 3.5). They applied the run chart rules and found no signal of improvement. But they did not let that stop them from calculating a regression line for their data (see Figure 3.39). The trend line implies a slight decrease in STAT times, but there is no evidence that this is any more than just a result of the random month-to-month variation in the data. This is a misuse of the trend line.

What about autocorrelated data? A basic assumption in using a run chart is that the data for each subgroup are independent; that is, the data from one subgroup does not help us predict another period. Sometimes process operations or data collection procedures result in data that are not independent from subgroup to subgroup. This phenomenon is called **autocorrelation**.[12] This relationship between the plotted points would make all the probability-based run chart rules invalid. Rely on only the visual analysis when studying a run chart with autocorrelated data. (See more on working with autocorrelated data for Shewhart charts in Chapter Eight).

A common example in a clinical setting is analyzing data that is stored in a computerized registry for patients with chronic diseases such as diabetes, asthma, or cardiovascular disease. Typically these patients visit the clinic every two to four months and clinical tests and observations are done to monitor their health status. In some clinics, the average value or overall percentage of the various measures in the registry are summarized each month and used to monitor the performance of the clinic for that particular population of patients (see case study at the end of Chapter One for an example of this practice). The autocorrelation problem occurs because the data for most patients are not updated each month; only the data for the patients who come in for a visit. If one-third of the patients come in during the current month and have their data updated, the monthly summary will use the same data as the previous month for two-thirds of the patients. If a few patients have a very high glycated hemoglobin test (HbA1c) those high levels will influence the data for subsequent time periods until the registry is updated with a newer HbA1c. This creates a relationship between the monthly measures, or autocorrelation.

Figure 3.40 shows a run chart for the average HbA1c values from a registry of about 130 adult patients with diabetes. Patients are scheduled to visit the clinic every three months, so about one-third visit each month and their registry values are updated. Because

---

[12]Montgomery, D. C., and Mastrangelo, C. M., "Some Statistical Process Control Methods for Autocorrelated Data," *Journal of Quality Technology*, 1991, *23*, 179–193.

FIGURE 3.40   Run Chart of Autocorrelated Data from a Patient Registry

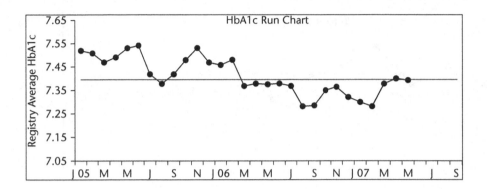

of the way the data are collected for this chart, autocorrelation was expected. The chart appears to indicate numerous nonrandom signals (shifts above, too few runs and a shift below the median). Are these really signals or the impact of autocorrelation due to use of the registry values? In analyzing autocorrelated data using a run chart do not apply any of the probability-based rules (shift, the number of runs or trend rule); rely solely on visual analysis of the run chart. In Chapter Eight, we will further discuss autocorrelation in the context of Shewhart charts.

Stratification with Run Charts

As described in Chapter Two, stratification is the separation and classification of data according to selected variables or factors. The object is to find patterns which help in understanding the causal mechanisms in the process. Stratification is a key strategy in learning from data. To stratify the data on a run chart, different symbols can be used to represent different variables in the process or groupings of the data. Figure 3.41 is an example of three run charts plotting harm rate. Chart A displays the overall harm rate per 1,000 patient days each month. There is no indication of change evident on this run chart. The second chart, chart B, displays the same data stratified by the two hospitals that compose this system. The data stratified by hospital reveals that hospital one has a much higher rate of harm that does hospital two. The harm data also was collected in a way that allowed these data to be stratified by shift. Chart C displays this stratification by shift. Day shift accounts for most of the harm occurring in their organization. Stratification using a run chart can help us learn about the impact of causal factors involved in the variation we see in process or outcome.

Multi-Vari Run Charts. The concept of stratification on a run chart can be extended to include study of multiple variables in the process. This technique has been called "**multi-vari.**"[13] Where a simple run chart graphs the effect of time on our measure, the multi-vari chart allows us to display and learn from classification variables other than time such as different protocols, clinicians, treatment locations, facilities, demographic groups, or any combination of these.

---

[13]Seder, L. A., "Diagnosis with Diagrams-Part I and II," *Industrial Quality Control*. 1950, Jan–Feb; Vargo, J. J., "Multi-Vari, the Neglected Problem-Solving Tool," *ASQC Quality Congress Transactions*, 1988, 329–337.

FIGURE 3.41   Stratification Using a Run Chart

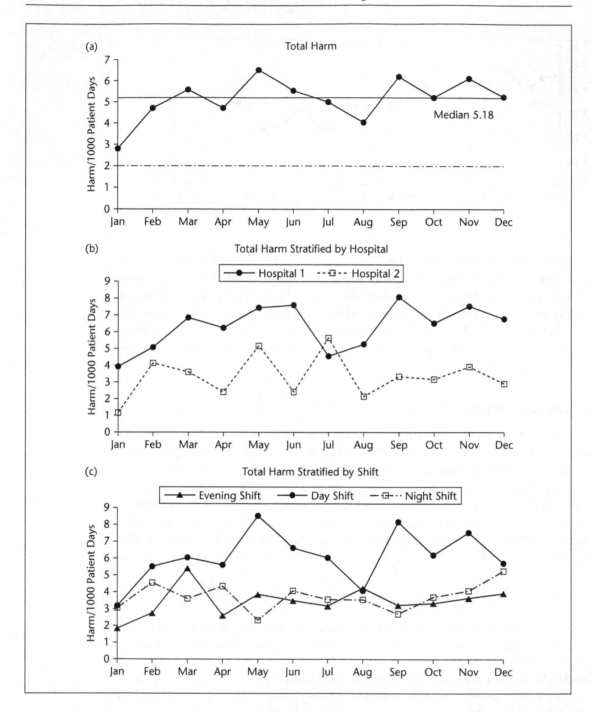

By stratifying the harm data as they did in Figure 3.41 the organization learned that the day shift had a much higher rate of harm than did the evening or night shift. By using a multi-vari run chart the team could simultaneously display variation in more than one characteristic. A multi-vari run chart allowed this team to display the variation related to hospital and to shift each month simultaneously. The multi-vari run chart data are shown in Table 3.5.

The chart in Figure 3.42 reveals that Hospital One is very different from Hospital Two but only on day shift. Hospital One's harm rate on the other two shifts is very similar to

Table 3.5 Harm Rate Data for Multi-Vari Chart

Month	Shift	Hospital 1 Harm Rate Per 1,000 Patient Days	Hospital 2 Harm Rate Per 1,000 Patient Days
Jan	D	1.972	1.654
	E	1.030	0.840
	N	0.894	0.320
Feb	D	3.060	2.366
	E	0.870	1.393
	N	1.128	0.938
Mar	D	3.960	2.723
	E	1.033	1.205
	N	1.828	1.606
Apr	D	3.960	2.130
	E	1.421	1.460
	N	0.856	1.110
May	D	4.960	2.721
	E	1.098	2.433
	N	1.360	1.348
Jun	D	4.960	2.721
	E	1.098	2.433
	N	1.360	1.348

FIGURE 3.42   Multi-Vari Chart

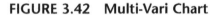

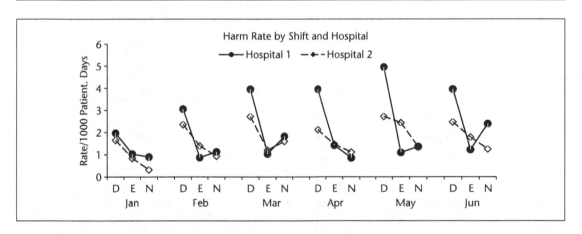

Hospital Two's rate. Using the multi-vari chart to display the impact of multiple variables can aid us in focusing our improvement efforts in the most fruitful arenas.

Using the Cumulative Sum Statistic with Run Charts

The run chart used in conjunction with the cumulative sum (CUSUM)[14] statistic can yield some important information about changes in the average operating level of a process. The **CUSUM statistic** is the sum of the differences between the data points and a selected

---

[14]Wadsworth, H. M., Stephens, K. S., and Godfrey, A. B·, *Modern Methods for Quality Control and Improvement*, New York: Wiley, 1986, Chapter 8.

Associates in Process Improvement, *Improvement Handbook*. Austin, TX: API, 1998, Chapter 22.

Table 3.6 Patient Satisfaction CUSUM Using Process Average as Target

Month	% Sat (X)	Target (Average)	X-Target (Si)	CUSUM	CUSUM + Target
J-09	82	88.296	−6.296	−6.296	82
F	79	88.296	−9.296	−15.592	72.704
M	84	88.296	−4.296	−19.888	68.408
A	82	88.296	−6.296	−26.184	62.112
M	92	88.296	3.704	−22.48	65.816
J	80	88.296	−8.296	−30.776	57.52
J	94	88.296	5.704	−25.072	63.224
A	78	88.296	−10.296	−35.368	52.928
S	83	88.296	−5.296	−40.664	47.632
O	84	88.296	−4.296	−44.96	43.336
N	92	88.296	3.704	−41.256	47.04
D	84	88.296	−4.296	−45.552	42.744
J-10	89	88.296	0.704	−44.848	43.448
F	88	88.296	−0.296	−45.144	43.152
M	93	88.296	4.704	−40.44	47.856
A	84	88.296	−4.296	−44.736	43.56
M	98	88.296	9.704	−35.032	53.264
J	92	88.296	3.704	−31.328	56.968
J	87	88.296	−1.296	−32.624	55.672
A	94	88.296	5.704	−26.92	61.376
S	93	88.296	4.704	−22.216	66.08
O	95	88.296	6.704	−15.512	72.784
N	91	88.296	2.704	−12.808	75.488
D	84	88.296	−4.296	−17.104	71.192
J-11	95	88.296	6.704	−10.4	77.896
F	92	88.296	3.704	−6.696	81.6
M	95	88.296	6.704	0.008	88.304

target. Instead of plotting the individual value, the run chart using the CUSUM technique displays the cumulative evidence of change. These charts can be used with both historical and real-time data to discover changes in a process. It's important to note that the analysis of the CUSUM run chart is purely visual. Neither the median nor the probability-based rules should be used in the analysis of the CUSUM run chart. For more advanced analysis of a CUSUM-type chart see Chapter Seven.

Table 3.6 contains data used with a CUSUM calculation. The CUSUM for the first period on the run chart is calculated by subtracting the target from the initial value. The CUSUM for the second period on the run chart is calculated by subtracting the target value from the second value and then adding this difference to the CUSUM from the first period. This procedure continues for each succeeding value. This technique can be accomplished using the following method:

1. Select the characteristic (measure) of interest to be charted (X).
2. Determine a desired target value or known process target (this could be a historical average) (T).
3. The cumulative sum statistic (S) is the sum of the deviations of the individual measurements from a target value, for example:

$$S_i = S_{i-1} + (X_i - T), \text{ where } S_i \text{ is the } i^{th} \text{ cumulative sum,}$$
$$X_i = \text{the } i^{th} \text{ observation,}$$
$$T = \text{Target (often from historical averages)}$$
$$S_i = \text{the } i^{th} \text{ cumulative statistic.}$$

4. Establish a scale with zero near the center that will accommodate all the CUSUM values in the series. Then, plot the CUSUM statistic in order of time (Note: sometimes the target is added to the initial CUSUM statistic to make the chart centered on the target instead of zero.)

For a measure from a process that is not changing and is running at the target level, the plot of data on a CUSUM chart will follow a horizontal pattern. Changes in the direction of this pattern will usually be explained by some change in the process under study. Table 3.6 contains patient satisfaction data. Each month the percent of patients scoring the organization as "Very Good" or "Excellent" was calculated.

The monthly patient satisfaction data were plotted on the run chart in Figure 3.43 using the traditional run chart. The team noted no signal of improvement using the run chart rules despite changes to their processes designed to improve patient satisfaction. Using a CUSUM run chart helped them see the cumulative performance of their process.

FIGURE 3.43   Run Chart and CUSUM Run Chart of Patient Satisfaction Data

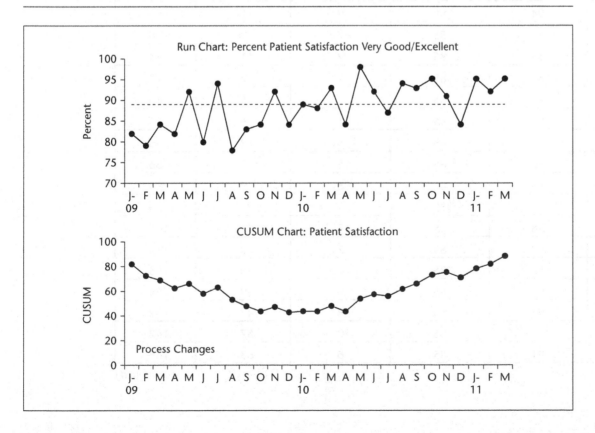

The percent patient satisfaction and the calculated CUSUM statistics for these data are shown in Table 3.6. The target value of 88.48, their average satisfaction level to date, was used in the calculation. The CUSUM chart in Figure 3.44 shows a gradual continued change from the target (zero line plus 88.48) after the introduction of process changes beginning in November despite some recent months this year with poor performance. The traditional run chart shows the same data, but the change in the patient satisfaction per month is not as easy to detect (none of the run chart rules are present). The power of the CUSUM run chart to visually show improvement in a process can be demonstrated by comparison of the run chart to the CUSUM run chart in Figure 3.43.

The CUSUM run chart may also be constructed using a performance target rather than current process average. The question this chart would answer is "How is our process performance relative to our performance target?" Table 3.7 shows the CUSUM calculations for the patient satisfaction process when using a target of 85%.

The CUSUM run chart in Figure 3.44 initially shows a flat slope indicating that performance is near the target. The slope starts to rise in October indicating that monthly

Table 3.7   Patient Satisfaction CUSUM Using Performance Goal of 85% as Target

Month	% Sat (X)	Target (Goal)	X-Target (Si)	CUSUM	CUSUM + Target
J-09	82	85	−3	−3	82
F	79	85	−6	−9	76
M	84	85	−1	−10	75
A	82	85	−3	−13	72
M	92	85	7	−6	79
J	80	85	−5	−11	74
J	94	85	9	−2	83
A	78	85	−7	−9	76
S	83	85	−2	−11	74
O	84	85	−1	−12	73
N	92	85	7	−5	80
D	84	85	−1	−6	79
J-10	89	85	4	−2	83
F	88	85	3	1	86
M	93	85	8	9	94
A	84	85	−1	8	93
M	98	85	13	21	106
J	92	85	7	28	113
J	87	85	2	30	115
A	94	85	9	39	124
S	93	85	8	47	132
O	95	85	10	57	142
N	91	85	6	63	148

(continued)

Table 3.7 Continued

Month	% Sat (X)	Target (Goal)	X-Target (Si)	CUSUM	CUSUM + Target
D	84	85	−1	62	147
J-11	95	85	10	72	157
F	97	85	12	84	169
M	95	85	10	94	179

FIGURE 3.44   CUSUM Run Chart with Performance Goal as Target

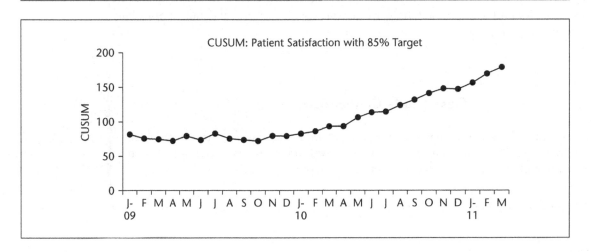

performance is now greater than the target of 85%. The process slope continues to climb indicating continued performance above the target.

SUMMARY

A run chart is easy to construct and simple to interpret. Because improvement is temporal, the run chart is the fundamental method to evaluate the impact of changes tested and, ultimately, the success of improvement efforts. This simplicity makes it one of the most important methods for communicating and understanding variation. Important uses of the run chart include:

- Displaying data to make process performance visible
- Determining whether our change resulted in improvement
- Determining whether we are holding the gain made by our improvement

  Some key ideas presented about run charts:

- The run chart is basically a visual tool. To go beyond visual analysis of a run chart we make use of other guidance and rules.
- Adding a median to the run chart and using some probability-based interpretive rules allows us to learn whether our process exhibits a nonrandom signal of change.

- There are a variety of modifications to the basic run chart that can be useful:
  - Putting multiple measures on the same run chart
  - Using an x-axis other than time
  - Using a real-time scale when time intervals are unequal
  - Adding a trend line to a run chart
- Stratification can be used with run charts to compare the variation of groupings of data.
- The CUSUM technique used with run charts allows us to detect small persistent changes to a process that we may be unable to note on the more basic run chart.
- The run chart fosters a great deal of learning about the performance of our process with minimal mathematical complexity. It's often also the first step toward developing a Shewhart chart. Chapter Four will introduce the Shewhart chart and provide a brief overview of the other tools in our tool kit for learning from variation: the Pareto chart, frequency plot and scatter plot. Chapter Five will provide substantial detail on Shewhart chart selection and use.

Case Study Connection

To learn more about the use of run charts in improvement work you may want to explore Case Study A. This case study illustrates the use of run charts with an improvement project. It also provides an example of the use of a family of measures all graphically displayed on a single page with run charts.

KEY TERMS

Astronomical point	Run chart
Autocorrelation	Runs
CUSUM statistic	Shift
Median	Signal of improvement
Multi-vari run charts	Trend

## CHAPTER 4

LEARNING FROM VARIATION IN DATA

Chapter Three described the use of the run chart, a graphical display of data plotted in time order. Because improvement is temporal, a run chart is almost always the beginning point for learning from data to facilitate improvement. This chapter goes more deeply into learning from variation in data for improvement. It will build on the use of the run chart and introduce other tools to learn from the patterns of variation in data. In this chapter we will address: concepts and theory about variation including the theory of special and common cause variation; strategies when working with special cause and with common cause variation; the Shewhart control chart; interpretation of the Shewhart chart; making and revising limits on Shewhart charts; stratification and rational subgrouping with Shewhart charts; and learning from variation using other tools, including the Pareto chart, frequency plot, and scatter plot.

THE CONCEPT OF VARIATION

One of the key strategies in improvement is to control variation. Often, when first presented, this concept sounds threatening to health care professionals whose job is to make judgments and treat the conditions of unique patients. So first we must differentiate intended versus unintended variation (Berwick, 1991).[1] **Intended variation** (often called purposeful, planned, guided, or considered) is an important part of effective, patient-centered health care. A physician, for example, purposely prescribes different doses of a drug to a child and an adult. Certainly, in a patient-centered health care system, it is desirable to have variation intended to best match patient preferences for communication style, interaction with family, and so forth.

Unintended variation is due to changes introduced into health care process that are not purposeful, planned, or guided. The changes can come from decisions made, but usually they show up through equipment, supplies, environment, measurement, and management practices. Often, health care professionals are not even aware that the changes are happening as care is delivered. This is the variation that creates inefficiencies, waste, rework, ineffective care, errors, and injuries in our health care system. Walter Shewhart (Shewhart, 1931) focused his studies on this unintended variation.[2] He found that reducing unintended variation in a process usually resulted in improved outcomes and lower costs.

---

[1]Berwick, D. M., "Controlling Variation in Health Care: A Consultation with Walter Shewhart," *Medical Care*, 1991, *29*(12), 1212–1225.

[2]Shewhart, W. A., *Control of Quality of Manufactured Product*, New York: D. Van Nostrand Company, 1931. [Reprinted by the American Society for Quality Control, 1980.]

A fundamental concept for the study and improvement of processes, due to Walter Shewhart (1931), is that variation in a measure of quality has its origins in one of two types of causes:

Common Causes—those causes that are inherent in the system (process or product) over time, affect everyone working in the system, and affect all outcomes of the system.

Special Causes—those causes that are not part of the system (process or product) all the time or do not affect everyone, but arise because of specific circumstances.

(Note: Shewhart initially used the terms *assignable* rather than *special* and *chance* rather than *common* to describe these two types of causes. Deming (1986) popularized the common and special cause nomenclature).[3]

A system that has only common causes affecting the outcomes is called a **stable system**, or one that is in a state of statistical control. A stable process implies that the variation is predictable within statistically established limits. This does not mean that the stable system is performing well; it may be stable but producing very undesirable results. A system whose outcomes are affected by both common causes and special causes is called an **unstable system**. An unstable system does not necessarily mean one with large variation. It means that the magnitude of the variation from one time period to the next is unpredictable. It is important to note that special causes may be good or bad news.

This distinction between common and special causes of variation is fundamental to developing effective improvement strategies. When a measure is stable—that is, it exhibits only common cause variation—it means that we are seeing only variation inherent in the current process design for this measure. Our improvement strategy then will involve:

- Realizing that since that the process is performing as well as possible, to make it perform better will require process redesign.
- Identifying aspects of the process to change.
- Testing those changes using the Plan-Do-Study-Act (PDSA) cycle. (See Chapter 1 regarding PDSA cycle.)
- Implementing successful changes using the PDSA cycle.

When we become aware that there are special causes affecting a process or outcome measure, it means that something not typically part of the process design is affecting the process. In this case it is feasible and economically sound to learn from the special cause. Our improvement strategy then will involve:

- Identifying when the special cause occurred.
- Learning from the special cause.
- Taking action based on the special cause.

Special cause may be unfavorable or favorable. For example, we may begin using a new medical device only to find that many patients using it get infections. When we see undesirable special cause the logical action is to remove the special cause and make it difficult for it to occur again. Other times, the special cause produces a favorable result, so the appropriate action is to make it a permanent part of the health care process. For example, a new employee takes a particular type of x-ray in a different way from the established employees' method. We note that their x-ray retake rate is far lower than that of the other employees and constitutes favorable special cause. We study their approach and adopt it as the new standard technique for all x-ray technicians.

---

[3]Deming, W. E., *Out of the Crisis*, Chapter. 11, Cambridge, MA: MIT Center for Advanced Engineering Study, 1986.

As special causes are identified and removed, the process becomes stable. Deming gives several benefits of a stable process:[4]

- The process has an identity; its performance is predictable.
- Costs and quality are predictable.
- Productivity is at a maximum and costs at a minimum under the present system.
- The effect of changes in the process can be measured with greater speed and reliability. PDSA tests of change and more complex experiments can be efficiently used to identify changes that results in improvement.
- A stable process provides a sound argument for altering specifications that cannot be met economically.

Note that in improvement projects, we are often introducing changes into a stable process, hoping to produce a signal of a special cause that indicates an improvement in the process.

Besides providing these basic concepts of variation, Dr. Shewhart also provided the method for determining whether a system is dominated by common or special causes.[5] This method is called the Shewhart chart and will be discussed later in this chapter. Figure 4.1 illustrates the central role of a Shewhart chart in guiding strategies and tactics in

FIGURE 4.1   Using Shewhart Charts to Give Direction to an Improvement Effort

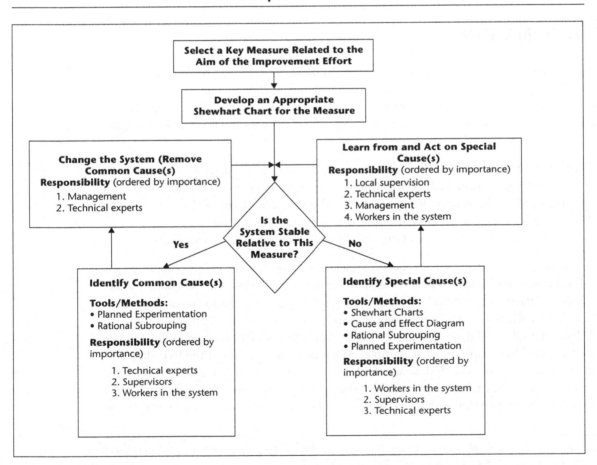

[4]Ibid., 340.

[5]Shewhart, W. A., *Statistical Method from the Viewpoint of Quality Control* (W. E. Deming [ed.]), Washington, D.C.: The Graduate School, The Department of Agriculture, 1939.

an improvement effort. We introduced the Model for Improvement in Chapter One. The second question in this model is "How will we know a change is an improvement?" In Figure 4.1 the first step in answering this question is developing a measure related to the aim of the improvement work. The second step in Figure 4.1 involves selecting and creating the appropriate Shewhart chart. Interpretation of this Shewhart chart will allow the user to answer question two of the Model for Improvement. In addition, interpretation of the Shewhart chart will aid in answering the third question in the Model for Improvement, "What changes can we make that will lead to improvement?" If special cause is identified on the Shewhart chart the appropriate action is to investigate the special cause and take appropriate action to either use or prevent the special cause depending on whether it was a favorable or unfavorable special cause. If solely common cause is identified on the Shewhart chart improvement will require redesign of process(es) that have an impact on the project aim. The use of the Plan-Do-Study-Act (PDSA) cycle is associated with working to improve a stable system, one exhibiting solely common cause variation. The Plan-Do-Study-Act cycle is used extensively to test and then implement changes to improve a stable system.

Why are we focusing so much of the rest of this book on the use of Shewhart charts? Mohammed et al.[6] summarized our feelings succinctly in the summary of their 2001 article: "The case for the control chart to guide action has been presented. Its guidance has proved immensely useful to industry over the past 50 years; it is time for it to be integrated into clinical governance." We want to provide the understanding, guidance, and examples to make Shewhart's theories and methods more available to those who work in health care environments.

DEPICTING VARIATION

How can we make learning from variation in data more prominent in health care organizations? Effective visual presentations of data, instead of tabular displays, provide the most opportunity for learning to take place. In Chapter Two Figure 2.26 introduced five fundamental tools to learn from variation in data. All of these tools rely on a visual display to gain insights from variation in data:

- Run Chart: Study variation in data over time; understand the impact of changes.
- Shewhart Chart: Distinguish between special and common causes of variation.
- Frequency Plot: Understand location, spread, shape, and patterns of data.
- Pareto Chart: Focus on areas of improvement with greatest impact.
- Scatter Plot: Analyze the associations or relationship between two variables.

A good graphic display of data encourages learning from the data. Insights can be gained that don't come from looking at tables of numbers or a statistical summary. The example at the beginning of the run chart chapter illustrated this point. To further make the point, Anscombe (1973) developed another revealing example of the importance of the visual display.[7]

Table 4.1 tabulates data on waiting times and patient satisfaction rating for four clinics (data modified from Anscombe's example). What do you learn about the four data sets from study of the table? Each data set of 11 pairs of waiting time and satisfaction rating has the same average for both waiting time and satisfaction. An analysis (regression analysis[8]) to evaluate the linear relationship between wait time and satisfaction rating results in the

---

[6]Mohammed, M., Cheng, K., Rouse, A., and Marshall, T., "Bristol, Shipman, and Clinical Governance: Shewhart's Forgotten Lessons," *The Lancet*, 2001, *357*, 463–467.

[7]Anscombe, F. J., "Graphs in Statistical Analysis," *American Statistician* 1973, *27*, 17–21.

[8]Mosteller, F., and Tukey, J., *Data Analysis and Regression*. Reading, MA: Addison-Wesley, 1977.

Table 4.1 Wait Time and Satisfaction Data from Four Clinics

	Clinic 1		Clinic 2		Clinic 3		Clinic 4	
Week	Average wait time (minutes)	Average patient rating	Average wait time (minutes)	Average patient rating	Average wait time (minutes)	Average patient rating	Average wait time (minutes)	Average patient rating
1	40.0	3.98	40.0	3.43	40.0	4.27	32.0	4.71
2	32.0	4.53	32.0	3.93	32.0	4.62	32.0	5.12
3	52.0	4.21	52.0	3.63	52.0	1.63	32.0	4.15
4	36.0	3.60	36.0	3.62	36.0	4.45	32.0	3.58
5	44.0	3.84	44.0	3.37	44.0	4.10	32.0	3.77
6	56.0	3.02	56.0	3.95	56.0	3.58	32.0	4.48
7	24.0	4.38	24.0	4.94	24.0	4.96	32.0	5.38
8	16.0	5.87	16.0	6.45	16.0	5.31	76.0	1.75
9	48.0	2.58	48.0	3.44	48.0	3.93	32.0	5.22
10	28.0	5.59	28.0	4.37	28.0	4.79	32.0	4.05
11	20.0	5.16	20.0	5.63	20.0	5.14	32.0	4.56
Number of weeks	11	11	11	11	11	11	11	11
Overall average	36.00	4.25	36.00	4.25	36.00	4.25	36.00	4.25
Standard deviation	13.27	1.02	13.27	1.02	13.27	1.02	13.27	1.02
Correlation: (r statistic)	0.82		0.82		0.82		0.82	
Regression: intercept/slope	6.50	−0.062	6.50	−0.062	6.50	−0.062	6.50	−0.062
Regression standard error	0.62		0.62		0.62		0.62	
P-value for regression	0.0022		0.0022		0.0022		0.0022	

FIGURE 4.2   Scatter Plots for Data in Table 4.1

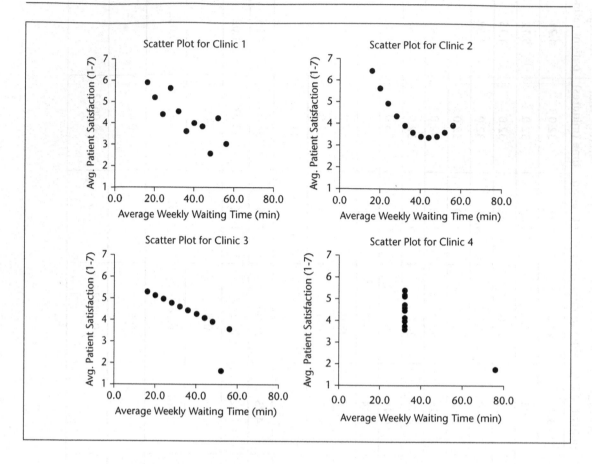

same relationship (intercept, slope, and correlation coefficient all identical) for each data set. Are the data from the four clinics different? What are the data trying to tell us?

Figure 4.2 shows four scatter plots for the data from each of the four clinics. These plots quickly tell us that the four data sets are very different, each with different things to tell us about the relationship between the average wait time and patient satisfaction rating:

● Clinic 1: A typical pattern that might be expected with the statistics from the table.
● Clinic 2: An almost perfect nonlinear parabolic relationship. Satisfaction at first decreased with increasing wait time, but after wait time exceeded 40 minutes, satisfaction began to increase.
● Clinic 3: A perfect linear relationship with decreasing satisfaction directly related to increasing wait time. But there is one special cause (week 3 when patients were very unhappy).
● Clinic 4: No relationship, as wait time is usually constant at 32 minutes (except week 8 with very high wait time of 76 minutes and low patient satisfaction).

This example illustrates the power of the graphical display of data.[9] The run chart was discussed in Chapter Three. The next section will discuss the Shewhart Chart, and then the end of the chapter will discuss frequency plots, Pareto charts, and scatter plots.

---

[9]Guthrie, B., Love, T., Fahey, T., Morris, A., and Sullivan, A., "Control, Compare and Communicate: Designing Control Charts to Summarize Efficiently Data from Multiple Quality Indicators," *Quality Safety in Health Care*, 2005, *14*, 450–454.

INTRODUCTION TO SHEWHART CHARTS

The **Shewhart chart** is a statistical tool used to distinguish between variation in a measure due to common causes and variation due to special causes. The name used by Shewhart and other authors to describe the chart is "control chart." But this name is misleading because the most common uses of these charts in improvement activities are to learn about variation and to evaluate the impact of changes. Also the word "control" has other meanings often associated with specifications or targets. A more descriptive name might be "learning chart" or "system performance chart." We will use the term "Shewhart chart" in this book. The references below summarize the current use of Shewhart charts in health care applications.[10]

Figure 4.3 shows a typical Shewhart chart. Shewhart charts created with equal subgroups size (each subgroup or "dot" contains the same number of data values) will have straight upper and lower limits as in Figure 4.3. Certain types of Shewhart charts are appropriate when subgroup size is unequal (one subgroup may have contained 20 cases, then next 35, the following 18, and so on). A Shewhart chart made with unequal subgroup sizes will have varying limits as in Figure 4.4. These varying limits are due to adjustments in the limit calculation so it is appropriate for each varying subgroup size.

Chapter Three was focused on the run chart. Although the Shewhart chart may look like an extension of the run chart, it actually uses different theory in its construction and interpretation. When should a run chart be used rather than a Shewhart chart? A run

FIGURE 4.3   Example of Shewhart Chart for Equal Subgroup Size

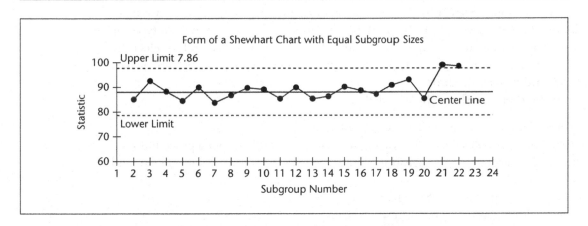

[10]Benneyan J., Lloyd, R., and Plsek, P., "Statistical Process Control as a Tool for Research and Healthcare Improvement," *Quality and Safety in Health Care*, 2003, *12*, 458–464.

Finison, L. J., Finison, K. S., Bliersbach, C. M. et al., "The Use of Control Charts to Improve Healthcare Quality," *Journal for Healthcare Quality*, 1993, *15*(1), 9–23.

Thor, J., Lundberg, J., Ask, J., Olsson, J., Carli, C., Harenstam, K., and Brommels, M., "Application of Statistical Process Control in Healthcare Improvement: Systematic Review," *Quality and Safety in Health Care*, 2007, *16*, 387–399.

Woodall, W. H., "The Use of Control Charts in Health-care and Public-health Surveillance," *Journal of Quality Technology*, 2006, *38*(2).

Mohammed M., Worthington, P., and Woodall, W., "Plotting Basic Control Charts: Tutorial Notes for Healthcare Practitioners," *Quality and Safety in Health Care*, 2008, *17*, 137–145.

FIGURE 4.4 Example of Shewhart Chart for Unequal Subgroup Size

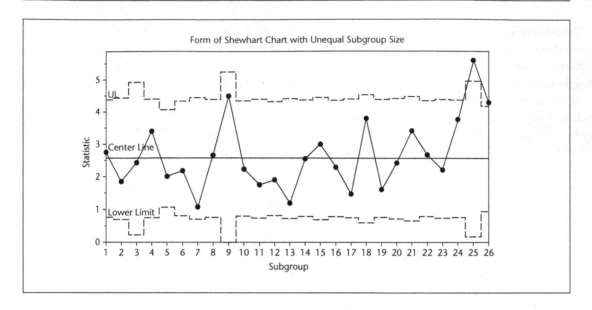

chart is useful when we don't yet have a great deal of data and we want to rapidly detect signals of improvement. In addition, because it is not a complex tool, the run chart may be more readily accepted in some circumstances. The run chart makes the amount of process variation visible, aids in detecting improvement, and helps to determine whether improvement has been maintained. But it cannot reliably distinguish special from common cause variation. Only a Shewhart chart can aid in distinguishing between these two types of variation. The Shewhart chart, by being able to distinguish between the two types of variation, enables us to determine process stability, process capability, and to select the appropriate improvement strategy. Typically, when enough data are available a Shewhart chart is preferable to a run chart.

The method of Shewhart charts includes:

- Selection of a measure and a statistic to be plotted
- A method of data collection: observation, measurement, and sampling procedures
- A strategy for determining subgroups of measurements (including subgroup size and frequency)
- Selection of the appropriate Shewhart chart
- Criteria for identifying a signal of a special cause

Shewhart charts include a center line and an upper and lower limit. Shewhart[11] called the limits of the chart "three-sigma" limits and gave a general formula to calculate the limits for any statistic to be charted. Let S be the statistic to be charted, then

$$\text{the center line: CL} = \mu_s$$
$$\text{the upper limit: UL} = \mu_s + 3 * \sigma_s$$
$$\text{the lower limit: LL} = \mu_s - 3 * \sigma_s$$

where μ_s is the expected value of the statistic and σ_s is the estimate of the standard deviation (or standard error) of the statistic. Shewhart emphasized that statistical theory can

---

[11]Shewhart, W., *The Economic Control of Quality of Manufactured Product*, D. Van Nostrand Company, New York, 1931, 299. [Reprinted by ASQC, Milwaukee, WI, 1980.]

furnish the expected value and standard deviation of the statistic, but empirical evidence justifies the width of the limits (the use of "3" in the limit calculation).

The challenge for any particular situation is to develop appropriate estimates of the expected value and standard deviation of the statistic to be plotted. Appropriate statistics have been developed for Shewhart charts for a wide variety of applications. Each type of Shewhart chart has its own formula with the most appropriate statistics used for that formula. Chapter Five will address the details of selecting and using specific types of Shewhart charts.

The rationale for the use of Shewhart's three-sigma limits includes:

- The limits have a basis in statistical theory.
- The limits have proven in practice to distinguish between special and common causes of variation.
- In most cases, use of the limits will approximately minimize the total cost due to over-reaction and underreaction to variation in the process.
- The limits protect the morale of workers in the process by defining the magnitude of the variation that has been built into the process.

Some authors overemphasize the statistical basis for Shewhart charts. Deming addressed this point directly: "It is wrong (misuse of the meaning of a control chart) to suppose that there is some ascertainable probability that either of these false signals [fail to identify or cause investigation where there is not one] will occur. We can only say that the risk to incur either false signal is very small."[12] In addition, Dr. Deming emphasized that: "It is a mistake to suppose that the control chart furnishes a test of significance—that a point beyond a control limit is 'significant.' This supposition is a barricade to understanding."

Shewhart referenced Tchebycheff's inequality to put probability bounds on the limits.[13] Tchebycheff's inequality can be used to show that the probability for making a mistake of identifying a special cause for a stable process (Mistake 1 or Type 1 error) each time the three-sigma limits are used, regardless of the distribution of data, is less that 11%. He also referenced the Camp/Meidell Criteria (distribution of data are unimodal and monotonic), which indicates that probability for a Type 1 error is less than 4.9% for three-sigma limits. So, even though there is a statistical rational for the control chart, Shewhart concluded that: "Obviously, the basis for such limits must be, in the last analysis, empirical."[14]

Constructing a Shewhart chart does not have to be a complicated process. Anyone can get started by selecting a measure and plotting it in on a run chart (Chapter Three). When enough data become available, a center line and upper and lower limits can be calculated. Software is readily available to do the calculations and present the charts graphically. But in complex situations, the effective use of Shewhart charts requires careful planning to develop and maintain the chart. There are a number of issues related to measurement and sampling that must be resolved prior to beginning a Shewhart chart. The type of data for each variable to be charted will determine the appropriate type of chart to use. The next section discusses selecting the appropriate chart for various types of data.

Note that the Shewhart chart is not related to the calculation of confidence intervals that many health care researchers are familiar with. Chapter Eight provides additional insights into the difference between limits on a Shewhart chart and confidence intervals.

---

[12]Deming, W. E., *The New Economics*, 2nd ed., Boston: MIT Center for Advanced Studies, 1994, 176–177.

[13]Shewhart, *The Economic Control of Quality of Manufactured Product*, 176–177.

[14]Ibid., p. 276.

INTERPRETATION OF A SHEWHART CHART

The Shewhart chart provides a basis for taking action to improve a process (or system). A process is considered to be stable when there is a random distribution of the plotted points within the limits. For a stable process, action should be directed at identifying the important causes of variation common to all of the points. If the distribution (or pattern) of points is not random, the process is considered to be unstable and action should be taken to learn about the special causes of variation.

There is general agreement among users of Shewhart charts that a single point outside of either limit is an indication of a special cause of variation. However there have been many suggestions for systems of rules to identify special causes that appear as nonrandom patterns within the limits. Figure 4.5 contains five rules which are recommended for general use with Shewhart charts. These rules are consistent in the sense that the chance of occurrence of Rules 2 through 5 in a stable process is approximately equal to the chance of Rule 1 occurring in a stable process. The occurrence of any one of the rules is a clear indication of the presence of a special cause. To declare a process stable (the process exhibits only common cause variation) requires that none of these rules are violated.

When applying the rules, the following guidelines will help with consistent interpretation of charts:

- A point exactly on a limit is not considered outside the limit (Rule 1).
- A point exactly on the center line does not cancel or count toward a run (the run in Rule 2 is also commonly called a shift).
- Ties between two consecutive points do not cancel or add to a trend (Rule 3).
- When Shewhart charts have varying limits (due to varying numbers of measurements within subgroups), Rule 3 should be used with caution. Theoretically, it is not correct but it still gives useful information in practice.

FIGURE 4.5 Rules for Determining a Special Cause

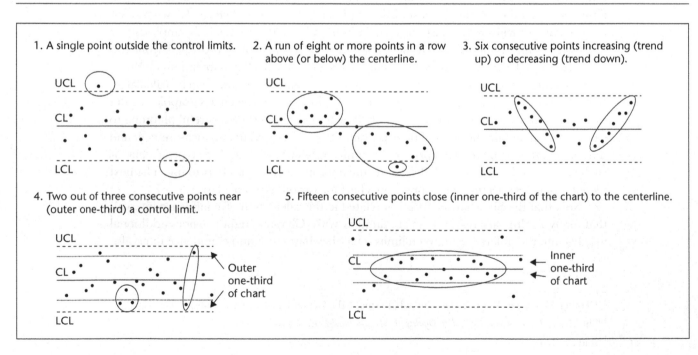

- When there is not a lower or upper limit on one side of the center line (for example, on a standard deviation chart with fewer than six measures in a subgroup or on a P chart with 100% as a possible result for the process), Rules 1 and 4 do not apply to the side missing the limit.

The five rules are designed to rapidly detect special cause occurring in the system that generated the measure. While they work as a system, each rule is useful to identify different types of special causes. Rule 1 quickly identifies sudden changes in the measure. Rule 2 identifies small, sustained changes (like a small improvement to a process). Rule 3 detects a small, consistent drift in a process (trend). Rule 4 adds additional sensitivity to detect changes that have not yet triggered Rule 1 or Rule 2. Rule 5 is especially useful in detecting a reduction of variation with an I chart, or for detecting improper subgrouping with an $\overline{\text{X}}$ chart.

Special circumstances may warrant use of some additional tests given by Nelson.[15] Deming emphasizes that the most important issue is the necessity to state in advance what rules to apply to a given situation.[16]

For improvement activities, these five rules can be used to provide evidence of an improvement to a process or system. These rules also provide evidence of "losing" gains previously made in a system. Figure 4.6 illustrates this important application of the special cause rules.

In this example, a hospital improvement team did some great work to improve patient satisfaction scores during 2004 and early 2005. Shewhart limits for the improved process were calculated using data from the 20 months after full implementation (May 2004 through December 2005). These limits were extended into 2006. In July 2006, as special cause (Rule # 1) was detected. Investigations of this special cause revealed there had been some slippage back into old procedures used prior to the improvement team's work.

As stated earlier, the Shewhart chart provides a basis for taking action to improve a process.

FIGURE 4.6   Detecting "Losing the Gains" for an Improved Process

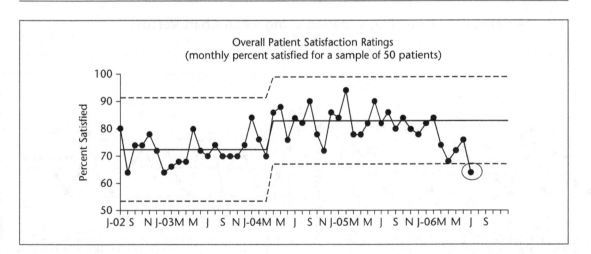

[15]Nelson, L., "The Shewhart Chart—Test for Special Causes," *Journal of Quality Technology*, 1984, *16*(4), 237–239.

[16]Deming, W. E., *Out of the Crisis*, Chapter 11.

In developing the method, Shewhart emphasized the importance of the economic balance between looking for special causes when they do not exist and overlooking special causes that do exist. Table 4.2 illustrates the impact of these two mistakes.

Mistake 1: To react to an outcome as if it came from a special cause, when actually it came from common causes of variation.

Mistake 2: To treat an outcome as if it came from common causes of variation, when actually it came from a special cause.

Marshall et al. describe a study conducted to determine the impact of making Mistake 1 in using Shewhart charts, versus other approaches, to review health care performance data.[17]

Figure 4.7 illustrates the ability of the Shewhart chart to detect special causes of variation in the data when a run chart does not have the ability to do so. Run charts are very useful in improvement but are not the appropriate tool to determine process stability. The Shewhart chart is the tool best suited to this purpose.

Table 4.2   Balancing the Mistakes Made in Attempts to Improve

ACTION	ACTUAL SITUATION	
	When No Special Cause Is Occurring in System	**When a Special Cause Is Occurring in System**
Take action on individual outcome (special)	− $ (Mistake 1)	+ $
Treat outcome as part of system; work on changing the system (common)	+ $	− $ (Mistake 2)

FIGURE 4.7   Depicting Variation Using a Run Chart Versus a Shewhart Chart

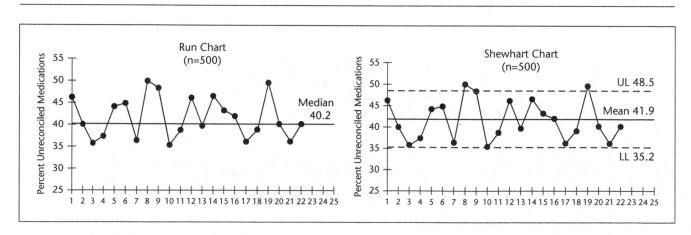

[17]Marshall, T., Mohammed, M., and Rouse, A., "A Randomized Controlled Trial of League Tables and Control Charts as Aids to Health Service Decision Making." *International Journal for Quality in Health Care*, 2004, *16*(4) 309–315.

The Shewhart chart method is useful in all phases of an improvement project using the Model for Improvement as a road map:

1. What are we trying to accomplish?

    Existing Shewhart charts for measures of a health care process can be used to decide whether an improvement effort should be focused on fundamental changes (for a common cause process or system) or to fixing the current system or process (for a process or system exhibiting special cause). See Figure 4.8. The capability of the process (as defined by the Shewhart chart) can be compared to benchmarks or targets to identify gaps in performance and set priorities for improvement.

2. How will we know that a change is an improvement?

    The Shewhart chart method provides a formal way to decide whether observed variation in a measure of quality should be attributed to changes made or to other causes of variation in the system (Figure 4.9).

FIGURE 4.8   Shewhart Charts Common Cause and Special Cause Systems

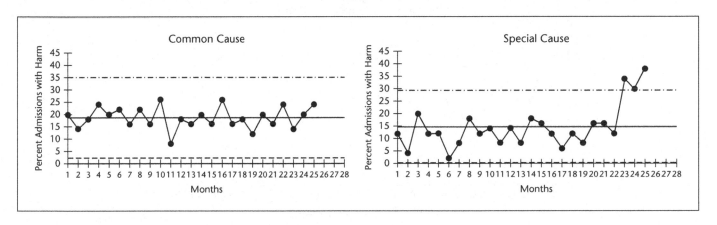

FIGURE 4.9   Shewhart Chart Revealing Process or System Improvement

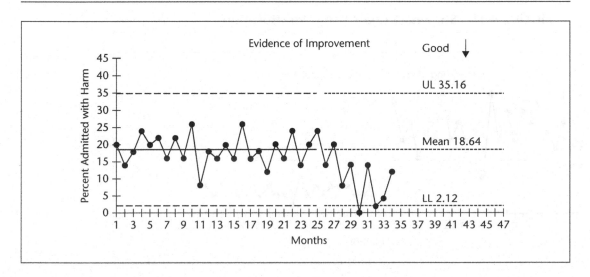

3. What changes can we make that will result in improvement?

The Shewhart chart can help an individual or team decide whether the focus for the next PDSA cycle should be on identification, understanding, or removal of common causes of variation (fundamental redesign of the system) or rather should focus on understanding and taking action on special causes of variation (fixing the current system). It can also be used to detect causes of variation which can then lead to ideas for change. Rational subgrouping and stratification are approaches used with Shewhart charts to aid in developing ideas for change. Figure 4.10 illustrates a Shewhart chart using rational subgrouping and Figure 4.11 a Shewhart chart using stratification to provide clues for improvement. Stratification and rational subgrouping are addressed in more depth later in this chapter.

FIGURE 4.10   Shewhart Chart Using Rational Subgrouping

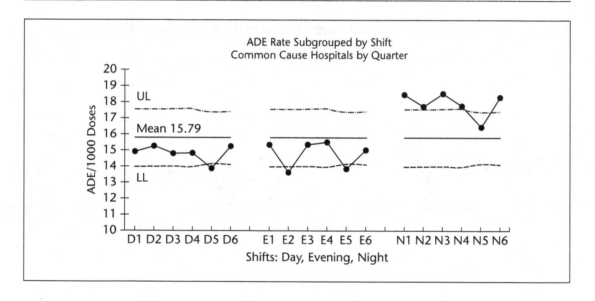

FIGURE 4.11   Shewhart Chart Using Stratification

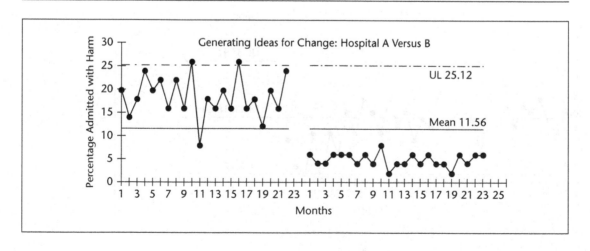

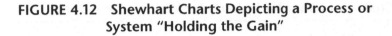

FIGURE 4.12   Shewhart Charts Depicting a Process or
System "Holding the Gain"

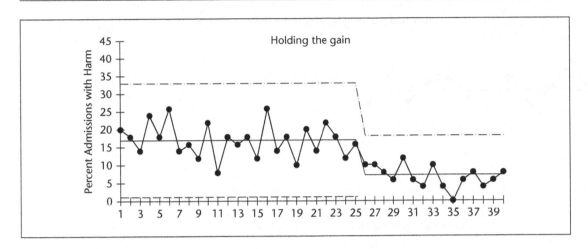

Another important use of a Shewhart chart is for "holding the gain" once an improvement effort is completed (Figure 4.12). Shewhart charts can be maintained for the key measures used in the improvement effort. These maintenance charts will provide signals of special causes if the process ever begins to deteriorate or revert to practices used before the improvement was made.

ESTABLISHING AND REVISING LIMITS FOR SHEWHART CHARTS

Limits for a Shewhart chart should be established using 20 to 30 subgroups from a period when the process is stable. When time is used to define the subgroups, this means one month of daily measures, six months of weekly measures, two years of monthly measures, or five years of quarterly measures. When new improvement efforts are initiated, going back in time to get baseline data is usually a good strategy. When this is not possible (for example with a new measure that an improvement team creates), it would still be very useful to have some limits to get feedback in an improvement effort. For most types of Shewhart charts fewer than 20 subgroups may be used to calculate **trial limits**. Use these trial limits until 20 data points become available then update the limits. These trial limits may be used to detect special cause which may be evidence of improvement or of undesirable unintended consequences in the process. If a special cause is evident when the chart is analyzed using limits constructed from only a few subgroups, it will likely stay a special cause when additional data are added to create more robust limits. The set of charts at Figure 4.13 illustrates this approach.

In this example, a run chart was updated each month as data became available. After 13 months, trial limits were calculated to see if there were any signals of improvement in the waiting times. These trial limits were extended and used for eight more months. At this point a total of 20 data points were available and the limits were recalculated. In this example, with only common cause variation, the limits based on 20 points are similar to the trial limits.

Note that with attribute charts, p, c, and u charts, as well as the $\overline{X}$ and S chart for measurement data, accurate trial limits may be made with as few as 12 data points. For the Individuals chart (I chart) and the t chart (time between rare events) it is important that limits be constructed with 20 or more subgroups. Trial limits are frequently *not useful* for I charts nor for t charts (the t chart is based on the I chart).

FIGURE 4.13   Run Charts and Shewhart Charts for Waiting Time Data

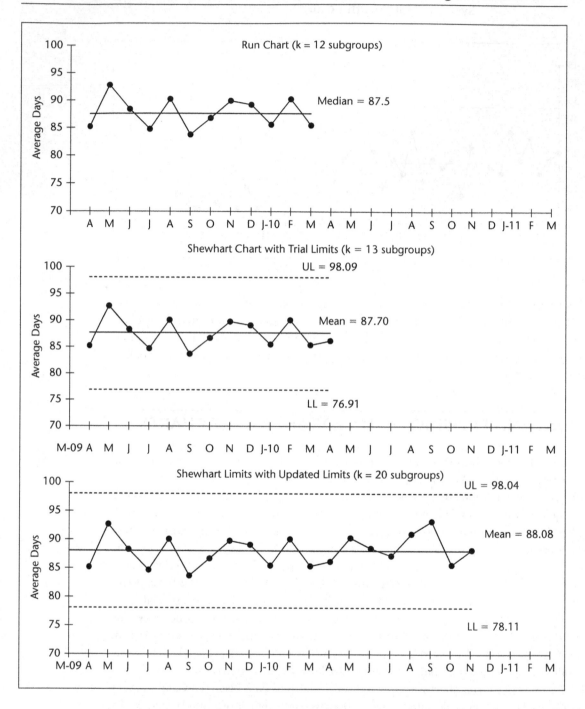

A good technique in using a Shewhart chart to detect improvement is to create **initial limits** using 20 or more data points and, if the baseline data are stable, freeze and extend these initial limits and center line into the future. Special cause in new data being added to the chart will be detected more rapidly because the new data are not influencing the center line or the limits. See Figure 4.14. Note that when the Shewhart chart is working with uneven subgroup sizes the limits will vary appropriately with the subgroup size as seen in Figure 4.4. As we cannot know the subgroup size of future subgroups in this instance, we suggest freezing and extending the center line but not the limits with Shewhart charts for unequal subgroup size.

**FIGURE 4.14   Improper and Proper Extension of Baseline Limits
on Shewhart Chart**

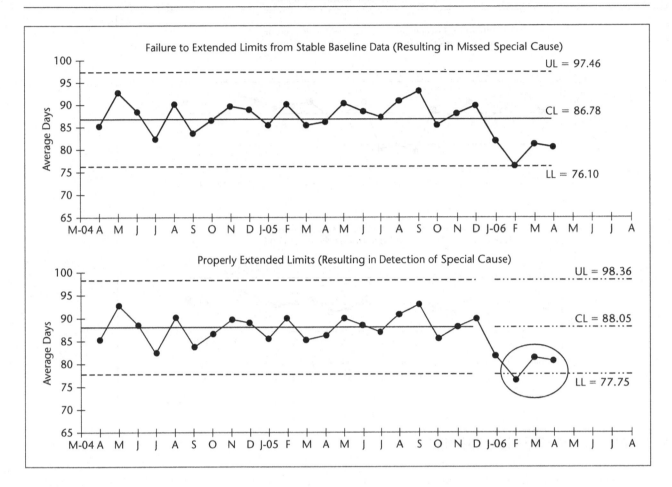

If it is desirable to extend the limits after they are calculated, any points affected by special causes should be removed from the baseline limits calculation and the limits recalculated. The limits should only be extended when they are calculated using data without special causes. The limits on the first graph in Figure 4.15 include special cause data in the calculation of the limits. The improvement team would involve subject matter experts in identifying and taking appropriate action related to the special cause. Only after that should recalculation of the limits be discussed.

When recalculating the limits so that they can be extended, the special cause data should be not be used, but it is usually desirable to leave the data points affected by special cause on the chart. One way to do this is to "cause" or "ghost" the data points affected by the special cause as seen in the second graph at Figure 4.15. "Ghosting" here means leaving the data visible on the graph but excluding it from the calculation of the mean and limits. The limits revised by this technique will reflect only the common cause variation in the process and may now be extended into the future.

Shewhart charts are most useful when displaying 20 to 80 data points. When there is not enough reported data to calculate limits, consider alternative data collection plans. For example, separate five monthly data points into 21 weekly data points. Or separate the data from the 4 weekly averages from last month into 30 daily values. When dealing with a great deal of data consider aggregation. For example, aggregate 180 daily data points into 26 weekly subgroups of data. Or convert two years of weekly data into 24 monthly data points.

FIGURE 4.15   Dealing with Special Cause Data in Baseline Limits

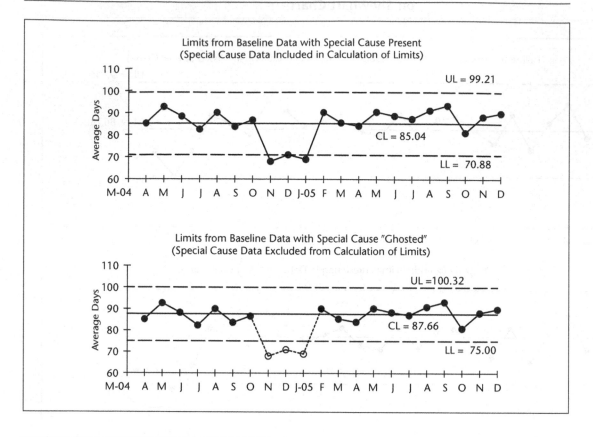

WHEN DO WE REVISE LIMITS?

Revision of the limits should be done when the existing limits are no longer useful. There are four circumstances when the original limits should be recalculated:

1. When trial limits have been calculated with fewer than 20 to 30 subgroups. In this case, the limits should be recalculated when 20 to 30 subgroups become available as seen in Figure 4.13.
2. When the initial Shewhart chart has special causes and there is a desire to use the calculated limits for analysis of data to be collected in the future. In this case, limits should be recalculated without using the data associated with the special causes (see previous example, Figure 4.15).
3. When improvements have been made to the process and the improvements result in special causes on the Shewhart chart. Center line and limits should then be calculated for the new process as seen at Figure 4.16. If there are fewer than 12 data points in the new process, display it as a run chart. Update it and create limits when the new process has 12 or more data points.
4. When the Shewhart chart remains unstable for an extended period of time (20 or more subgroups) and approaches to identify and remove the special cause(s) have been exhausted. Limits should be recalculated to determine if the process has stabilized at different operating levels as shown at Figure 4.17.

The date on which the limits were last calculated (if not obvious on the chart) should be a part of the ongoing record for the Shewhart chart. It is sometimes useful to add a notation (such as vertical lines on the chart) to indicate subgroups used to calculate limits.

FIGURE 4.16 Recalculating Limits After Special Cause Improvement

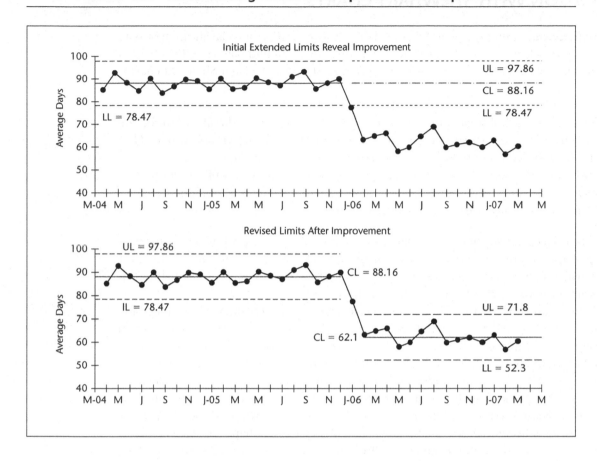

FIGURE 4.17 Recalculating Limits After Exhausting Efforts to Remove Special Cause

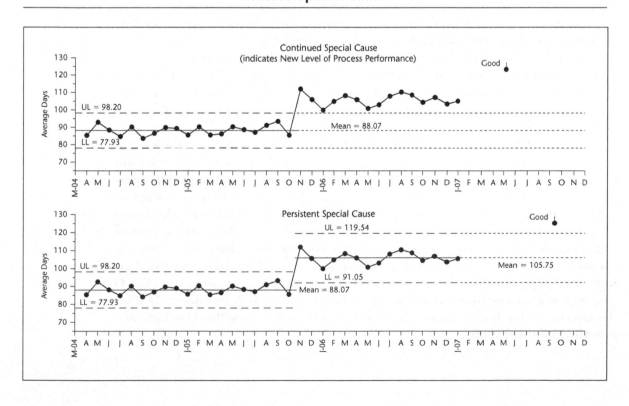

STRATIFICATION WITH SHEWHART CHARTS

Stratification, as introduced in Chapter Two, is the separation and classification of data according to selected variables or factors. The objective is to find patterns which help in understanding the causal mechanisms in a process. Stratification on a Shewhart chart is done in two different ways:

1. Plotting a symbol (instead of the usual • or x) to indicate a classification for the measurement or statistic being plotted. For example, plot the symbol A, B, or C to indicate which of the three clinics the measurements came from.
2. Ordering the measurements, or subgroups of measurements, by stratification variables such as laboratory, physician, patient classification, procedure type, shift, department, and so forth, to investigate the importance of these factors.

The concept of stratification is directly related to rational subgrouping (organizing a group of measurements into meaningful subgroups to form data points for the Shewhart chart) which is discussed in the next section. Figure 4.18 illustrates the concept of stratification with a Shewhart chart, specifically, an I chart.

The measure is the time (hours) to receive a specific genetic analysis from outside laboratories. The first Shewhart chart in Figure 4.18 shows a usual individual chart in the time order that the laboratory analyses were requested. The second graph shows the same Shewhart chart with a special plotting symbol representing the particular laboratory (A, B, or C). The third graph shows an individual chart with the same data reordered so that they are sequenced by the testing laboratory. The limits are much tighter for this chart because the common cause variation is calculated using variation within a laboratory rather than between laboratories (see further discussion of I charts in Chapter Five). The difference in turn-around time for each of the three laboratories is clear on this last Shewhart chart stratified by laboratory.

Figure 4.19 show a second example of using stratification with a Shewhart chart (specifically an I chart) for intake times in a community psychiatric clinic.

The measure on the charts is the time in minutes to run the intake process for new patients coming to the community substance abuse treatment center. The first chart shows a stable process with an average of over 90 minutes to conduct the intake interviews with wide limits from 0 to almost 200 minutes. Why are the limits so wide? The intake interviews are conducted by four different providers. The second chart shows the same Shewhart chart with the points identified with a symbol for each provider (stratification of the data points).

The third Shewhart chart is an individual chart with the same data reordered so that it is sequenced by each of the four providers. The limits are much tighter for this chart (27 to 150 minutes). The intake times for Providers A and C are around the average of 90 minutes. The average time for Provider B is higher, noted by special causes on the high side of the chart. The times for Provider D are significantly lower with all eight of the cases below the center line and one point below the lower limit. The treatment center may be able to develop some strategies to reduce the intake interviewing times by studying the methods used by provider D. Of course, we should be aware that this chart indicates that provider D is faster, not necessarily better overall. For example, provider D may be faster because his interviews are less comprehensive, which may adversely affect the success rate for those admitted. Still, this stratification does show that D is faster, and is worthy of further study.

FIGURE 4.18   Stratification of Laboratory Data with a Shewhart Chart

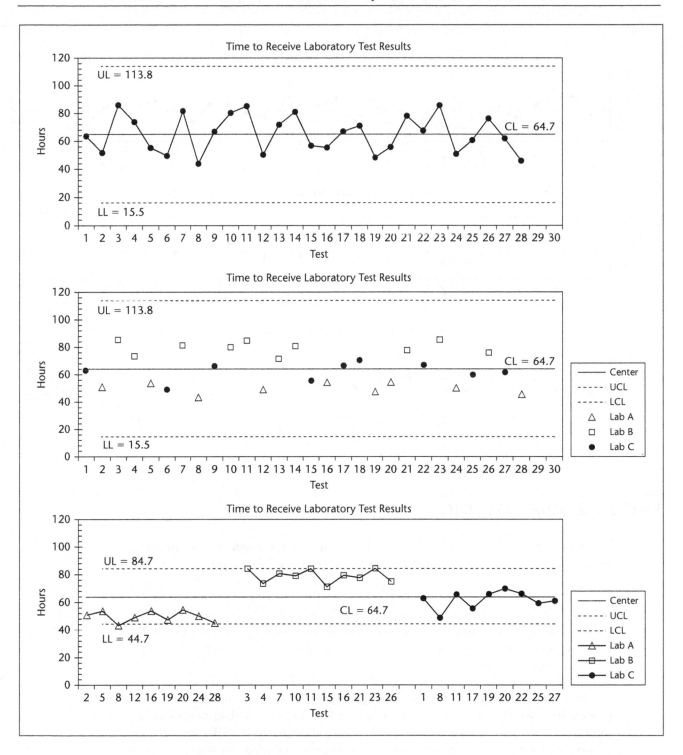

FIGURE 4.19   Stratification of Intake Process Data with a Shewhart Chart

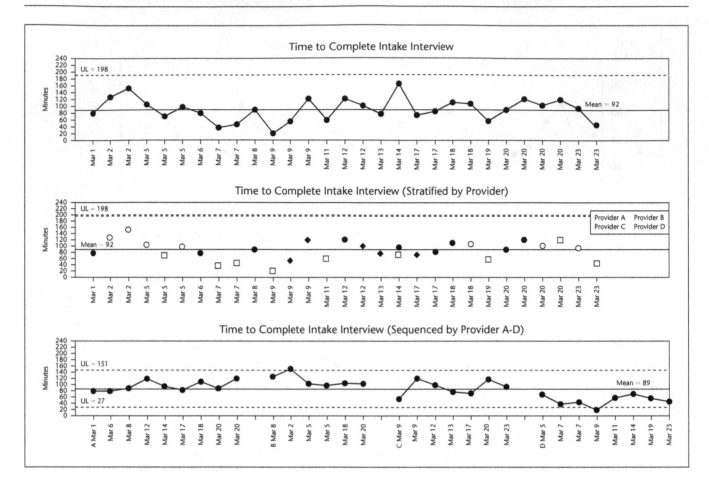

RATIONAL SUBGROUPING

The concept of subgrouping is one of the most important considerations in using the Shewhart chart method. Shewhart said the following about subgrouping:

> Obviously, the ultimate object is not only to detect trouble but also to find it, and such discovery naturally involves classification. The engineer who is successful in dividing his data into rational subgroups based upon rational hypotheses is therefore inherently better off in the long run than the one who is not thus successful.[18]

Shewhart's concept of **rational subgrouping** involves organizing data from the process in a way that is likely to give the greatest chance for the data in each subgroup to be alike and greatest chance for data in other subgroups to be different. The aim of rational subgrouping is to include only common causes of variation within a subgroup, with all special causes of variation occurring between subgroups.

The most common method to obtain rational subgroups is to hold time "constant" within a subgroup. Only data taken at the same time (or for some selected time period)

---

[18]Shewhart, *The Economic Control of Quality of Manufactured Product*, 299.

are included in a subgroup. Data from different time periods will be in other subgroups. This use of time as the basis of subgrouping allows the detection of causes of variation that come and go with time.

As an example of rational subgrouping, consider a study planned to reduce late payments. Historical data from the accounting files will be used to study the variation in late payments. What is a good way to subgroup the historical data on late payments? The data could be grouped by billing month, receiving month, payer, or service line. Knowledge or theories about the process should be used to decide which of these subgrouping strategies would lead to the best learning. Some combination of time (either receiving or billing month) and one or more of the other variables in the process would be a reasonable way to develop the first chart. A few examples of rational subgrouping strategies in health care are:

Measure (Situation): Possible Rational Subgrouping Strategies

Adverse Drug Events: units, shifts, drug category, method of administration

Length of Stay: diagnostic group (DRG), provider, unit, categories of patient age

Nosocomial Infections: location, type of organism, method of transmission

Diabetes Control: care options, provider, patient characteristics

Falls (long-term care): unit, risk level, age, sex, or other patient characteristics

Medication Compliance: housing situation, diagnosis, provider, geographic location

After selecting a method of subgrouping, the user of the Shewhart chart should be able to state which sources of variation in the process will be present within subgroups and which sources will occur between subgroups. The specific objective of the Shewhart chart will often help determine the strategy for subgrouping the data. For example, if the objective is to evaluate differences between several different types of hip prostheses, then only data from a single type of hip prosthesis should be included in data within a subgroup.

Figure 4.20 shows a Shewhart chart (specifically a U chart) for the Adverse Drug Event (ADE) rate for a multihospital system. The systemwide ADE rate was stable but not performing at a desirable level.

The team working on this project theorized different causes of variation and then determined ways to change the subgrouping of the data to study various theories. One theory was that ADEs occurred more frequently on certain days of the week. Figure 4.21 shows the same data rationally subgrouped by day of the week. The data for the first six-month period are grouped by day of the week, and then repeated for the next two six-month periods. Six-month subgroups were chosen to result in a total of 21 subgroups (to create a readable Shewhart Chart with effective limits).

There was no evidence that any day of the week was special cause in their system. Another theory they voiced was that ADEs occurred more frequently on certain shifts. They decided to subgroup their data by day shift (D), Evening (E) or night (N) shift, for each of the six quarters in the data set, resulting in a total of 18 subgroups. Figure 4.22 shows this chart.

When rationally subgrouping their data by shift, night shift showed up as special cause in their system. See Chapter Nine where this example is expanded for additional details of their investigation into the special cause on evening shift.

The team also wondered if the rate of ADEs varied substantially by type of medication administered. They decided to rationally subgroup the ADE data by medication.

FIGURE 4.20   Shewhart Chart with Aggregate Data

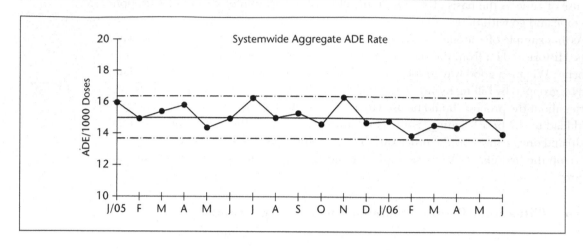

FIGURE 4.21   ADE Data Rationally Subgrouped by Day of the Week

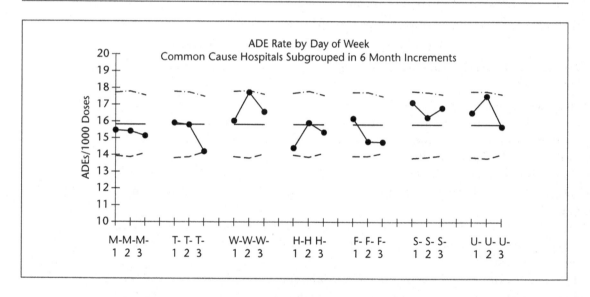

FIGURE 4.22   ADE Data Rationally Subgrouped by Shift

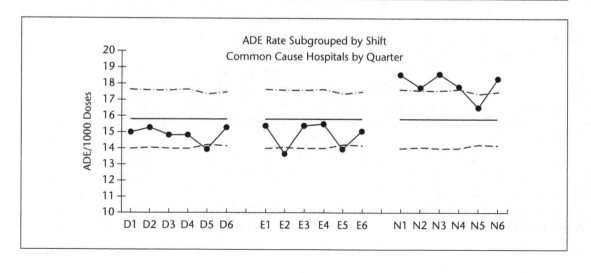

FIGURE 4.23   Shewhart Chart with Data Rationally Subgrouped by Medication

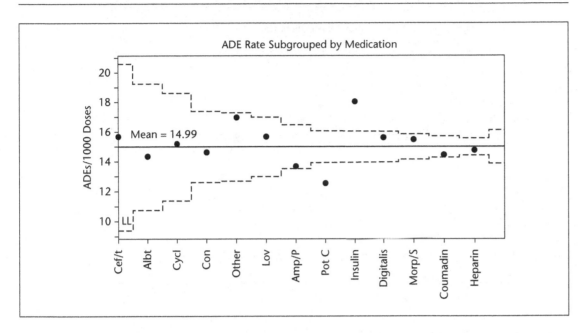

Figure 4.23 displays the results of the rational subgrouping. The team discovered special cause revealing a very low rate of ADEs related to potassium chloride. They were elated as they had worked hard to reduce ADEs related to this medication. They also noted another special cause with a high rate of ADEs related to insulin administration. This presented the team with an additional opportunity to focus their improvement work.

Both stratification and rational subgrouping are key strategies to for drilling down into aggregate data for learning and improvement. Chapter Nine will develop these topics further.

SHEWHART CHARTS WITH TARGETS, GOALS, OR OTHER SPECIFICATIONS

A common issue with the use of Shewhart charts is confusion between limits on the Shewhart chart and goals, targets, or benchmarks. This confusion can result in the wrong improvement strategy being used. We advise analysis of the Shewhart chart for special or common cause variation first in order to determine the appropriate improvement strategy. After this analysis, we can then consider how the process performance compares to the customer's need expressed as a target, goal, or specification. The method to do this is called a capability analysis and is presented in Chapter Five. An example of this approach is described in the following example.

A large government-funded payer of health care wanted to ensure that most of the money they managed went directly for patient care, not to overhead or administrative costs. They tracked the percentage of their budget going to direct patient care monthly. Figure 4.24 shows their monthly data.

The leadership team recognized that a special cause in the last few months (two out of three consecutive months in the outer third of the limits, and the most recent month below the lower limit) had occurred, indicating that a lower percentage of their budget

FIGURE 4.24 Shewhart Chart Meeting Goal But Unstable

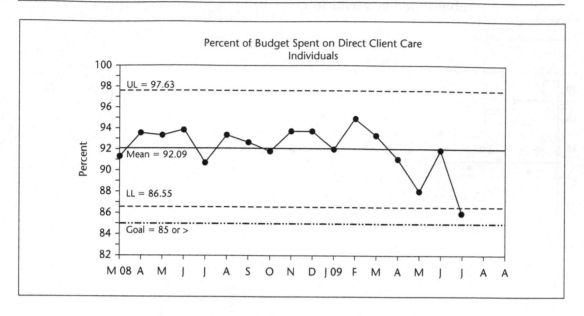

was going to direct patient care. As they investigated the special cause they discovered that some offices had decided to upgrade furnishings in the workplace and were exceeding budgeted levels for this endeavor. This leadership team had a goal of 85% or more of budget allocated to direct patient care. Some of the newer leadership team members insisted on including the goal as a line on the graph. When the newer team members reviewed the chart, they questioned why any action needed to be taken. After all, each month this process met the goal of 85%. Why be concerned?

Those more experienced in understanding variation explained that the process was exhibiting a special cause. Irrespective of the goal, the process was not stable, not predictable. Things were getting worse. The special cause indicated to the leadership that something had changed, and that it was time to take action, even though the goal was still being met.

A second example of using goals with Shewhart charts involves a long-term care leadership team that recently started using a Shewhart chart to track the number of falls for their community of residents as seen at Figure 4.25. The team had a goal of fewer than eight falls per month. When they reviewed the chart they noted no special cause. The number of falls was stable, which meant that all the variation was inherent in their current system.

They recognized that the process was stable and the number of falls was predictable within limits (up to 14 falls per month). But with three months above the goal of eight or fewer falls, they knew that some fundamental changes to their care processes were needed to make sure every month stayed below the goal. They put together a team who studied some novel approaches used by other organizations to reduce falls. They gathered a list of ideas to start testing in their organization and got to work.

The leadership team did experience some struggles before they came to the decision to use a common cause strategy and redesign their care processes. The goal line on the chart led to one of the leaders insisting that they investigate the cause of the three "high points above the goal line." After some discussion the leaders understood that every data set will likely have some high and some low data. That does not make those data special cause. They realized that they were about to make Shewhart's Mistake 1, treating

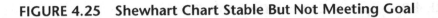

FIGURE 4.25   Shewhart Chart Stable But Not Meeting Goal

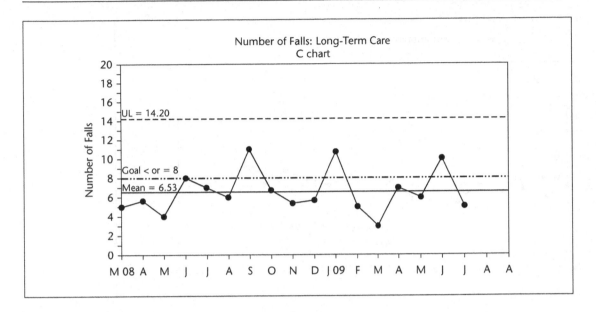

common cause variation as if it were special, as described in Table 4.2. Rather than go investigate the points that were high and ignore the rest of the data, they needed to learn from all the data so they could understand and redesign fundamental processes in order to improve.

Goals, targets, and specifications are important for focus and building will for change. Often they express the needs of customers. They can be thought of as the voice of the customers in the room. However, in order to make improvements to meet a goal, it's important to know whether to take a common or special cause improvement strategy. Should the focus be on redesigning some aspect(s) of a process? Or is something special going on in the process that needs to be investigated and addressed first? For this reason, analysis of the Shewhart chart for special or common cause variation is useful as a first step in order to determine the appropriate improvement strategy. After this analysis, we can then consider how the process performance compares to the customer's need and incorporate that knowledge into our planning. Chapter Five describes the methods to do this for the various types of Shewhart charts (capability analysis).

SPECIAL CAUSE: IS IT GOOD OR BAD?

It depends. Special cause may be evidence of improvement. It may also be evidence of process degradation, or even of an unintended consequence of a change that the improvement team is testing. A hospital was working to more appropriately discontinue prophylactic antibiotics within 24 hours of their start. Figure 4.26 shows their Shewhart chart for this measure.

In this situation they were testing changes and hoping to see special cause in the desired direction. By June of 2009 they saw evidence of special cause with two out of three consecutive points in the outer third of the limits or beyond. This special cause continued in July with an additional point outside the upper limit. The team was excited with the good news that their tests of change were resulting in improvement; these were good special causes!

FIGURE 4.26   Special Cause in Desirable Direction

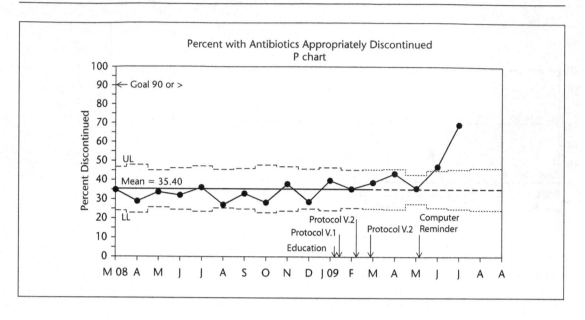

FIGURE 4.27   Shewhart Chart with Special Cause in Undesirable Direction

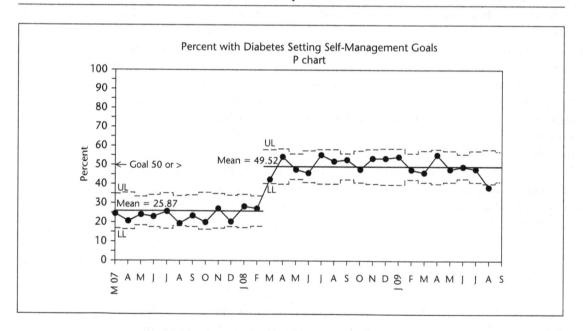

Another organization was monitoring the percentage of people with diabetes in their care who were using self-management goals. Two years earlier they had worked hard to increase the percentage of patients actively engaging in self-management and had been quite successful in almost doubling the percentage of patients. But recently their process exhibited a special cause with the August 2009 data point below the lower limit. Their Shewhart chart is in Figure 4.27. The special cause indicated that they were not maintaining the gain they had made to their clinic system. It was time to step in, determine what was happening in the process, and correct the situation. In this case, the special cause signal was bad news as their process was no longer stable.

As discussed in Chapter Two, putting all of an improvement team's focus on a single measure as evidence of improvement can lead to erroneous conclusions. One aspect of the system may be improved only to make things worse in another. A hospital was working to reduce length of stay (LOS). The changes they tested resulted in special cause in the desired direction (reduction in LOS). Figure 4.28 shows the Shewhart chart for their measure.

Fortunately, this team thought to also track unplanned readmissions. They noted that while LOS was improving, unplanned readmissions showed special cause to the bad (in an undesirable direction) as seen in Figure 4.29. They needed to test changes to LOS that would not worsen unplanned readmission. Special cause needs to be considered in context before determining whether it is good or bad for the system as a whole.

FIGURE 4.28   Shewhart Chart for LOS

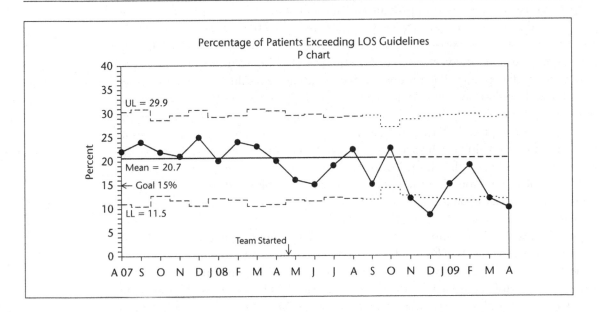

FIGURE 4.29   Percent of Patients with an Unplanned Readmission

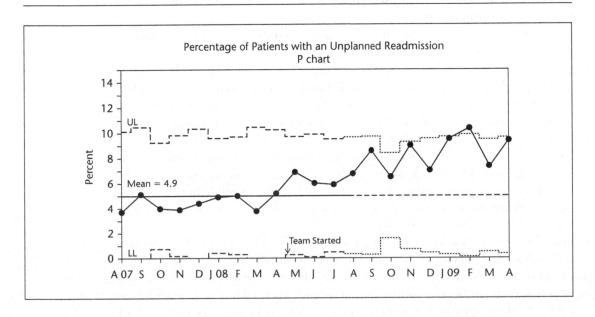

OTHER TOOLS FOR LEARNING FROM VARIATION

Figure 2.26 in Chapter Two showed five visual tools to learn from variation in data. Chapter Three described the run chart in detail, and Shewhart charts will be further explored in Chapters Five through Nine. The use of frequency plots, Pareto charts, and scatter plots is the focus for the remainder of this chapter. These tools were defined in Table 1.4 in Chapter One and have been used in some of the examples in previous chapters. The important concept of stratification introduced in Chapter Two will be illustrated with each of these tools.

Frequency Plot

A **frequency plot** is designed to present information about the location, spread, and shape of a particular measure. A frequency plot is constructed by putting the scale of the measure of interest on the horizontal axis and then number of occurrences of each value (or groups of values) on the vertical axis. A frequency plot should usually be developed from 30 or more data points. The number of data points at each value can be represented by bars, stacked symbols, or lines. When bars are used, the graph is often called a histogram. When dots are used to display the number of each unique value in the data set, the graph is called a dot plot. A stem-and-leaf plot is a type of frequency plot where whole numbers are used to define the horizontal axis and the decimal value (1, 2, 3, and so on) is plotted as the symbol on the chart. Figure 4.30 illustrates these three ways to view data using a frequency plot. Note that these three views each exhibit the data a bit differently. The histogram places the data in bars of cells of equal intervals. The dot plot displays a dot for each value and does not aggregate the data in cells. The dot plot is less useful when displaying data with a large number of unique values. It is better suited to a set of data with a few values possible. See Figure 4.31 for a more effective dot plot.

The stem-and-leaf plot displays each piece of data. In the first stem in Figure 4.30 we see a 0, then the numbers in the leaf are 4, 5, 5, and so forth. This means we had someone fall who was 4 years old, two who were 5, and so on. The second stem is a 1 with the leaf being 0, then another 0 and so on. Looking at the stem-and-leaf plot of people who fell, we can readily tell that we had four people who were 10, another four who were 11, two who were 12, and one who was 19.

The frequency plot is most useful after examining a run chart or Shewhart chart for stability. For a stable measure, the frequency plot can be used to summarize the capability of the process performance for the measure (see Chapter Five for discussion of capability). The frequency plot is useful for finding patterns in the data such as rounding errors, missing values, and truncation, and favorite values of the measure. Useful information about measures with an unusually shaped distribution can also be seen from a frequency plot (see previous examples in Chapter Two, Figures 2.7, 2.16, 2.18, and 2.19).

To construct a frequency plot for data on a continuous scale, the range of data for the measure of interest is divided into 5–20 cells, defined by intervals encompassing the total range of the measure. The more data that are available, the more cells can be used. For discrete data, such as patient satisfaction data using a 1–5 scale, the cells can be defined by the possible values of the discrete measure.

The concept of stratification is important when using frequency plots. Stratification can be used by breaking the bar for each interval according to the number of occurrences for each level of the stratification variable. If symbols (for example, dots) are stacked instead of a bar, then a different symbol should be used for each level of the stratification variable. Another approach is to make separate frequency plots for each level of

FIGURE 4.30 Histogram, Dot Plot, and Stem-and-Leaf Plot for Age at Fall

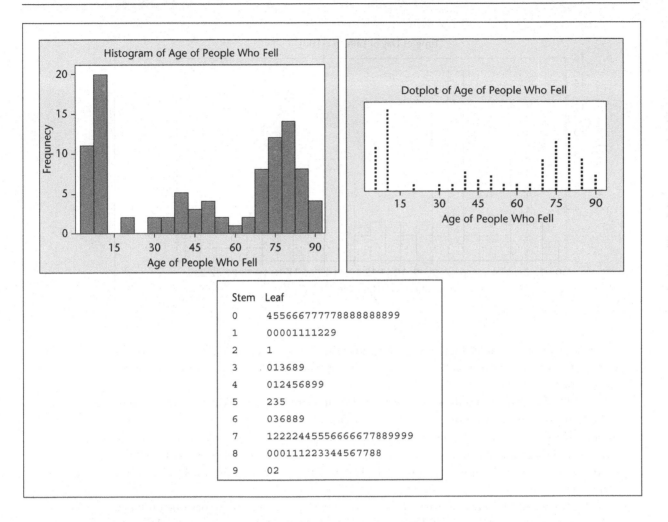

Stem	Leaf
0	455666777778888888899
1	00001111229
2	1
3	013689
4	012456899
5	235
6	036889
7	12222445556666677889999
8	000111223344567788
9	02

FIGURE 4.31 Example of a Dot Plot of Patient Satisfaction Data (Scale 1–7)

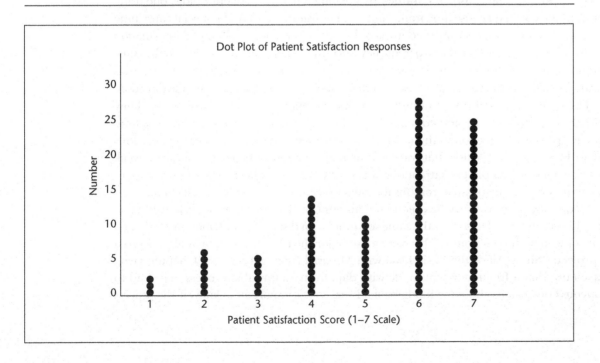

FIGURE 4.32   Histogram of Total Falls by Time of Day

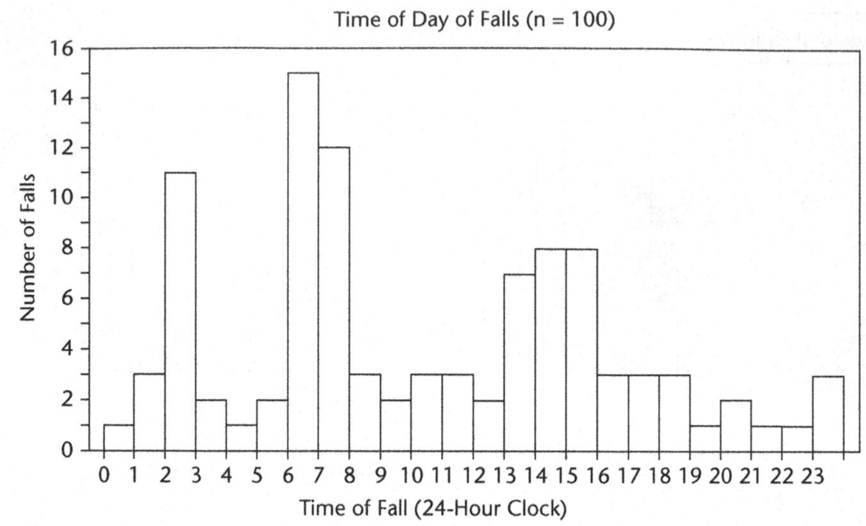

Time of Day of Falls (n = 100)

the stratification variable. Figure 4.32 illustrates this latter approach for a frequency plot displaying total hospital data for the time of day at which a patient fell. These data show several peaks.

To develop improvement strategies, the QI team wanted to stratify the data by patient age (those 50 and under, those 51 and above) to look at the time of day when the two age groups were experiencing falls (Figure 4.33). The stratified frequency plot of falls by age showed that patients under 50 years of age had a wide range of distribution of the time of day with falls peaking in the afternoon. For patients older than 50, most of the falls were during the night.

If a Shewhart chart reveals that a process was stable, but at some point became unstable, the frequency plot may be a useful tool in learning about the difference between the common cause and special cause time frames. By creating a pair of frequency plots, one using data from the common cause time frame and another using data from the special cause time frame, the two time frames can be contrasted. It may be possible to gain useful information from the differences between the two frequency plots. In tracking patient satisfaction the clinic team noted that satisfaction had been stable until the most current week. Figure 4.34 reveals that in week 20 the average satisfaction exhibited a special cause in an undesirable direction.

The team suspected that waiting time strongly influenced patient satisfaction. They decided to stratify the data and compare the waiting time during the common cause time frame for patient satisfaction to the waiting time during the special cause time frame. This view, at Figure 4.35, revealed that waiting time had been much longer in the recent week when special cause in patient satisfaction was noted. The team decided to do some more work to determine the possible reasons for longer recent waiting times in the clinic.

Frequency plots are very flexible in the amount of data that can be displayed. The vertical axis can be scaled so that the same size graph can display the distribution of 20 data points or a million data points. This can be useful for the first step in data analysis from a QI project: "Show All of the Basic Data with Minimal Aggregation" (see Chapter Two). Please note that a frequency plot made with data from an unstable process may lead to erroneous conclusions about the fundamental issues so it is important to know if the process

FIGURE 4.33 Histogram of Time of Falls Stratified by Age

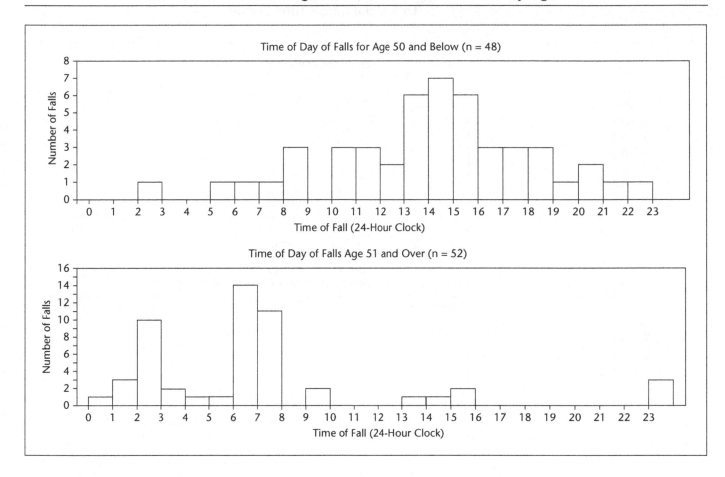

FIGURE 4.34 Shewhart Chart Tracking Average Patient Satisfaction

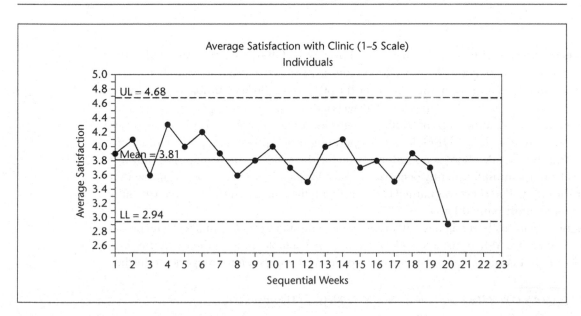

FIGURE 4.35 Frequency Plots Comparing Common Cause to Special Cause Time Frame

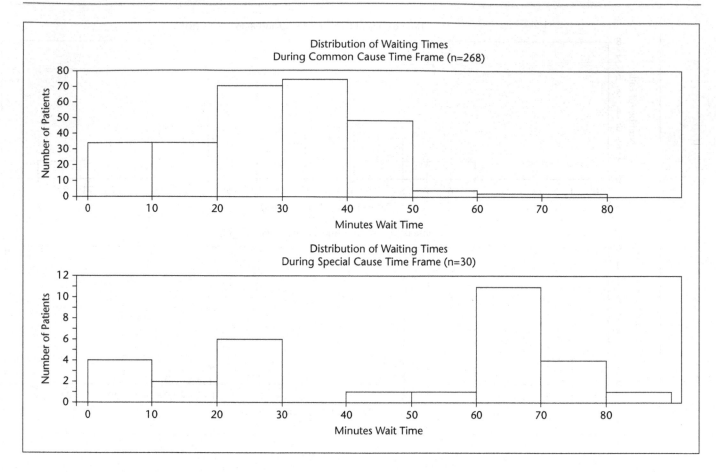

under study is stable prior to creating a frequency plot. This means that a Shewhart chart should be constructed and analyzed prior to deciding to construct the frequency chart.

Pareto Chart

A **Pareto chart** is shown in Figure 4.36. The Pareto Chart for attribute data is the equivalent of the frequency plot for a continuous measure. It is most useful to help focus improvement efforts and is a manifestation of the 80/20 rule (80% of problems are related to 20% of the categories). Problems, errors, defects, adverse drug events, patient complaints, and so forth can often be organized into categories or classifications. Typical categories for the horizontal scale are DRG, location, operating room, procedure, physician, failure mode, and the like. As there is no natural scale for the order of the categories, they are ordered from the most frequently occurring to least frequently occurring on the horizontal axis of the chart. The chart was named by Juran[19] with the name coming from a nineteenth-century economist named Pareto.

A useful Pareto chart will have 30 or more incidents. Charts with just a few data points can be misleading. When just a few observations are available, present the categories in a table. Data for a Pareto chart are occurrences of interest grouped into categories to further

---

[19]Juran, J., *Quality Control Handbook,* 3rd ed., New York: McGraw-Hill, 1979, 2–17.

FIGURE 4.36 Example of Pareto Chart

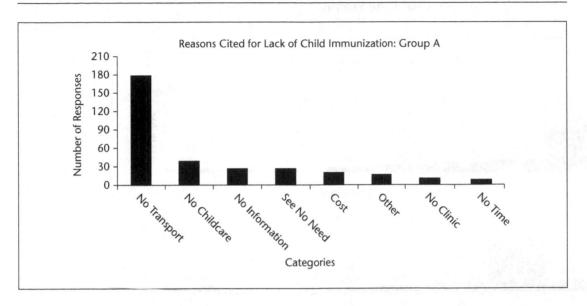

describe the occurrence of interest. On the horizontal axis, arrange the categories from those with the most occurrences to those with fewest occurrences. Then graph a bar to identify the number of occurrences in each category. Following the 80/20 rule (or Pareto principle), the categories on the left side of the graph are called the "vital few" while the rest are considered the "useful many."

A QI team working to improve immunization rates believed that the cost of the immunizations was the biggest barrier to improvement. After obtaining information from parents whose children were not up-to-date on their immunizations, they created the Pareto chart in Figure 4.36. In studying the Pareto chart they realized that reducing the cost of immunizations was unlikely to lead to improvement in immunization rates. They decided to focus on meeting transportation needs.

When interpreting a Pareto chart, one should be cautious to ensure that the categories related to the measure of interest are not assumed to be *causes*. It may be useful to construct a Pareto chart of patient falls by nursing unit; however, it does not mean nursing units are the *causes* of the falls. Nursing units are merely one way of categorizing our information about patient falls. Some other factor, or more likely some combination of several factors, may be responsible for the falls patients are experiencing and may cut across all nursing units. Also in interpreting a Pareto chart, we need to remember it is a display of all the data without knowledge of the cause of variation (common or special cause variation). A Pareto chart made with data from an unstable process may lead to erroneous conclusions about the fundamental issues so it is important to know if the process under study is stable prior to creating a Pareto Chart. This means that a Shewhart chart should be constructed and analyzed prior to deciding to construct the Pareto chart.

The Pareto chart is a useful tool with which to contrast and learn about the difference between a common cause and special cause time frame evident on a Shewhart chart. A clinic working to understand and improve patient satisfaction had noted a special cause in week 20 as noted in Figure 4.34. Figure 4.37 shows the Pareto chart they used to contrast sources of patient dissatisfaction noted on the patient surveys from the common cause time frame and the special cause time frame. They discovered that during the common cause time frame problems with parking were the major source of dissatisfaction for patients.

FIGURE 4.37   Pareto Chart Comparing Common Cause to Special Cause Time Frame

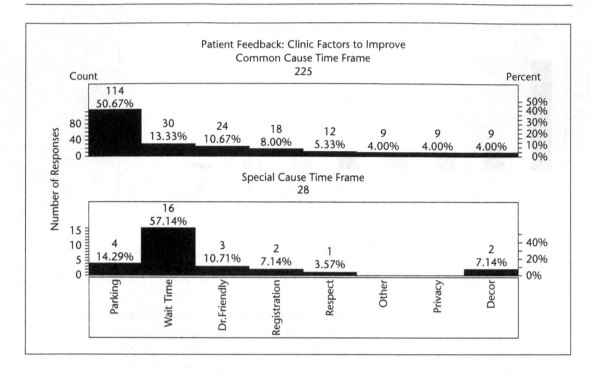

During the special cause time frame dissatisfaction with wait time had surfaced as their major source of dissatisfaction.

Stratification is useful with a Pareto chart. A team working to reduce medication harm wanted to learn from their existing data related to Adverse Drug Events (ADEs) that resulted in harm to patients. They displayed the ADEs by type of medication on a Pareto Chart (top left graph in Figure 4.38). The Pareto chart revealed a preponderance of ADEs related to anticoagulants and sedatives. The team wondered if this was true on the different types of nursing units. They decided to stratify their data by surgical units, medicine units and intensive care units. The three additional Pareto charts in Figure 4.38 reveal the important differences in the preponderance of drugs associated with an ADE resulting in harm between these types of units.

When developing run charts and Shewhart charts for attribute data (Chapter Two), developing an accompanying Pareto chart(s) for various categories of the classification or incident being evaluated on the time-ordered charts is almost always a good strategy. Pareto charts are also important tools in drilling down into aggregate attribute measures. Chapter Nine will illustrate this important role of the Pareto chart in drill-down strategies.

Scatter Plots

The **scatter plot** is illustrated in Figure 4.39. It is a tool for learning about associations or relationships between two variables.[20] If a cause-and-effect relationship exists between the variables, the scatter plot will show this relationship. The patterns on the charts indicate if two variables are associated.

---

[20]Cleveland, W., and McGill, R., "The Many Faces of a Scatterplot," *Journal of the American Statistical Association*, 1984, *79*(388).

FIGURE 4.38   Pareto Charts Stratified by ADE Type and Location

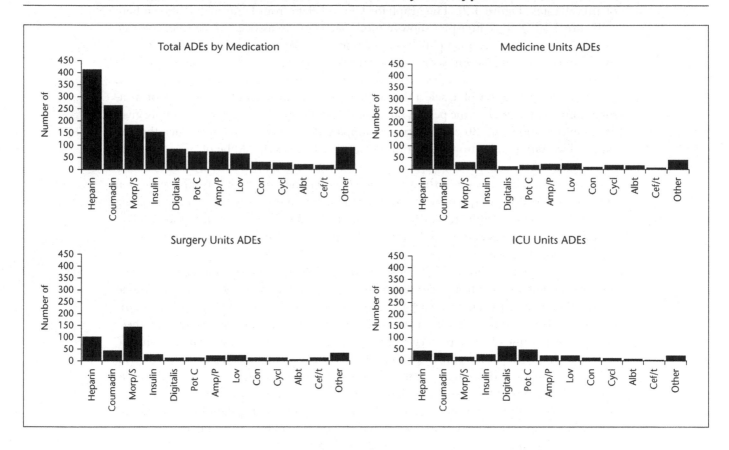

**FIGURE 4.39   Scatter Plot of Patient Satisfaction Versus
Wait Time (from Figure 4.2)**

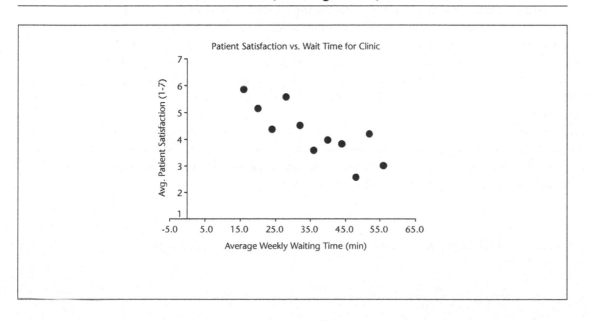

Scatter plots were used to illustrate the importance of plotting all data at the beginning of this chapter (Figure 4.2). The graph for Clinic 1 data from Figure 4.2 is shown here in Figure 4.39. This scatter plot shows a moderate negative association between average weekly wait time and average patient satisfaction scores for the same week. As wait times increase, patient satisfaction scores go down. The graph shows the association; subject matter expertise is required to develop cause-and-effect theories about these two measures.

To develop a scatter plot, select the two measures of interest and record pairs of measures (same patient, same time period, same clinic, and so forth). A scatter plot typically gives useful information with 30 or more paired samples. Plot the pairs on a scale such that the range of variation takes up the full range of data. The axes should be of approximately equal length for each variable (square graph). The correlation statistic (r) can be calculated as a statistical measure of the association between the two variables and a regression analysis can be done to quantify the relationship between two variables after examining the scatter plot (see Table 4.1 for the calculations for the scatter plot in Figure 4.39).[21] Stratification can be accomplished with a scatter plot by plotting different symbols to represent a third stratification variable.

For illustration purposes, Figure 4.40 shows six different patterns that one might find on a scatter plot, ranging from a strong positive (plot A) and negative (plot C) associations to no association (plot E). The two variables plotted are patient satisfaction and time with the provider during a clinic visit. Of course, in this example it would be hard to come up theories to explain some of these patterns! The correlation coefficient (r) is shown on each plot.

As with the frequency plot and Pareto chart, the scatter plot may be a useful tool with which to contrast and learn about the difference between a common cause and special cause time frame evident on a Shewhart chart. By creating a pair of scatter charts, one using data from the common cause time frame and another using data from the special cause time frame, we can contrast the two time frames and enhance our understanding of the variation in the process and its potential implications.

Stratification strategies are useful for learning with scatter plots. A behavioral health organization was experiencing sick leave use by the case managers that made it difficult to accomplish all of their case management work. They wanted to improve case management continuity and decrease sick leave costs. Some case managers stated that they thought sick leave use was related to heavy caseloads. Other case managers disagreed. The team created a scatter plot relating average weekly caseload for each case manager over the past three months and the number of days of sick leave used by that case manager in the past three months. This scatter plot is the first chart in Figure 4.41. From the scatter plot, it looked like the higher the caseload, the higher the sick leave use. The team decided to stratify these data by the department in which the case manager worked. The second scatter plot in Figure 4.41 used a different symbol to represent each department.

The stratified view in Figure 4.41 revealed that the positive relationship between caseload and sick leave is occurring in Department A. Departments B and C did not seem to show higher sick leave use associated with their higher caseloads. Stratifying the data led the team to focus their improvement efforts more appropriately.

---

[21]Draper, N., and Smith, H., *Applied Regression Analysis*, 3rd ed., New York: Wiley-Interscience, 1998.

FIGURE 4.40   Interpreting Patterns on the Scatter Plot

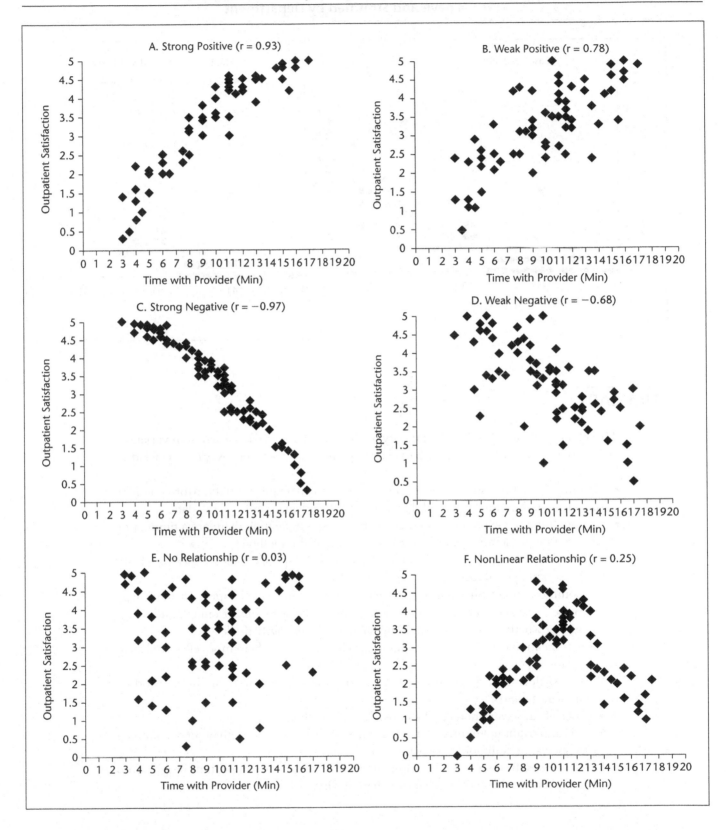

FIGURE 4.41 Scatter Diagrams Total Case Load Versus Sick Leave and Stratified by Department

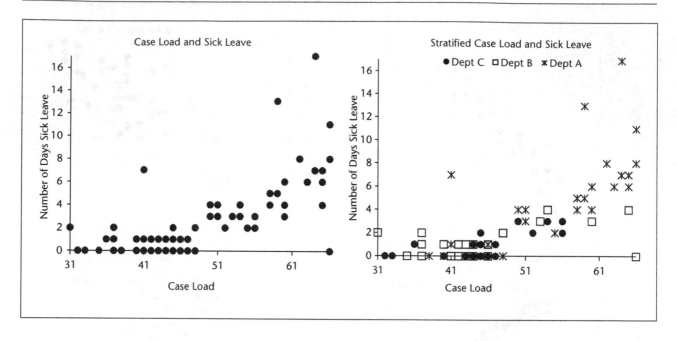

SUMMARY

This chapter discussed Shewhart's theory of variation, basic tools to learn from variation, and introduced the use of the Shewhart chart in improvement activities. Key points included:

- Graphical methods should always be used when learning from data. More complex statistical analysis might be useful, but only after studying graphs of the data.
- Although the Shewhart chart appears to be a very simple tool, there are a number of important considerations in making effective use of this method:
  - Shewhart charts are based on three-sigma limits and specific rules are used for identification of special causes on a Shewhart chart.
  - Common uses of Shewhart charts include determining which improvement strategy to use (special or common cause), providing evidence of improvement, and determining whether a process is holding on to gains previously made.
  - Stratification can be used with Shewhart charts to make them more effective learning tools.
  - The ordering and grouping of data are an important part of the method of Shewhart charts.
  - Special cause variation can be either "good" or "bad."
  - It is important not to mix up targets and goals for a measure with an understanding of special or common cause variation.
- Pareto charts, frequency plots, and scatter plots can provide important insights into data, especially when used with a run chart or Shewhart chart.

Case Study Connection

Several of the Case studies in Chapter Thirteen illustrate the concepts addressed in this chapter. **Case Study C** illustrates the use of a Shewhart chart to track the impact of a change. It also highlights the use of disaggregation, stratification, and rational subgrouping techniques to learn about the process. **Case Study F** addresses using Shewhart charts as a central part of an improvement effort. It also illustrates updating and revising Shewhart chart limits. **Case Study G** illustrates the use of Shewhart charts with routine financial data. It highlights the value of posing questions and using the appropriate Shewhart chart to aid in answering that question. In addition, it provides an example of the use of additional statistical process control tools, in this instance, scatter plots.

KEY TERMS

Common cause

Frequency plot

Initial limits

Intended variation

Mistake 1

Mistake 2

Pareto chart

Rational subgrouping

Scatter plot

Shewhart chart

Special cause

Stable system

Stratification

Trial limits

Unintended variation

Unstable system

## CHAPTER 5

UNDERSTANDING VARIATION USING SHEWHART CHARTS

The concept of variation was introduced in Chapter Four and five tools to learn from the variation in data were presented: Shewhart charts, Pareto charts, run charts, frequency plots, and scatter plots. This chapter further develops the Shewhart chart method as a more formal way to learn from variation and to guide the development of our improvement strategy. By studying this chapter, the reader will learn to select the appropriate Shewhart chart for the data available. This journey will begin by distinguishing between classification, count, and measurement data. Once the distinction between the types of data is clear, a Shewhart Chart Selection Guide (see Figure 5.1 and the chart at the back of the book) will aid the reader in determining which type of Shewhart chart to select. This chapter will also discuss such issues as the amount of data recommended for construction of a useful Shewhart chart, rational ordering, funnel limits, and the concept of process capability.

The Shewhart chart provides an operational definition of the two types of causes of variation in a measure:

Common Causes: Those causes that are inherent in the system (process or product) over time, affect everyone working in the system, and affect all outcomes of the system.

Special Causes: Those causes that are not part of the system (process or product) all the time or do not affect everyone, but arise because of specific circumstances.

SELECTING THE TYPE OF SHEWHART CHART

The selection of the specific Shewhart chart depends on the type of data to be analyzed. As discussed in Chapter Two, data are documented observations or measurements. The availability of data offers opportunities to obtain information and knowledge through inquiry, analysis, or summarization of the data. Data can be obtained by perception (such as observation) or by performing a measurement process. Various classifications of types of data were presented in Chapter Two. In particular, three categories of data commonly associated with Shewhart charts were presented:

- Classification data (**attribute** data)
- Count data (**attribute** data)
- Continuous data (**variable** data)

Continuous data have the following characteristics:

Are quantitative data and use some type of measurement scale.

Do not need to be a whole number when collected, may include decimal places.

Typically are biological measures, time, money, physical measures, perception data recorded on a scale (for example, Likert scale) or throughput (workload, productivity).

In health care, workload or productivity often use a numerical scale (for example, number of patients admitted, number of clinic visits, number of resident days, and number of childhood immunizations provided in the county). Although the numerical scale for workload data and Likert scales for perception data usually yield discrete data (data that are whole numbers when collected), they are still best treated as continuous data.

Classification and count data are often grouped together as attribute data to distinguish them from continuous data. Attribute data are:

Qualitative data sometimes involving judgment (what is an "error," what is "late").

Must be a whole number when collected (discrete data) and data are collected as a category or a count.

For classification data, units of interest are classified into or recorded in one of two categories. Examples of these categories are conforming units/nonconforming units, go/no-go decision, on-time/late appointment, in compliance/not in compliance. In contrast, for count data, we do not focus on a unit. Instead we count incidents that are unusual or undesirable, such as the number of mistakes, medication errors, complications, infections, patient complaints, or accidents.

Figure 5.1 contains a summary of the frequently used Shewhart charts for the different types of data. At the back of the book, you will find a more detailed version of this diagram to aid in chart selection. Learning to select the correct Shewhart chart for your data is an important skill as each has a different formula for computing the limits. The charts on the left side of Figure 5.1 are for attribute data: the C chart or U chart for count data and the P chart for classification data. The charts on the right side are for continuous data: the I chart or the set of $\overline{X}$ and S charts. Each of these different charts assumes a different distribution. Assumptions about the distribution are used to calculate sigma and therefore the upper and lower limits for each chart. The appendix to this chapter contains formulas to calculate the center line and limits for the different types of charts.[1]

---

[1] *Guide for Quality Shewhart Chart, Z1.1, Shewhart Chart Method of Analyzing Data, Z1.2. Shewhart Chart Method of Controlling Quality During Production, Z1.3*, Milwaukee, American Society for Quality Control, 1985.

FIGURE 5.1 Shewhart Chart Selection Guide (Short Form)

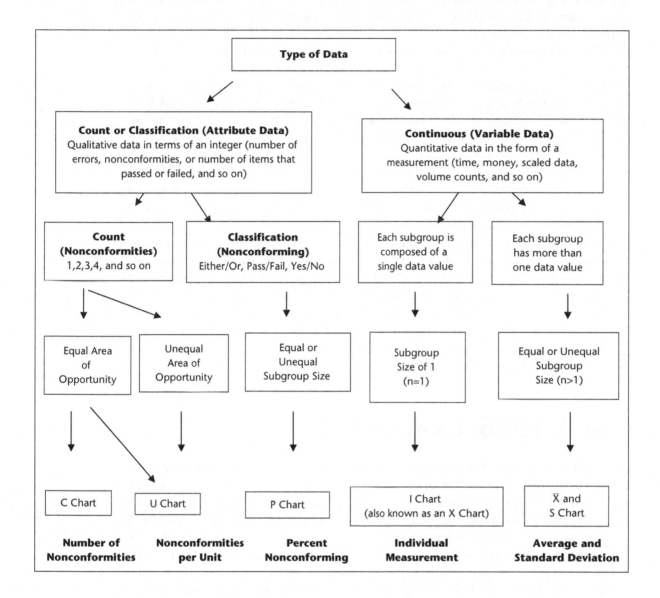

Two chart selection mistakes are common. One mistake frequently seen is inappropriately treating attribute data expressed as a percent or rate as continuous data. This error is made because the scale appears "continuous" (for example, we can have a number like 86.4% or a rate of 1.47) to the person selecting the type of Shewhart chart. If data expressed as a percentage or rate are attribute in nature (that is, qualitative classification of units or counts of unusual or undesirable events), the data are attribute and should not be placed on a Shewhart chart for continuous data. Examples of attribute data commonly confused for continuous data include percentage of patients experiencing harm during their care or the rate of serious falls per occupied bed day. Attribute data will be a whole number when individual data elements are collected. Dividing that whole number by a denominator results in a percent or rate. That does not make this data continuous data. See Chapter Nine (under I Chart section), for an illustration of the impact of making this error.

The second common error in chart selection is that of treating the count of workload or throughput, such as hospital census, the number of visits to a clinic, or the volume of lab tests completed as attribute data. We use the number scale to produce a lot of important data in health care processes. Workload, which could be measured in dollars, weighed, or counted, is still workload. These count data should be treated as continuous data because of their intent; they are productivity or workload data and belong on Shewhart charts for continuous data.

It is important to note that the method to develop limits on Shewhart charts for continuous data require an analysis of process variation. A narrowing of the limits on a Shewhart chart for continuous data is reflective of reduced variation in the data used to calculate those limits. Limits on Shewhart charts for attribute data *do not* reflect reduced variation in the limits. Rather, the width of the limits is determined by a combination of the center line and the subgroup size. If the limits on a Shewhart chart for attribute data become narrower, it is due to this increased subgroup size or the change in the center line rather than to a reduction in variation in the data used to calculate the limits. So the concept of "reduced variation" means very different things on attribute versus continuous Shewhart charts.

The remainder of this chapter describes the construction and interpretation of the basic types of Shewhart charts.

SHEWHART CHARTS FOR CONTINUOUS DATA

As discussed in Chapter Two, many measures are made on a continuous scale using some kind of measurement device (laboratory instrument, clock or calendar, meter readings, survey instrument, financial scale, and so on). The I chart or the $\bar{X}$ and S charts are appropriate for any of these characteristics measured on a continuous scale. The data placed on an I chart may generally represent all types of distributions of data. In general, there is little need to be concerned about distributions being normal with Shewhart charts. The I chart does have a few issues regarding distribution. These issues are discussed later on in this section. Table 5.1 lists some situations where a Shewhart chart for continuous data might be appropriate.

I CHARTS

One of the most flexible and useful Shewhart charts is the chart for individual measurements, or the **I chart**.[2] In the literature, this type of chart is also called an X chart, Xmr chart, and Individuals chart. The Shewhart chart for individuals is useful when:[3]

---

[2]Nelson, L. S., "Shewhart Charts for Individual Measurements," *Journal of Quality Technology*, 1982, *i*(3), 172–173.

[3]Rigdon, S., Cruthis, E., and Champ, C., "Design Strategies for Individuals and Moving Range Control Charts," *Journal of Quality Technology*, 1993, *25*(3), 274–287.

Table 5.1 Applications of Shewhart Charts for Continuous Data in Health Care

Area	Application	Measure	Possible Subgroup Strategy	Chart
Overall	Chronic care	Number in registry	Month/specific disease/provider	—
	Satisfaction	Employee satisfaction score	Employee categories	$\bar{X}$ and S
	Satisfaction	Patient satisfaction ratings	Month/unit provider/DRG	$\bar{X}$ and S
	Financial	Revenue ($)	Week/service line/ DRG	—
		Accounts receivable	Week/payer	—
ED	Access	Waiting time	Day of week/time of day	$\bar{X}$ and S
	Productivity	Visit time	Provider/shift/type patient	$\bar{X}$ and S
		Patients seen/hour	Month/provider	$\bar{X}$ and S
ICU	Productivity	Number of bed turns	DRG/provider/age	—
		Average LOS	Month/ DRG /payer	$\bar{X}$ and S
Surgery	Workload	Number of surgeries	Week/provider/procedure/location	—
	Timeliness	Minutes from scheduled time	Day/location/provider	$\bar{X}$ and S
Outpatient	Workload	Number of patient visits	Day/provider	—
	Diabetic care	Average HbA1c	Month/care option/provider	$\bar{X}$ and S
Long-Term Care	Workload	Number of resident days	Month/unit/payer	—
	Quality care	Number of medication doses	Day/shift/staff category	—
		Hours of social activity	Week/resident/sex/age	$\bar{X}$ and S
Behavioral Health	Workload	Number of client visits	Day/provider/type visit/location	$\bar{X}$ and S
	Satisfaction	Client rating of provider	Month/client category/diagnosis	$\bar{X}$ and S
	Care Process	Days sobriety	Program/patient characteristics	$\bar{X}$ and S

- There is no rational way to organize the data into subgroups (recall discussion of rational subgrouping in Chapter Four).

  Example: Corporate provides data at the end of each month regarding total monthly revenue. Monthly revenue is simply one number, the total revenue earned that month. Because each individual measure—in this case monthly revenue—is plotted on the chart, there is no opportunity to organize the data using different subgrouping strategies.

- Measures of performance of the process can only be obtained infrequently.

  Example: The number of minutes from decision to administer a thrombolytic agent to the time the agent is started is collected for each patient requiring thrombolysis. The department only cares for one or two patients requiring thrombolysis each month.

- The variation at any one time (within a subgroup) is insignificant relative to the between subgroup variation.

  Example: A dentist obtains a full-mouth x-ray once each year for her patients. She generally does not repeat the x-ray two or three times at one sitting to learn from the variation between retakes. Each x-ray is typically obtained once. The important variation is *between* x-rays year to year.

Examples of situations and data where a Shewhart chart for individuals can be useful include patient-specific clinical measures, monthly accounting data, laboratory test data, forecasts, and budget variances. Often the frequency of data collection cannot be controlled for these situations and types of data.

Automated instrument readings such as oxygen saturation, heart rate, blood pressures, and the like often have minimal variation at any one time, but will change over time. When there is a natural drift in the measure, the short-term variation can be insignificant relative to variation over time. Shewhart I charts can often be useful in these cases.

Some advantages of the I chart (compared to other types of Shewhart charts):

- No calculations are required when plotting data points on the chart.
- Plotting is done each time a measurement is made, providing immediate feedback as data become available. Study of the process does not have to wait for additional measurements for averaging or other calculations.
- As only one chart is required for each measure, charts for multiple measures of performance can be grouped on one form for presentation purposes to facilitate evaluation of a process.
- The capability of a process can be evaluated directly from the limits on the chart.

Because of these advantages, the I Chart is sometimes selected when another type of Shewhart chart is more appropriate. The I chart is less sensitive than other Shewhart charts with larger subgroup sizes in its ability to detect the presence of a special cause. Sometimes, data analyzed with an I chart will indicate a stable process, but the same data analyzed with a more appropriate chart ($\bar{X}$ and S, P chart, or C chart discussed in later sections) will clearly indicate the presence of special causes. This point is further developed in Chapter Six. Besides this lesser sensitivity, there are some other disadvantages to using an I chart to study variation in data:

- Because each individual measure is plotted on the chart, there is no opportunity to focus on different sources of variation through subgrouping (see Chapter Four discussion of rational subgrouping).

- All sources of variation are combined on one chart, sometimes making identification of the important sources of variation difficult.
- The I chart is sensitive to a nonsymmetric distribution of data and may require data transformation to be used effectively. Transforming data was introduced in Chapter Two and is further discussed in Chapter Eight.

The "**moving range**" (**MR**) (the difference between consecutive data values) is the statistic used to determine the common cause variation for an I chart. The rationale for using the moving range to determine the process variation for the I chart is that pairs of consecutive measurements are more likely to be affected by similar causes than are results at other points in time. Limits should be established on the basis of common cause variation only. Individual moving ranges that are inflated by special causes are screened prior to calculating the limits for the I chart. This minimizes the effect on the limits of special causes on the initial data set. Alternatively, direct calculation of the standard deviation using all the data causes the limits to be inflated with special causes as well as common cause variation. Beware that various software programs use this inappropriate approach to calculating limits for I charts.

To develop an I chart, the most recent 20 to 30 measurements should be used. More than any other chart, this minimum number of subgroups is important since each subgroup has only one data value. The symbol for the number of measures used to calculate limits is "k," which is also the number of subgroups. The individual measurements are plotted on the I chart and the average of the individual data values is used for the center line of the chart. The "moving ranges" of consecutive measurements are used to estimate the variation of the process and to develop limits for the I chart. The moving range is calculated by pairing consecutive measurements. The range is calculated for each set of two measurements by subtracting the low value from the high value. Each individual measurement is considered twice in the calculation of the moving ranges. Because a "previous" measurement is not available for the first measurement in the set, only k − 1 moving ranges can be calculated. After screening for special causes in the MRs, the average of the moving ranges (MR_{bar}) is used for limit calculations. Formula and steps for developing a Shewhart chart for individuals are given in the Appendix 5.1.

Because the I chart of individual measurements contains all the information available in the data, it is not necessary to plot the moving ranges. However, plotting the moving ranges can sometimes make an increase or decrease in the variation of the process more obvious than on the I chart. If the moving ranges are plotted, only Rule 1 (discussed in Chapter Four) should be used to evaluate the MR chart for special causes since the plotted points are not independent. We recommend not displaying the MR chart because of the complexity of interpretation.[4]

Examples of Shewhart Charts for Individual Measurements

A large organization was concerned about the amount of infectious waste it produced. They decided to use an I chart to display the waste data and created a team to test changes to reduce waste. The data and I chart calculations are shown in Table 5.2. Their initial I chart follows at Figure 5.2.

---

[4]Boes, K., Does, R., and Schurink, Y., "Shewhart-Type Control Charts for Individual Observations," *Journal of Quality Technology*, 1993, 25(3), 188–198.

Table 5.2 Data and Calculations for Infectious Waste I Chart

Month	Infectious Waste (#) per Patient Day (I)	Moving Range (MR)
J-07	6.8	*XXX*
J	6.7	0.10
A	6.86	0.16
S	6.63	0.23
O	6.86	0.23
N	7.61	0.75
D	6.99	0.62
J-08	7.48	0.49
F	6.96	0.52
M	7.22	0.26
A	7.27	0.05
M	7.19	0.08
J	7.58	0.39
J	7.46	0.12
A	6.6	0.86
S	6.97	0.37
O	7.05	0.08
N	7.41	0.36
D	7.91	0.50
J-09	6.38	1.53
F	6.69	0.31
Total	148.62	8.01
Average	7.077	0.40

1. Calculate the k − 1 moving ranges.

2. Calculate the average of the moving ranges (MR_{bar})

$$MR_{bar} = \frac{\sum MR}{k-1} = \frac{8.01}{(21-1)} = \frac{8.01}{20} = 0.40$$

3. Calculate the $UL_{MR} = 3.27 * MR_{bar}$. $UL_{MR} = 3.27 \times 0.40 = \underline{1.308}$

4. Remove any moving range bigger than the UL_{MR} and recalculate the average moving range (MR_{bar}). [Note: This recalculation should be done only once.] *In this example one*

moving range (J-07) exceeded the upper limit of the moving range chart. The new average moving range is:

$$\frac{(8.01 - 1.53)}{19} = \frac{6.48}{19} = 0.34$$

5. Calculate the average of the individual data (I_{bar}). This is the center line (CL) on the I chart.

$$CL\ (I_{bar}) = \frac{\sum I}{k} = \frac{148.62}{21} = 7.077$$

6. Calculate limits:

$UL = I_{bar} + (2.66 * MR_{bar})$ $LL = I_{bar} - (2.66 * MR_{bar})$
$UL = 7.077 + (2.66 * 0.34)$ $LL = 7.077 - (2.66 * 0.34)$
$UL = 7.077 + .904$ $LL = 7.077 - .904$
$UL = \mathbf{7.98}$ $LL = \mathbf{6.17}$

Note: Steps 3 and 4 above are critical when there are special causes in the data used to calculate the limits.[5] Many software programs for Individual charts skip step 3 and 4 of the above I Chart calculation procedure. These steps are necessary to assure that the control limits are not impacted by special cause variation. See Chapter Six for further discussion of this issue.

As the team continued to test and implement changes, special cause in the desired direction became evident. After awhile the team has enough data to create new limits for the improved process. Figure 5.3 shows the I chart displaying limits for the process before improvement and a second set of limits for the improved process. This view allows the team to show others the impact of their improvement work and to track the process to determine if the improvement is sustained.

FIGURE 5.2   I Chart with Initial Limits for Volume of Infectious Waste

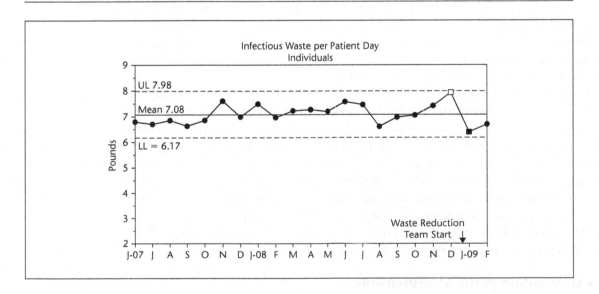

[5]Nelson, L. S., "Control Charts for Individual Measurements," *Journal of Quality Technology*, 1982, *14*(34).

FIGURE 5.3   I Chart Updated with Two Limits

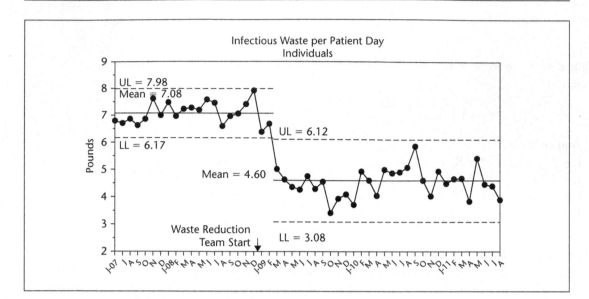

Rational Ordering with an Individual Chart

The concepts of rational ordering and subgrouping were introduced in Chapter Four. The major disadvantage of the individual Shewhart chart is that all the sources of variation in the process are included in the one chart. There is no opportunity to use the concept of rational subgrouping, as associated with the $\overline{X}$ and S charts for continuous data, to isolate and evaluate different sources of variation.

Usually the data for an I chart will be analyzed in a natural time order. But in some situations a time order is not relevant. For example, if the data consist of quarterly productivity data for 30 primary care clinic providers, an I chart could be used to identify special causes. In cases like this, the preference though is to obtain another data point (possibly from the previous quarter, or disaggregate the quarterly data into monthly data) for each individual and then use an $\overline{X}$ and S chart with subgroups of n = 2 or 3. If this is not possible, an I chart can be used, but the individual data must first be ordered in some rational way to compute the moving ranges (for example, from least experienced to most experienced provider or some such rational scheme).

A rational ordering of the data for the individual chart should be done based on the knowledge of the subject matter expert. For example, if experience was thought to be a factor that could affect the productivity data, the data should be ordered by experience of the providers on the horizontal axis. If the volume of visits completed was thought to affect the score, the data could be arranged by the volume during the quarter (or for the previous year). The appropriate order will depend on the objective of the chart or the questions that need to be answered. If no rational ordering is possible, the data could be ordered in a haphazard manner, such as alphabetical order, and plotted on a run chart. The calculation of limits in these cases may not be useful and can be misleading. If limits are necessary, the previous strategies to develop an $\overline{X}$ and S chart should be followed.

Effect of the Distribution of the Measurements

The limits for an I chart are more sensitive to the shape of the distribution of the measurements than limits on $\overline{X}$ charts. In most cases found in practice, the limits still provide a good economic balance between overreacting and underreacting to variation in the process.

Exceptions to this are when the data range over more than an order of magnitude (10, 100, 1,000, and so on) or when the data are highly skewed in one direction (for example, many measurements of time, including length of stay). The measurements can be transformed prior to developing the Shewhart chart to alleviate these situations. Common transformations are the logarithm for multiple order of magnitudes and the square root for skewed data. Chapter Eight contains further discussion of transformations with Shewhart charts.

Alternatives to the Shewhart chart for individuals include moving average and range charts, cumulative sum (CUSUM) Shewhart-type chart, and the exponentially weighted moving average chart. See Chapter Seven for further discussion of these other types of charts.

Example of Individual Chart for Deviations from a Target

An individual Shewhart chart is often used to evaluate data that has different target values, and is therefore expected to vary from measurement to measurement according to the different targets. Examples are the measurement of hours worked on a project for different groups of employees, variation from target staffing level, volume of ED workload for planning purposes, or financial data used to study planning tools such as budgets, forecasts, and schedules. The following example shows how to handle these data with an individual chart.

A forecast of costs is made three months in advance for each department in the hospital. The budgets are used for planning purposes and it is desirable to have them as accurate as possible. Because of fluctuations in operations, the budget (target) varies from month-to-month. Each month, the budget and the actual can be compared to evaluate the accuracy of the forecast. The percentage difference is calculated and used as a measure of forecast accuracy. As data are only available once a month, an individual chart is used to study the accuracy.

Figure 5.4 shows the Shewhart chart for a two-year period. Each month the budget, which had been forecasted two months in advance, is subtracted from the actual expenditure.

This difference is divided by the forecasted budget and multiplied by 100 to calculate the percentage difference. The percent difference is used to develop the I chart. It is important to retain the + (over budget) or −(under budget) sign with the percent difference. The center line at −1.44% indicates that on the average, the actual expenditures have been 1.44% under budget. The common cause variation is about + or −17% of budget. There is a special cause (22% over budget) in July 2005 that should be investigated.

FIGURE 5.4   Individual Shewhart Chart for Budget Variances

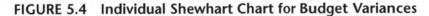

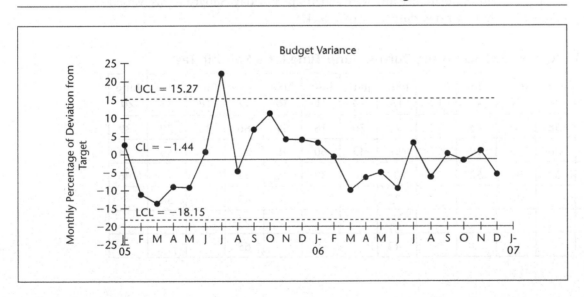

$\overline{X}$ and S Shewhart Charts

When continuous data are obtained from a process, it is sometimes of interest to learn about both the average performance of the process and the variation about the average level. For example, it may be useful to learn about the average length of stay (LOS) per month for a particular diagnosis and the variation among the cases comprising that average. In these cases, a set of two Shewhart charts are often used to study the process: the $\overline{X}$ **chart** and the **S chart**.

The collection of data for the construction of $\overline{X}$ and S Shewhart charts (pronounced X bar and S chart) requires that the data be organized in subgroups. A **subgroup** for continuous data is a set of measurements that were obtained under similar conditions or during the same time period. The subgroup size may vary for the $\overline{X}$ and S chart. The $\overline{X}$ chart contains the averages of each subgroup and the S chart the spread (standard deviation) between the measurements within each subgroup. These averages and standard deviations are usually plotted over time.

Subgroup sizes can be as low as two or three measures for the $\overline{X}$ and S charts. They can also handle large subgroup sizes which are often useful for data in administrative databases. Appendix 5.1 describes the formula to calculate the limits for $\overline{X}$ and S charts where the center line for the $\overline{X}$ chart is the weighted average of the subgroup averages and the S chart is calculated using the weighted average of the individual standard deviations. Because of the complexity in calculation and the varying limits, these charts are almost always done using a spreadsheet or other computer software.

The equations for the limits on the $\overline{X}$ and S chart are:

$$\overline{X} \text{ chart:} \quad UCL = \overline{\overline{X}} + (A_3 * S_{bar}) \quad\quad LCL = \overline{\overline{X}} - (A_3 * S_{bar})$$

$$S \text{ chart:} \quad UCL = (B_3 * S_{bar}) \quad\quad LCL = (B_4 * S_{bar})$$

The definition of the terms and the factors A3, B3, and B4 (which depend on the subgroup size) are tabulated in Appendix 5.1. Note that some software programs calculate the center line for the S chart using the pooled value of the subgroup standard deviations. If this statistic is used, the limits on the average chart will be more sensitive to special causes in the S chart, so this approach is not generally recommended.

Table 5.3 shows the data and Figure 5.5 shows the $\overline{X}$ and S chart for a test that was typically run less than 10 times per day in the radiology laboratory. It was desirable to have a turn-around time of less than one hour. Data were collected for the last two weeks to understand the current performance and were subgrouped by day. Subgroup size varied between three to six tests per day during the two weeks.

Table 5.3   Radiology Laboratory Turn-Around Time for a Specific Test

	June 7	June 8	June 9	June 10	June 11	June 12	June 13	June 14	June 15	June 16	June 17	June 18	June 19	June 20
Test 1	105	50	58	67	73	57	78	76	18	39	86	32	70	39
Test 2	54	105	26	52	59	64	96	49	60	45	27	47	56	34
Test 3	79	85	38	92	62	24	107	40	39	35	91	57	40	146
Test 4	49			46			72				49		34	
Test 5	31						27				23			
Test 6							43				65			

FIGURE 5.5   X̄ and S Shewhart Chart for Radiology Test Turn-Around Time

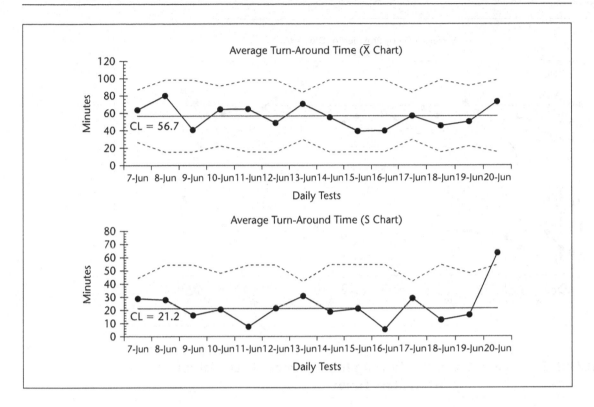

The S chart for the turn-around times shows a special cause on June 20th which indicates the variation in the process was greater during that period. The average on June 20th appeared pretty much like that of other days, but the variation within that day's samples was special cause on the S chart, indicating an unusual spread among the test times, some very high or very low test times, or both. Something special happened that day. The team decided that they needed to investigate the special cause on June 20th.

Figure 5.6 shows X̄ and S charts for the length of stay for patients admitted with a particular DRG. The data are subgrouped by both quarter (first and second quarter) and provider (provider number for the ten providers who admitted patients during this time period). The number of patients admitted by a particular provider and quarter ranged from 16 to 41. The X̄ chart shows a special cause associated with provider 66 for both quarters (Rules 1 and 4). The patients admitted by this provider have longer lengths of stay than would be expected from this DRG. The S chart indicates a special cause in the second quarter for provider 45. Note that the averages for provider # 45 do not look unusual. The S chart would point to something special about some of the patients admitted by provider 45. The X̄ and S charts in Figure 5.6 were constructed using the formula in Appendix 5.1.

A third example of the X̄ and S chart looks at start times for a specific type of surgical cases. For each surgery, there is a scheduled time to start. The actual time is recorded and the deviation (actual − scheduled) in minutes is calculated. A negative time indicates the surgery actually started early, whereas a positive time indicates it started late. The data are subgrouped by week, with 7 to 21 surgeries during the week.

Figure 5.7 shows the initial X̄ and S chart for this measure. Both the Average chart and the Standard Deviation chart (displaying variation within a week) show special cause signals. The center line for the average chart is 13.1, indicating an average of 13 minutes

FIGURE 5.6   X̄ and S Shewhart Subgrouped by Provider

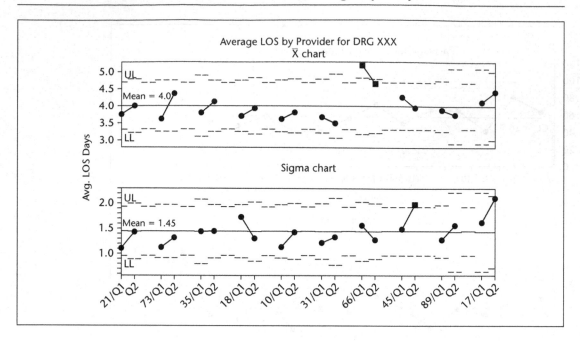

FIGURE 5.7   X̄ and S Charts Showing Improvement in Deviation
from Start Times

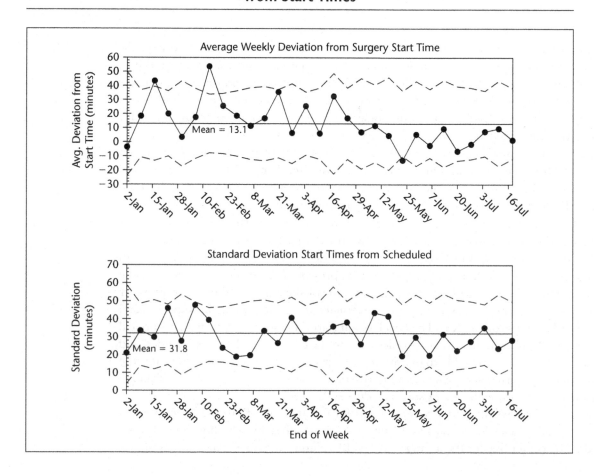

late start for these surgeries during this time period. The data for the last 12 weeks indicate an improvement with the average closer to 0 (that is, starting on time). The control limits should next be updated to reflect this success.

An alternative to the $\bar{X}$ and S chart that can be used when the subgroup size is constant is the $\bar{X}$ and R chart. Since the $\bar{X}$ and S charts can be used for both constant and variable subgroup size, we do not discuss the $\bar{X}$ and R chart here (see Chapter Seven for discussion, including formula).

Shewhart Charts for Attribute Data

Chapter Two described the two types of attribute data:

Classifications of units: each unit is classified as conforming or nonconforming, pass/fail, blue/not blue, go/no-go, and so on.

Count of incidents: a count of the number of nonconformities, defects (complications, infections, errors) accidents, trips, telephone calls, and so on.

In order to select the best Shewhart chart and to develop it correctly, it is important to be clear about which type of attribute data that will be used. To develop an attribute Shewhart chart, a subgrouping strategy must first be determined. The *subgroup size* (n) is the number of units tested, or inspected, for *classification data*. The subgroup size is called the *area of opportunity* for the incident to occur when working with *count data*. There are three commonly used Shewhart charts for attribute data, depending on the type of attribute data and the constancy of the subgroup size. Table 5.4 summarizes these charts.

Traditional Shewhart chart selection guides reference the NP chart. The NP chart is a Shewhart chart for classification data in which the subgroup size is constant. In health care, we rarely describe classification data as numbers, but rather use percentages. Typically we are using data from the process in its natural increments, such as the number of surgeries with complications that month, no-shows from all of the appointments in Clinic A that week. As the P chart will perform well for subgroup sizes that are constant or subgroup sizes that vary, we find we rarely use the NP chart in health care and so do not include it here (it is presented in Chapter Seven as an option).

Subgroup Size for Attribute Charts

Careful consideration of the subgrouping strategy for an attribute chart is important for developing a useful Shewhart chart. Although the width of the limits on Shewhart charts for continuous data depends on the common cause variation in the data, the limits of an attribute chart depend solely on the process average and the subgroup size. In order to develop effective attribute Shewhart charts, two important characteristics

Table 5.4   Three Types of Attribute Shewhart Charts

Chart Name	Type of Data	Distribution	Statistic Charted	Subgroup Size
P Chart	Classification	Binomial	Percent nonconforming units (P)	Constant or may vary
C Chart	Count	Poisson	Number of incidents (C)	Constant
U Chart	Count	Poisson	Incidents per unit (U)	Constant or may vary

of these charts should be considered. First, in order to better monitor improvement in the process, the chart should have a lower control limit. Second, it is desirable to have the size of the subgroup large enough so that some nonconformities or nonconforming units are found in most subgroups. In order to develop a useful attribute chart, no more than 25% of the subgroups should have zero nonconforming units (plotting "0" on the chart). The size of a subgroup plays an important role in achieving these two characteristics.

The minimum subgroup size for an effective P chart depends on the average value of "p_{bar}" (the center line of the chart). A common guideline in the SPC literature for the p chart is $n > 300/p$. Using the Binomial distribution for different average p's (p_{bar}), Table 5.5 summarizes the minimum subgroup size required:

1. to expect less than 25% of the subgroups with a subgroup p = 0
2. based on the common guideline (n > 300/p)
3. to expect a lower control limit > 0

Table 5.5   Minimum Subgroup Sizes for Effective P Charts

Estimate of Average % Nonconforming Units (p_{bar})	Minimum Subgroup Size (n) Required to Have < 25% zero for p's	Minimum Subgroup Size Common Guideline (n>300/p)	Minimum Subgroup Size Required to Have LCL > 0
0.1	1400	3000	9000
0.5	280	600	1800
1.0	140	300	900
1.5	93	200	600
2	70	150	450
3	47	100	300
4	35	75	220
5	28	60	175
6	24	50	142
8	17	38	104
10	14	30	81
12	12	25	66
15	9	20	51
20	7	15	36
25	5	12	28
30	4	10	22
40	3	8	14
50	2	6	10

Note: for p>50, use 100-p to enter the table (e.g. for p = 70% use table p of 30%, for p = 99% use table p of 1%, and so forth.)

To use this table to design a P chart for classification data, first estimate the average percent nonconforming units for the measure of interest. Then find this percentage (0.1–50%) in the left end column and move across the table to find the recommended minimum subgroup size to meet your criteria on interest. Then develop a subgrouping strategy that would result in at least the number of units.

A QI team was planning a P chart for the percent unplanned readmissions based on discharges from one of the floor units. Based on previous hospital reports, they predicted the average would be about 8%. They average about 300 discharges per month. From Table 5.5, they found that:

They would need at least 17 discharges to get a P chart that would be at all useful.

They would need at least 38 discharges to follow the common guideline for P charts.

They would need a least 104 discharges to get a P chart with a lower control limit.

After reviewing this information they realized that a weekly P chart would have subgroups of 70–80 discharges. Though this weekly chart would be a useful P chart, it would not have a lower limit to quickly detect an improvement. They decided to subgroup the data in two-week periods and have a P chart based on about 140–160 discharges. They would calculate the percentage of readmissions at the end of each two-week period and update the P chart.

For count data, the Poisson distribution is used to develop the limits on the Shewhart chart. On a C chart, whenever the average number of counts (C_{bar}) is less than 9, there will not be a lower control limit. Also C_{bar} has to be greater than 1.4 to expect < 25% of the subgroup values to be zero. So in selecting the area of opportunity for collecting count data, select the time period, geographic area, or number of units to expect at least an average of 1.4 or more nonconformities to get an effective C Chart. If the QI team desires to have a lower limit for the C Chart, an area of opportunity that gives an expectation of more than nine nonconformities is needed.

The key guidelines for a C Chart to have a C_{bar} >9 in order to have a lower limit and C_{bar} >1.4 in order to avoid too many zeros, can also be used to design effective U charts. In U charts the area of opportunity is allowed to vary. So a "standard" area of opportunity (1 day, 100 admissions, 1,000 line days, 10,000 deliveries, 100,000 hours worked, 1,000,000 miles driven, and so forth) is set and the "number of standard areas" is determined for each subgroup.

In designing a subgrouping strategy for the U chart, pick a standard area of opportunity and an estimate of the current average rate. Then divide 9 by the average rate to get the minimum number of "standard areas of opportunities" required for the U chart to have a lower limit. Divide 1.4 by the average rate to get the minimum number of "standard areas of opportunities" required to have a useful U chart (not too many zeros plotted).

A QI team was chartered to reduce hospital-wide infection rates. They wanted to develop a U Chart for their baseline data from the past two years. Infection rates were currently reported monthly as x/1,000 patient days (that is, occupied bed days). The average rate for the past year was 2.5 infections per 1,000 patient days. To determine the minimum subgroup strategy, they divided 1.4 by 2.5 to get 0.56 standard areas of opportunities. So they developed a useful U chart with an expected opportunity of 560 bed days. This meant they could have separate monthly charts (or subgroups) for wards with more than 19 occupied beds. To get a U chart with a lower limit, they would need 3.6 (9 divided by 2.5) standard areas of opportunity. This would work well for the hospital-wide monthly chart because the hospital had 150 beds and typically had more than 4,000 occupied bed days each month.

When the attribute we are interested in studying is a relatively rare event, these guidelines can often not be met. In these cases, the basic Shewhart charts may not be useful to detect improvement. An alternative in these cases is to develop Shewhart charts for the time or number of units between events. Chapter Two (Figure 2.22) introduced the concept of transforming rare event data to time or cases between events. Chapter Three (Figures 3.28 through 3.32) showed how to develop a run chart for cases between data. Chapter Seven shows how to use alternative G charts or T charts for these situations with rare events.

The P Chart for Classification Data

The **P chart** is appropriate whenever the data are based on classifications made in two categories, for example patients who were either harmed during their hospitalization or not harmed during their hospitalization. Table 5.6 gives some examples where a P chart could be used. The P chart limits are based on a binomial distribution of the data. The primary assumptions required to use a P chart are:

Each unit can be classified into only one of two categories.

The occurrence of a unit having either of the two attributes is independent of the attributes of any of the other units. (This assumption is most often violated when defects occur in bunches.)

It is impossible for the numerator to be larger than the denominator (if 50 cases are reviewed, the maximum that can fail to meet criteria is 50).

The percentage of units in one of the categories (either the positive or the negative one, for example, the percentage of those with the pneumonia vaccine or the percentage of those without the vaccine) is then calculated and graphed to develop the chart. Typically, at least

Table 5.6   Example of P Chart Applications in Health Care

Area	Application	Statistic	Possible Subgroup Strategy
Overall	Mortality	% mortality	Month/diagnosis/patient characteristics
	Satisfaction	% in highest satisfaction category	Service line/location/service
	Financial	% bills > 30 days	Month/payer
ED	Access	% left without being seen	Month/day of week/shift/ethnic group
	Care process	% given ace inhibitor	Day/shift/provider/shift
ICU	Care process	% patients w/ventilator bundle	Week/physician/patient's sex
	Mortality	% mortality	Time/diagnosis/patient characteristics
Surgery	Care process	% antibiotic on time	Week/provider/day
	Care process	% antibiotic d/c in 24 hrs.	Week/provider/service
	Care process	% ASA level 3 patients	Month/provider/procedure
	Timeliness	% on-time start	Day/location/provider
Outpatient	Utilization	% keep follow-up appt.	Day/time of day/provider
	Diabetic care	% HbA1c of 7 or less	Month/care option/provider
Long-Term Care	Care process	% with complete care plan	Month/unit/care provider
	Medication delivery	% doses on-time	Day/shift/provider
	Quality of life	% residence in org. involved in social activity	Week/resident/sex/age categories/day of week/month/quarter
Behavioral Health	Effectiveness	% sober six months post rehabilitation program	Month/program/provider/client
	Satisfaction	% clients in highest satisfaction category	Month/client category/diagnosis/provider
	Care process	% adhering to medications	Month/program/provider/patient characteristics

Table 5.7   P Chart Patient Harm Data and Calculations

Months	Number of Patients w/Harm	Number of Charts Reviewed	Percent Harm (%)
F09	9	20	45
M	5	20	25
A	8	20	40
M	10	20	50
J	11	20	55
J	9	20	45
A	7	20	35
S	8	20	40
O	10	20	50
N	5	20	25
D	9	20	45
J10	8	20	40
Totals	99	240	495

20 subgroups are desirable for calculating the limits with at least 30 units in each subgroup. Larger subgroup sizes are needed when there is a low chance of occurrence in one of the categories (see Table 5.5). Appendix 5.1 gives the steps for calculating limits for a P charts.

Examples of P Charts

This example deals with a situation where a constant subgroup size is appropriate. The patient safety team needed to gather information on patient harm in their organization as they worked to reduce the percentage of patients harmed. Each month they reviewed the records of 20 people discharged from their hospital that month for evidence of harm using a global trigger tool to identify harm. This was a very high-level global measure (the team also worked with other measures appropriate for pilot unit outcomes and to their many process changes) related to their global safety measure. After 12 months they knew they had enough data to compute trial limits.

Table 5.7 contains the data collected each month and the calculations for their P chart with trial limits. Note that with charts for attribute data the width of the limits is not dependent on variation between subgroups but rather on the subgroup size. Narrowing of the limits on attribute charts is not reflective of reduced variation in the limits but rather of larger subgroup size. Wider limits are not indicative of increased process variation but of reduced subgroup size.

$$P_{bar} = \frac{\sum p}{k} = \frac{495}{12} = \underline{\mathbf{41.25}}$$

$$\sigma_p = \sqrt{\frac{P_{bar}*(100 - P_{bar})}{n}} = \sqrt{\frac{41.25*(100 - 41.25)}{20}} = \sqrt{\frac{41.25*58.75}{20}} = \sqrt{121.17} = \underline{11.007}$$

$$UL = P_{bar} + (3 * \sigma_p) \qquad\qquad LL = P_{bar} - (3 * \sigma_p)$$

$$UL = \underline{41.25} + (3 * \underline{11.007}) \qquad LL = \underline{41.25} - (3 * \underline{11.007})$$

$$UL = 41.25 + \underline{33.021} \qquad\qquad LL = 41.25 - \underline{33.021}$$

$$UL = \mathbf{74.27} \qquad\qquad LL = \mathbf{8.23}$$

FIGURE 5.8   P Chart of Percentage of Patients Harmed with Trial Limits

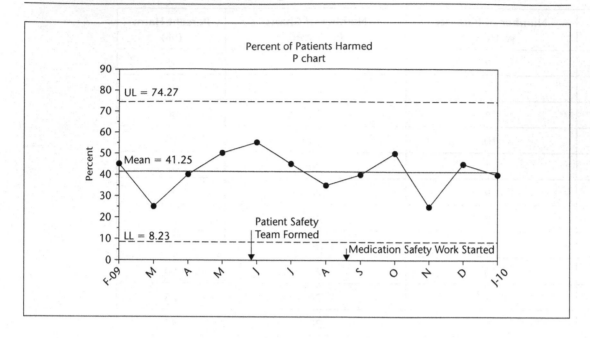

FIGURE 5.9   P Chart with Trial Limits Extended and Evidence of Special Cause

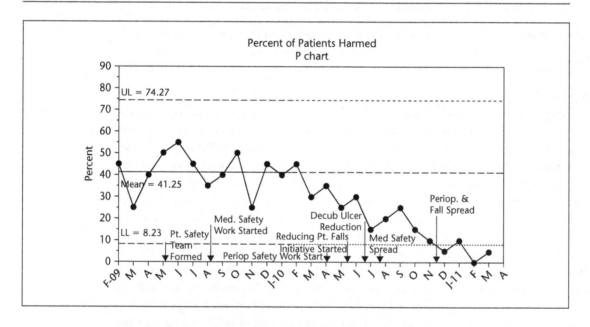

Note: if the calculation of the UL is greater than 100, then there is no UL. If the calculation for the LL is less than 0, then there is no LL.

Figure 5.8 shows the Shewhart chart for the percentage of patients harmed.

As they tested, and then spread a variety of patient safety initiatives special cause becomes evident on their chart at Figure 5.9. This special cause is evidence of improvement.

A common misconception in interpreting Shewhart attribute charts is to relate improvement directly to the width of the control limits. Figure 5.10 is an example of an organization that increased the percentage of patients with diabetes who used self-management goal setting from an average of 20% to an average of 50%. This was a huge accomplishment. Note that the limits did not become narrower in the time frame in which the improvement is evident. The limits for a P chart are dependent on the subgroup size. Narrowing on the limits on an attribute chart is not indicative of reduced variation in the process, nor is widening of the limits indicative of increased variation in the process.

An additional example deals with a situation in which the subgroup size is variable. It would be problematic to try to interpret the number of patients with an unplanned readmission without taking into account the number of patients discharged each month. A P chart is useful in this situation. A team working to reduce patient length of stay (LOS) decided to track a balancing measure, unplanned readmissions (Chapter Two addresses outcome, process, and balancing measures for improvement projects). This team tracked unplanned readmissions out of those discharged from the hospital each month. The data for unplanned readmissions follows in Table 5.8.

The team noted that as they worked successfully to reduce LOS, the P chart tracking unplanned readmissions, Figure 5.11, showed undesirable special cause. This unintended negative consequence of their improvement work required their attention. Improvement projects require outcome, process, and balancing measures. Shewhart charts are useful in tracking these key project measures.

A regional medical system wanted to track the percent of *Staphylococcus aureus* infections that were of the particularly dangerous methicillin-resistant *Staphylococcus aureus* variety (MRSA) over the last year in order to learn about system performance and variation between hospitals. Their data are shown in Table 5.9.

FIGURE 5.10   P Chart: Width of Limits Dependent on Subgroup Size

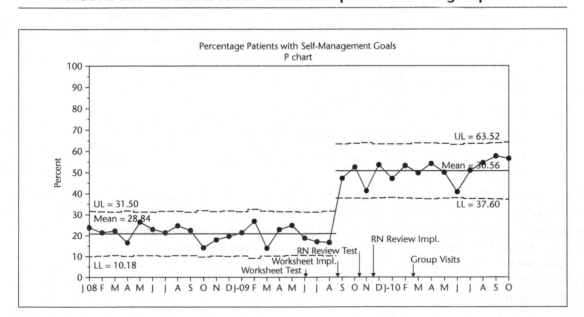

Table 5.8 Unplanned Readmissions Data

Month	Patients Admitted	Discharges
J09	19	688
F	12	643
M	10	411
A	23	678
M	20	999
J	16	735
J	7	647
A	18	678
S	14	312
O	16	717
N	12	680
D	14	733
J10	8	670
F	18	703
M	19	638
A	16	702
M	10	682
J	22	578
J	11	686
A	16	663
S	21	614
O	19	711
N	15	678
D	26	690
J11	22	392
F	37	861

They selected a P chart as the appropriate chart for their data and subgrouped the data by hospital to create the chart in Figure 5.12. They were able to detect three organizations with percentages of MRSA that were special cause; two high and one hospital low. This raised opportunities for targeted intervention and learning.

It is possible to create an adjusted P chart where the control limits are constant even when the subgroup size varies.[6] The plotted points are adjusted percentages, which users will not be familiar with, but the constant limits may be attractive.

---

[6]Rocke, D., "The Adjusted P Chart and U Chart for Varying Sample Sizes," *Journal of Quality Technology*, Vol. 22, No. 3, July 1990, 206–209.

FIGURE 5.11   P Chart of Percentage of Unplanned Readmissions

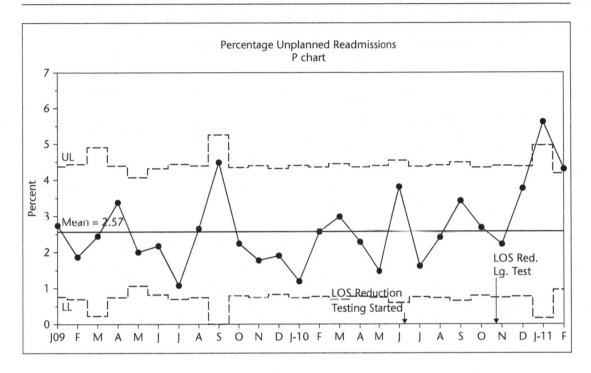

Table 5.9   MRSA Data

Hospital	Number of S. Aureus Infections	Number of MRSA
South	87	59
North	60	50
East	53	32
West	94	48
Mid	27	22
Capital	44	41
Plains	59	33
City	68	39
Central	39	22
University	44	30
General	52	26
Community	59	22
Regional	41	30

FIGURE 5.12 P Chart of Percentage of MRSA by Hospital

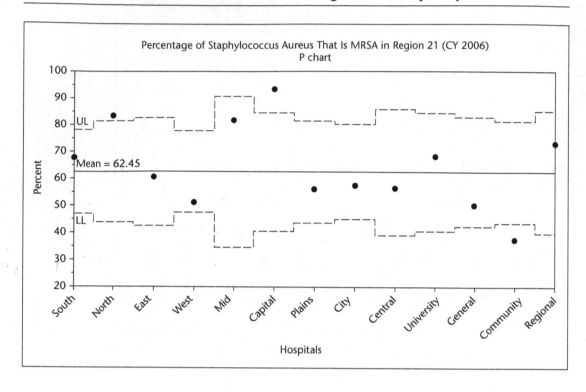

Creation of Funnel Limits for a P Chart

Funnel limits[7] may be created for any Shewhart chart with unequal subgroup size or area of opportunity ($\bar{X}$ and S, P, U charts). **Funnel limits** are created by sequencing the data on the Shewhart chart in order of subgroup size, rather than sequencing by time order or another sequencing strategy. To create funnel limits, the data are ordered from the smallest subgroup size to the largest, and then limits are calculated. Funnel limits will be wider with the smaller subgroup sizes and narrow as subgroup size increases. This gives the limits their "funnel" appearance which many users find much more appealing than the up and down of variable limits. The use of funnel limits is fairly intuitive for the viewer and may make it easier to interpret the chart. It allows for useful comparison of data from organizations differing in size. For example, funnel limits may make it readily apparent if all the special cause in MRSA is occurring in organizations with a large number of *Staphylococcus aureus* cases. Figure 5.12 could readily be formatted to make use of funnel limits (see Figure 5.13). This was accomplished by reordering the data on the chart from the hospital with the most cases of *Staphylococcus aureus* (the denominator) to the hospital with the least. Seeing the data displayed using funnel we see clearly that special cause in MRSA rates is not occurring only in organizations with a large number of cases of staphylococcusaureus. "Funnel charts" are currently being used to study performance using comparative databases that range across a wide variety of practice sizes.[8]

---

[7]Spiegelhalter, D., "Funnel Plots for Institutional Comparison," *Quality and Safety in Health Care*, 2002, *11*, 390–391.

[8]Gale, C., Roberts, A., Batin, P., and Hall, A., "Funnel Plots, Performance Variation and the Myocardial Infarction National Audit Project 2003–2004," *Biomedical Central Cardiovascular Disorders*, 2006, *6*(34).

Woodall, H., "The Use of Control Charts in Health-Care and Public-Health Surveillance," *Journal of Quality Technology*, 2006, *38*(2), 89–103.

FIGURE 5.13   P Chart of Percentage of MRSA with Funnel Limits

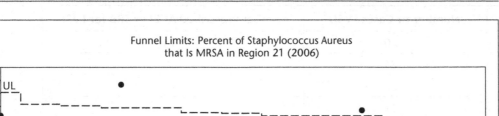

Figure 5.14 illustrates the use of funnel limits with data from a system tracking the percent compliance of organizations in prescribing ACEI or ARB medications for heart failure patients with LVSD. The data are sequenced from least to most number of cases to heart failure patients.

Table 5.10 contains the data ordered by subgroup size for the funnel chart in Figure 5.14. The number of cases per organization varied widely in the year studied. The data were ordered on the P chart by the number of cases and labeled by organization code/number of cases. Organization A saw 20 patients with LVSD, Organization F saw 26, and so on. This funnel P chart reveals that organizations J, C, and B are special cause with a low percentage of appropriate medication prescription for LVDS. Organizations O and P are special cause with a high percentage of compliance. This presents opportunities for systemwide learning and improvement.

C and U Charts for Counts of Nonconformities

When actual counts of incidents (called nonconformities) rather than classification of units are made, either a C chart or a U chart is usually the appropriate Shewhart chart. C and U charts limits are based on the Poisson distribution. Table 5.4 outlined the difference between count and classification data. Because the subgrouping method for counts is not always based on the selection of a certain number of units, a subgroup is defined as an **area of opportunity**, which is simply the region selected within which the count of occurrences or nonconformities will take place. An area of opportunity could be of any of the following three forms shown in Table 5.11:

To decide whether to use a C chart or a U chart, determine whether the area of opportunity will be constant or will vary for each subgroup of counts. For example, an area of opportunity could be the number of assessments performed each week. If the

Table 5.10 Data for Funnel Limits of ACEI/ARB Compliance for LVSD

Organization	Number of Cases LVSD	Number Prescribed ACEI or SRB for LVSD
A	20	14
F	26	18
D	29	20
G	31	28
J	40	32
S	47	31
K	66	60
H	68	59
O	77	76
L	85	74
C	99	71
R	140	129
E	150	138
N	155	128
Q	190	168
P	201	195
B	252	189
M	280	254
I	507	427

FIGURE 5.14 P Chart of Medication Compliance with Funnel Limits

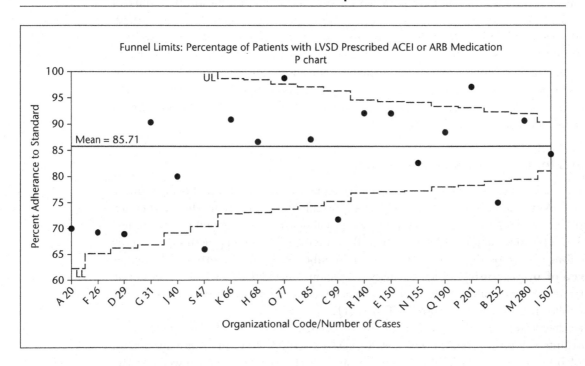

Table 5.11 Examples of Area of Opportunity for Counts Data

Form	Area of Opportunity	Example of a Measure
Number of Units	20 procedures	Number of errors per each group of 20 procedures
	10 patient charts	Number of coding errors per each group of 10 patient charts
	50 invoices	Number of coding errors per each group of 50 invoices
Space	1 square centimeter	Number of colonies in each sample of square centimeter
	3 milliliter sample of specimen	Number of white blood cells in 3 millimeter of blood sample
	5 square inches surface area	Number of defects in sample of 5 square inches of artificial skin
Time	One week	Number of rejected insurance claims each week
	One shift	Number of patient comments about waiting time in ER for each shift
	Three months	Number of employee needlesticks in each three-month time frame

number of missing items from these assessments is counted, the count would be distorted if the number of assessments performed varied from week to week. The C chart and U chart are discussed in the remaining part of this section. Table 5.12 lists examples of applications of C and U charts.

C Charts

The primary assumptions associated with use of a **C chart** are:

The incidents are a whole number when originally counted (discrete data).

An incident at any one place or time is independent of any other incident.

The region (area of opportunity), which determines the subgrouping for the count, is well defined and is constant for each subgroup. When a special cause is detected on a C chart it's wise to check this assumption and ascertain whether the area of opportunity remained constant.

The chance of an incident at any one place or time is small.

It is possible, even if unlikely, for the numerator to exceed the denominator (that is, it is possible to have more than 50 errors in 50 medical charts inspected). This would be the case in the example stated previously if 50 assessments were performed each week. The statistic plotted for a C chart is simply the total number of items missing (errors) from the assessments in each area of opportunity (50 assessments). It is not necessary for the area of opportunity to be exactly the same for each subgroup in order to use a C chart. The area of opportunity in any analysis can be considered constant if each region (number of units, time, or space), on which the counts are taken, is within 25% of the overall average subgroup size.

Table 5.12   C Chart and U Chart Applications in Health Care

Area	Application	Statistic	Area of Opportunity	Chart
Overall	Accuracy in reporting	Total number of errors	Documents each of which has about the same number of pages	C chart
		Number of errors per 1,000 pages (total # errors divided by total # pages/1,000)	Documents but total number of pages in each document differs	U chart
ICU	Safety	Number of infections	Each month when the number of occupied bed days is relatively constant	C chart
		Number of infections per 1,000 occupied bed days	Each month when the number of occupied bed days varies from month to month	U chart
Surgery	Safety	Total number of complications	Number of surgeries for a constant subgroup size (e.g., sample of 50 surgeries for each subgroup)	C chart
		Number of complications per 100 surgeries	All surgeries this month (when the # surgeries varies each month)	U chart
Inpatient Care	Satisfaction	Number of complaints per month	Month when the # admissions is about the same each month	C chart
		Number of complaints per 100 admissions	Month but the number of admissions varies from month to month	U chart
Lab	Accuracy	Total number of bacteria in sample	Total centimeters tested per subgroup always the same (e.g., 2 cm each subgroup)	C chart
		Number of bacteria per centimeter of sample	Centimeters and the # centimeters tested is different per subgroup	U chart
Outpatient	Safety	Total number of employee accidents	Each month (when the number hours worked is about the same each month)	C chart
		Employee accidents per 100,000 hours worked	Hours worked each month (and the number hours worked varies each month)	U chart

Once it has been determined that the area of opportunity will be constant for each subgroup, the steps to construct a C chart are described in the Appendix to this chapter. The limits for the C chart are simply:

$$CL = c_{bar} = \Sigma\, c \,/\, k \qquad UL = c_{bar} + (3*\sqrt{c_{bar}}) \qquad LL = c_{bar}(3*\sqrt{c_{bar}})$$

Where C = number of nonconformities in each subgroup and k = number of subgroups.

The following example illustrates some of the important points concerning construction of a C chart.

In an effort to improve employee safety in their organization, a large hospital decided to chart the number of employee needlesticks each month. Because approximately the same amount of hours was worked each month, the area of opportunity (total staff hours worked in one month) was constant and a C chart was utilized. Table 5.13 contains the data collected over a two-year period and the calculation of the C chart limits. Figure 5.15 shows the Shewhart chart for this data.

Table 5.13   Employee Needlestick Data and C Chart Calculations

Month	Number of Needlesticks—{c}
J-09	6
F	2
M	4
A	8
M	5
J	4
J	23
A	7
S	3
O	5
N	12
D	7
J-10	10
F	5
M	9
A	4
M	3
J	2
J	2
A	1
S	3
O	4
N	3
D	1

$c_{bar} = \Sigma\ c/k = 133/24 = 5.54$

$UL = c_{bar} + (3* \sqrt{c_{bar}})$ $LL = c_{bar} - (3* \sqrt{c_{bar}})$

$UL = 5.54 + (3* \sqrt{5.54})$ $UL = 5.54 - (3* \sqrt{5.54})$

$UL = 5.54 + 7.06$ $LL = 5.54 - 7.06$

$\mathbf{UL = 12.6}$ $\mathbf{LL = -1.52 = no\ lower\ limit}$

In July 2009, the reporting of 23 needlesticks resulted in a point above the upper limit. This special cause was the result of a severe nursing shortage combined with employee summer vacation taken during July. Less-experienced people and excessive overtime were

FIGURE 5.15   C Chart of Employee Needlesticks

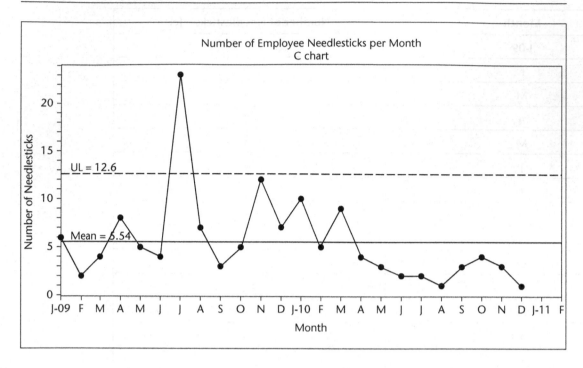

needed to achieve the normal number of hours worked for a month. There was also a run of 9 points in a row below the center line starting in April 2010. This indicated that the average number of reported needlesticks per month had been reduced. This reduction was attributed to a switch from standard to automatically retracting needles, which greatly reduced the number of needlesticks. The C chart assumes that the area of opportunity remains constant. When a special cause is noted on a C chart it's wise to check this assumption and ascertain whether the area of opportunity remained constant. If it had, and this improvement is sustained, the limits should be recalculated when sufficient data are available.

It should be noted that there is no lower limit in the Shewhart chart in this example. Therefore, a downward trend of 6 points or a shift of 8 or more points below the center line is required to demonstrate improvement. See the discussion at the beginning of this chapter on selecting the area of opportunity for a C chart. In this example, with a C_{bar} of 5.54, we would need 1.7 areas of opportunities to have a lower limit. Thus, combining data for two months would result in a C chart with a lower limit.

U Charts

The primary assumptions associated with the use of a **U chart** are:

The incidents being counted are whole numbers.

An incident at any one place or time is independent of any other incident.

The area of opportunity between subgroups may vary.

The chance of an incident at any one place or time is small.

It is possible, even if unlikely, for the numerator to exceed the denominator (that is, it is possible to have more than 50 errors in 50 medical charts inspected).

Counts that are made on areas of opportunity that differ cannot be compared directly as they are in a C chart. The u statistic (often called rate data) is calculated by dividing the count for each subgroup by the number of "standard areas of opportunity" in the subgroup. It should be noted that n used in the calculations of the limits for a U chart is defined as the number of standard areas of opportunity in a subgroup. Therefore, n for any group is calculated by dividing the area of opportunity for that subgroup by the size of the standard area of opportunity. Many times the standard area of opportunity is chosen so that the resulting u statistic will be whole numbers (for example, defects per 100 or 1,000 or 10,000).

The following example illustrates the use of a U chart. A hospital grew concerned about its use of flash sterilization during surgery when they became aware of the link between flash sterilization during surgery and infection. They were determined to reduce their use of flash sterilization during surgery. They had some baseline data providing the number of flash sterilizations during surgery each week and the number of surgeries that week. They selected a U chart because they were counting each flash sterilization (not just whether or not a surgery had a flash sterilization) and the area of opportunity (the number of surgeries that week) varied. Their data is shown in Table 5.14. The resulting U chart is shown in Figure 5.16. Note that each set of limits is based on the area of opportunity for *that* subgroup.

The team created and extended limits using the initial 20 weeks of baseline data. As they tested and expanded changes they noted special cause in the desired direction. After celebrating their improvement and discontinuing the team, the manager continued to track weekly flash sterilization use. The manager noted that the improvement was not sustained after the team disbanded. The manager found that although the changes tested were successful, they had not adequately considered how to build the changes into day-to-day

FIGURE 5.16   U Chart for Flash Sterilization

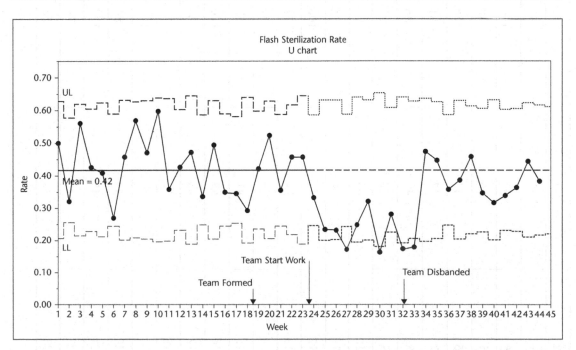

Table 5.14   Data for Flash Sterilization

Week	Number of Flash Sterilizations	Number of Surgeries
1	42	84
2	47	146
3	51	91
4	45	106
5	36	88
6	34	126
7	37	81
8	49	86
9	39	83
10	46	77
11	28	78
12	46	108
13	34	72
14	44	131
15	41	83
16	44	126
17	48	139
18	22	75
19	48	114
20	44	84
21	45	127
22	43	94
23	33	72

Week	Number of Flash Sterilizations	Number of Surgeries
24	43	130
25	19	81
26	19	82
27	22	127
28	19	76
29	26	81
30	11	67
31	29	103
32	13	75
33	15	84
34	37	78
35	38	85
36	47	131
37	32	83
38	45	98
39	36	104
40	26	82
41	37	109
42	39	107
43	39	88
44	36	94
45		

work by, for example, considering orientation of new personnel, routine communication flow, documentation needs, and policy clarification.

Health care works with a great deal of rate data. Whenever the rates are based on attribute count data, we should select a U chart. We often choose to display rates per 1,000 units, 10,000 units, or some other base. This is typically done when rates of error, harm or other occurrence are quite small and therefore somewhat hard to conceptualize or talk about. In addition, when the data are being compared across organizations it is often expressed to some common base such as 1,000 units of opportunity. Table 5.15 shows the number of adverse drug events (ADEs), the number of doses of medication dispensed that

Table 5.15   Adverse Drug Event (ADE) Data

Month	Number of ADEs	Number of Doses Dispensed	Units of 1,000 Doses Dispensed (# Doses/1,000)
M-05	50	17110	17.11
A	44	12140	12.14
M	47	17990	17.99
J	32	14980	14.98
J	51	21980	21.98
A	57	15320	15.32
S	43	12990	12.99
O	61	19760	19.76
N	30	8670	8.67
D	32	12680	12.68
J-06	41	20330	20.33
F	57	18550	18.55
M	31	14310	14.31
A	11	9730	9.73
M	3	11470	11.47
J	6	5390	5.39
J	9	21700	21.7
A	3	6370	6.37
S	10	22500	22.5
O	8	11170	11.17
N	9	10910	10.91
D	4	8760	8.76
J-07	9	11140	11.14
F	10	12300	12.3
M	13	17170	17.17
A	2	8910	8.91

FIGURE 5.17   U Charts for ADEs per 1,000 Doses Versus ADEs per Dose

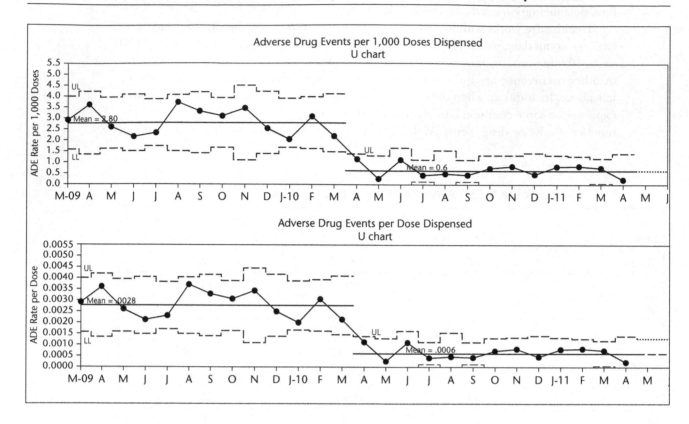

same month (area of opportunity). It also shows how they converted their ADE data to ADEs/1,000 doses dispensed. They did so by dividing the area of opportunity each month by 1,000. Their area of opportunity then became "units of 1,000 doses."

Figure 5.17 displays both the U charts for ADEs/1,000 doses and the U chart for ADEs/dose. Other than the scale on the vertical axis these charts are identical. The pattern of special cause becomes evident at the same time on each chart. The chart displaying ADEs/1,000 doses might be simpler for communication purposes. Many find it easier to discuss nearly 3 ADEs per 1,000 doses dispensed than to talk about 0.003 ADEs/per dose.

Creation of Funnel Limits for a U Chart

Another example of a U Chart is for an organization that wanted to compare the incident of patient complaints among their internal medicine clinics. Their data are at Table 5.16. They selected a U chart as the appropriate chart for their data and subgrouped the data by clinic to create the chart in Figure 5.18. They were able to detect one organization with a very low complaint rate (special cause). They raised an opportunity to learn. Was clinic F simply not reporting complaints or were they actually doing something different from the other clinics that resulted in fewer complaints?

Sequencing these data to create funnel limits (in order of the clinic with the greatest number of visits to the clinic with the least number of visits) provides another way to view

Table 5.16   Clinic Complaint Data

Clinic	Number of Complaints	Number of Visits
A	17	18003
B	11	13542
C	21	22891
D	21	12111
E	18	16167
F	21	43689
G	31	21007
H	22	17532
I	15	18209
J	11	14715
K	31	19024
L	25	18933
M	26	14328
N	32	19999
O	20	18634
P	17	15421
Q	26	19333

FIGURE 5.18   U Chart for Complaints per 1,000 Visits

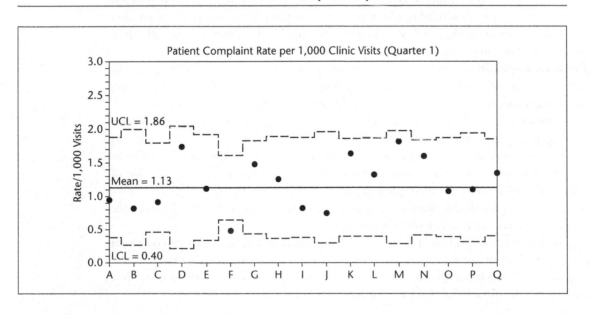

FIGURE 5.19   U Chart with Funnel Limits for Complaints per 1,000 Visits

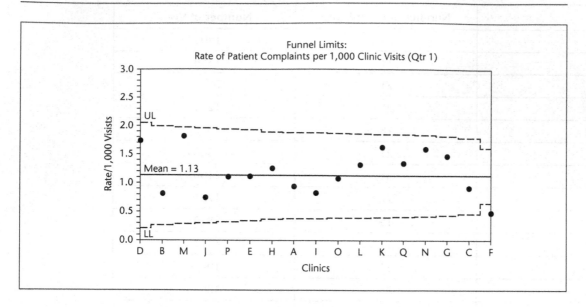

the data. See Figure 5.19. With the funnel limits it is readily apparent that Clinic F also has the largest number of patient visits. Even so, the rate of complaints is still special cause given their subgroup size.

PROCESS CAPABILITY

A capable process or system is one that is able to produce outcomes that meet agreed requirements, targets, specifications, or goals. These requirements may be in the form of customer specifications or internal requirements. For example, a health care system has requirements that patients should not have to wait more than 15 minutes to be seen after a scheduled appointment. A clinic's system would be capable if it could consistently meet this requirement for all patients.

Process capability is a prediction of future performance of the process. It can be stated as the range of outcomes expected for any measure of interest. Before considering capability, the process for the measure of interest must be stable (no special causes). This gives us a rational basis for the prediction. Thus, developing an appropriate Shewhart chart for the measure of interest is a prelude to a capability analysis. The process capability can be compared to the requirements or specifications for the measure. This is best done graphically. A number of indices have also been created to describe this comparison of capability to specifications (for example Cp, Cpk, and the Taguchi loss function[9]). These may be useful for a particular situation where everyone using the indices understand the process performance used to calculate the index.

Figure 5.20 shows a graphical depiction of four different situations that can occur for a capability analysis of continuous data. The process requirements in this figure are stated in terms of upper and lower specifications. In many situations in health care process, there is only one specification, either lower or upper.

---

[9]Wheeler, D. J., *Advanced Topics in Statistical Process Control*, Knoxville, TN: SPC Press, 1994, Chapter 8.

FIGURE 5.20   Capability Situations and Actions for Continuous Data

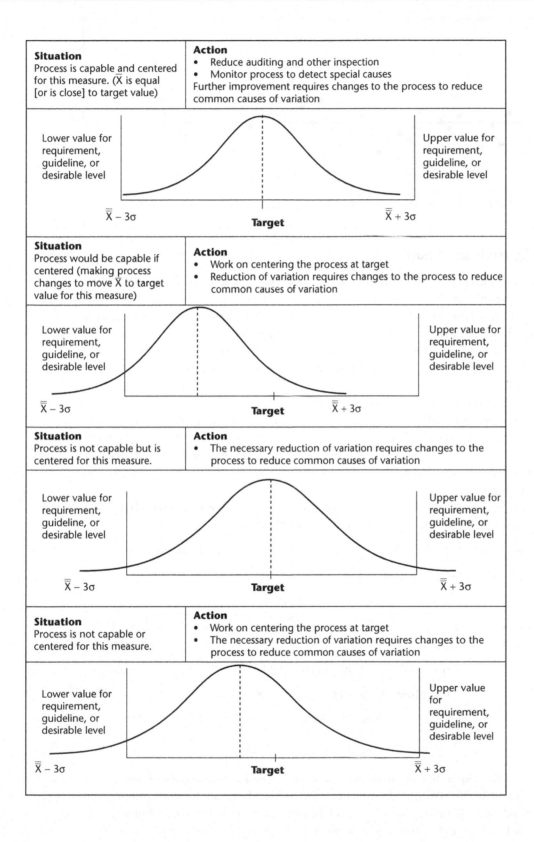

Situation
Process is capable and centered for this measure. ($\overline{\overline{X}}$ is equal [or is close] to target value)

Action
• Reduce auditing and other inspection
• Monitor process to detect special causes
Further improvement requires changes to the process to reduce common causes of variation

Lower value for requirement, guideline, or desirable level

Upper value for requirement, guideline, or desirable level

$\overline{\overline{X}} - 3\sigma$ **Target** $\overline{\overline{X}} + 3\sigma$

Situation
Process would be capable if centered (making process changes to move $\overline{\overline{X}}$ to target value for this measure)

Action
• Work on centering the process at target
• Reduction of variation requires changes to the process to reduce common causes of variation

Lower value for requirement, guideline, or desirable level

Upper value for requirement, guideline, or desirable level

$\overline{\overline{X}} - 3\sigma$ **Target** $\overline{\overline{X}} + 3\sigma$

Situation
Process is not capable but is centered for this measure.

Action
• The necessary reduction of variation requires changes to the process to reduce common causes of variation

Lower value for requirement, guideline, or desirable level

Upper value for requirement, guideline, or desirable level

$\overline{\overline{X}} - 3\sigma$ **Target** $\overline{\overline{X}} + 3\sigma$

Situation
Process is not capable or centered for this measure.

Action
• Work on centering the process at target
• The necessary reduction of variation requires changes to the process to reduce common causes of variation

Lower value for requirement, guideline, or desirable level

Upper value for requirement, guideline, or desirable level

$\overline{\overline{X}} - 3\sigma$ **Target** $\overline{\overline{X}} + 3\sigma$

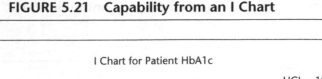

FIGURE 5.21 Capability from an I Chart

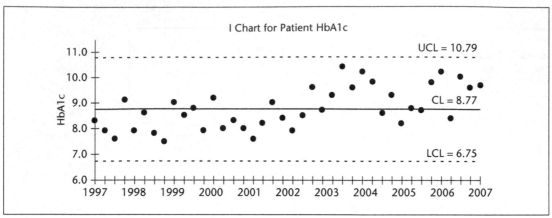

Process Capability from an I Chart

Most Shewhart charts plot some statistic that summarizes individual data values from the process (for example, average, standard deviation, percentage, rate, and so on). The exception is the I chart, where the individual data values are plotted. Because of this, determining process capability is straightforward for an I chart. Once the limits are determined and the process is found to be stable, the upper and lower limits define the capability of the process. Future results are expected to fall within these limits unless some change is made to the process.

For example, the I chart of patient HbA1c values in Figure 5.21 has a lower limit of 6.75 and the upper limit is 10.79. These limits define the capability of the process and can be directly compared to guidelines or specifications. If the requirements for this patient were an HbA1c from 6 to 11, we would say the stable measurement for this patient is capable of meeting the requirement. If the requirement is for it to be less than 8 this process would be deemed incapable.

To relate the use of the I chart limits to capability analysis for $\bar{X}$ and S charts, the common cause variation can be determined for an I chart by:

$\sigma = MR_{bar}/1.128$ (1.128 is the d_2 factor for n = 2 to convert a range to a sigma)

Then the capability could be calculated as:

$$\bar{X} - 3\sigma \quad \text{to} \quad \bar{X} + 3\sigma$$

The average moving range for the data was 0.76 and the center line ($\bar{X}$) was 8.77. Using these values, we can calculate the capability:

$$\sigma = MR_{bar}/1.128 = 0.76/1.128 = 0.673$$

$$\text{Capability} = \bar{X} - 3\sigma \quad \text{to} \quad \bar{X} + 3\sigma$$

$$= 8.77 - 3(0.673) \quad \text{to} \quad 8.77 + 3(0.673)$$

$$= 6.75 \quad \text{to} \quad 10.79$$

Note that this capability calculation is the same as the lower and upper limits of the I chart (6.75 and 10.79). We would predict that future HbA1c values for that patient could range from 6.8 to 10.8 unless there is a special cause. The fact that the capability can be read directly from the I chart is an advantage of this type of Shewhart chart.

Capability of a Process from $\overline{X}$ and S Chart (or R chart)

The $\overline{X}$ and S charts display process performance for averages. Averaging smooths some of the individual variation in the data. The 3 sigma limits on an $\overline{X}$ and S chart are limits for the *averages* being charted (for example, average waiting time per week, average cost for knee replacements each month). If we want to determine capability we want to know how long any *individual* might wait, or what cost we can expect for an *individual* knee replacement.

Capability analysis is done to translate the information about the performance of the process on the $\overline{X}$ and S chart to the expectations for an individual patient. If the process is stable, only common cause variation is evident on both the $\overline{X}$ chart and the S chart (or $\overline{X}$ and the R chart if using that chart), then the process capability can be determined. The center line of the $\overline{X}$ and the center line of the S (or R) charts are the two key statistics needed to determine capability. In addition, the capability formula uses a constant, c4, which is dependent on subgroup size. The table for c4 can be found on the $\overline{X}$ and S formula sheet Appendix 5.1. The factor d_2 for the range chart in given in Chapter Seven. Capability analysis:

1. Compute the standard deviation of the process from $\overline{X}$ or R_{bar} from a stable chart:

$$\sigma = S_{bar}/c_4 \text{ or } = R_{bar}/d_2 \text{ (use median n to choose c4 factor)}$$

2. Use the $\overline{X}$ center line to compute the practical minimum of the process:

$$\text{Minimum} = \overline{\overline{X}} - 3\sigma$$

3. Compute the practical maximum of the process:

$$\text{Maximum} = \overline{\overline{X}} + 3\sigma$$

4. The process capability of $\overline{\overline{X}} - 3\sigma$ to $\overline{\overline{X}} + 3\sigma$ can then be compared to process specifications or requirements. Often this range is sketched as a distribution as shown in Figure 5.20.

The $\overline{X}$ and S chart for turn-around time in the example shown in Figure 5.5 has a special cause signal on the S chart in the last subgroup June 20). Therefore, we are not ready to calculate the capability of the process. An investigation showed that one of the times recorded on that day was associated with a repair of the centrifuge. Figure 5.22

FIGURE 5.22 Capability from an $\overline{X}$ and S Chart with Revised Limits

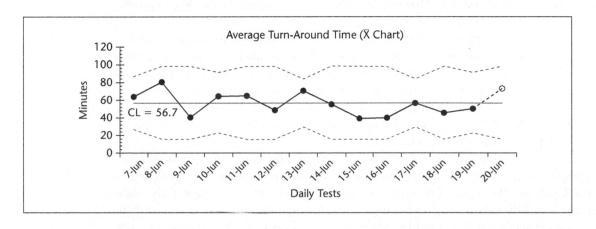

shows the $\overline{X}$ with limits appropriately recalculated after removing that last subgroup from the calculation of the mean and limits. (Chapter Four discusses when to revise limits using a Shewhart chart).

The process is now stable (both charts) and the capability can be determined. The team thought their process was doing pretty well. After all, the average turn-around time (TAT) was less than 60 minutes. Their goal was to complete the each test within 90 minutes. To understand the performance for individual tests, they calculated process capability as shown here:

1. Calculate the standard deviation σ (using the c_4 value for median subgroup size, $n = 3$)

$$\sigma = S_{bar}/c_4 = 20.5/0.886 = 23.1$$

2. Calculate the practical minimum:

$$\text{Minimum} = \overline{\overline{X}} - 3\sigma = 56.7 - 3\,(23.1) = -12.7 \text{ (practical minimum 0)}$$

3. Calculate the practical maximum:

$$\text{Maximum} = \overline{\overline{X}} + 3\sigma = 56.7 + 3(23.1) = 126.1$$

So the current capability of the process for turn-around time was 0 to 126 minutes, or about 0 to 2 hours. As the requirement was for turn-around time to be less than 90 minutes, this process is not capable of meeting the current requirements. Work will need to be done to redesign the process to reduce the average, reduce the variation, or both.

Capability of a Process from Attribute Control Charts

After a process is considered to be stable, based on the study of the attribute control charts, the capability of the process can be determined. The capability of a process is a prediction of future measurements of the measure from the process. For continuous data, capability focuses on the range of individual measurements. With attribute data, capability analysis is not directed at individual measurements, but rather at specific subgroups of measurements that are of interest.

Capability from a P Chart

For characteristics studied using the P chart, the center line (p_{bar}) is often used to express the capability. Thus, for a stable characteristic with a center line of 12%, the capability is expressed as 12%. The process would be expected to produce 12% nonconforming items in the future if it continued to operate in the current manner. Capability could also be expressed as 88% ($100\% - \overline{p}$) conforming units.

Often it is useful to express a range for p that might be expected over a given number of units. The control limits provide one such range, if the number of units of interest is equal to the subgroup size. For example, a P chart is constructed using a sample of 100 randomly selected active patient charts in the hospital each month and the percentage without complete documentation determined. The center line is 12% and the limits are 2.2% (LL) to 21.8% (UL), the process is stable. These Shewhart limits give a prediction of the range of p for samples of 100 charts.

There may be other number of units besides the subgroup size which are of interest, for example, a typical day's census on the unit or in the hospital. If the average census is about 500 patients, the range of percent incomplete charts expected on a typical day might be of interest. This prediction can be made using the control limits based on n = 500. Using the formula for a p chart found in Appendix 5.1 a "process capability" range of 7.6%

FIGURE 5.23   Capability from a P Chart with a Subgroup Size of 20

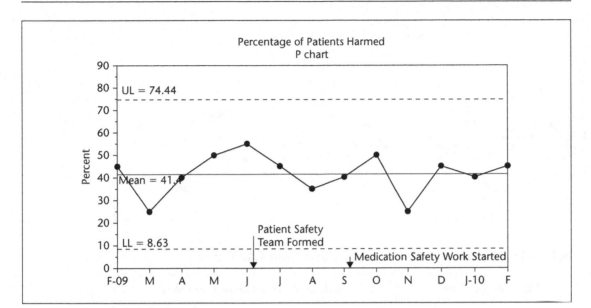

(the LL for p_{bar} = 12% and n = 500) to 16.4% (the similar UL) is found. Thus 12% incomplete charts would be expected when the census is 500, but on any given day it could range from 7.6% to 16.4% incomplete.

Figure 5.23 shows a stable P chart for "percent of patients harmed" based on a subgroup of 20 randomly selected charts. The center line is 41.4%. The capability based on sampling 20 charts each month is from 8% to 74% (that is, the control limits for the chart). What if we decided to sample 50 charts per month from this stable system? Using the control limit calculations for the P chart with P_{bar} = 41.4 and n = 50, we can calculate a capability of 27–62% of patients harmed.

What if we were only able to sample 10 charts one month? Then the capability would be from 0 to 88%.

Capability from a C or U Chart

Determining the capability of a process, when a C or U chart is used to monitor a measure is similar to determining capability from a P chart. The center line (c_{bar} or u_{bar}) is the capability. Also, it is often of interest to know the range of incidents expected for a given area of opportunity.

For example, consider a hospital with an average of two employee accidents per month. A C chart was used to monitor the accidents with c_{bar} = 2 and the UCL = 6.2. If the process is stable, the hospital would expect two accidents per month, but in any one month there could be no accidents (no LL) or as many as six accidents (UL = 6.2).

For the ICU infection example in Figure 5.24, the process is stable with u_{bar} = 7.2 infections per 100 admissions (100 admissions = standard unit for this example to determine area of opportunity).

The limits depended on the number of admissions during any given month (in this example, there is not a lower limit for any of the months). From u_{bar} it is easy to compute the expected number of infections for any given number of admissions. For example, in 200 admissions the expected number of infections is:

Expected number of infections per 200 admissions = 7.2 infections/100 admissions × 2
= 14.4 infections

FIGURE 5.24   Capability from a U Chart for ICU Infections

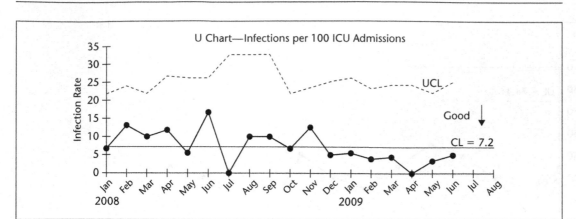

Table 5.17   Summary: Methods for Describing Capability

Chart	Estimate of Sigma	Method for Describing Capability
I	$\sigma = MR_{bar}/1.128$	$\bar{X} - 3\sigma$ to $\bar{X} - 3\sigma$
$\bar{X}$ and S	$\sigma = S_{bar}/c_4$	$\bar{\bar{X}} - 3\sigma$ to $\bar{\bar{X}} + 3\sigma$
P	$\sigma p = \sqrt{p_{bar} * (100 - p_{bar})}/\sqrt{n}$	p_{bar} or $100 - p_{bar}$ OR $p_{bar} +/- 3\sigma$ for the specific value of n of interest
C	$\sqrt{c_{bar}}$	c_{bar} or $100 - c_{bar}$ OR $c_{bar} - 3\sigma$ to $c_{bar} + 3\sigma$
U	$\sqrt{u_{bar}}/\sqrt{n}$	u_{bar} OR $U_{bar} +/- 3\sigma$ for the specific value of n of interest

To find the expected range of infections for months with 200 admissions, simply compute the usual control limits for a C chart, see Appendix 5.1, with:

$$c_{bar} = 14.4$$
$$UL = c_{bar} + (3\sqrt{14.4})$$
$$LL = c_{bar} - (3\sqrt{14.4})$$

That is, on average, there will be about 14 infections per 200 admissions, but any given month with 200 admissions, the number of infections would range from 3 to 26. For a one week period with 50 admissions, we would expect 0 to 9 infections. For a period with 500 admissions, we would expect the number of infections to range from 18 to 54 infections.

Table 5.17 summarizes methods to calculate process capability for each type of chart.

SUMMARY

The Shewhart chart method is a way to make the concept of common and special causes operational. The Shewhart chart is a statistical tool used to distinguish between variation in a process due to common causes and variation due to special causes. The Shewhart chart is the only tool that can ascertain whether a system is stable and therefore predictable, or unstable and thus unpredictable. Although the Shewhart chart appears to be a very simple tool, there are a number of important considerations in making effective use of this method:

Appropriate use of Shewhart charts involves understanding the type of data we are working with and then selecting the appropriate type of Shewhart chart for that data.

There are standard formulas and rules to use with all Shewhart charts to obtain appropriate 3-sigma upper and lower limits for the chart. Calculation forms for the various types of charts are included in this chapter.

The individual or I chart is one of the easiest type of Shewhart charts to construct and interpret.

Funnel limits may be made for any Shewhart chart with a variable subgroup size ($\bar{X}$ and S, P, U charts)

The capability for a measure of a process can be determined after establishing stability using a Shewhart chart.

Shewhart charts have universal applicability. To make improvement more efficient and effective, all individuals and groups in an organization should have knowledge of the concepts of common and special causes of variation and the use of Shewhart charts to differentiate between these causes.

Case Study Connection

To deepen understanding of the concepts and methods in this chapter a number of case studies may be of interest to the reader:

Case Study B illustrates the use of data to support improvement project in a Radiology Department. This case study addresses using rare event data, capability analysis, and examples of updating charts after improvements have been made.

Case Study C illustrates the use of a Shewhart chart to track the impact of a change. It also highlights the use of disaggregation, stratification, and rational subgrouping techniques to learn about the process.

Case Study F addresses using Shewhart charts as a central part of an improvement effort. It also illustrates updating and revising Shewhart chart limits.

Case Study G illustrates the use of Shewhart charts with routine financial data. It highlights the value of posing questions and using the appropriate Shewhart chart to aid in answering that question. In addition, it provides an example of the use of additional statistical process control tools; in this instance, scatter plots.

KEY TERMS

Area of opportunity

Attribute data

C chart

Classification data

Common cause variation

Continuous data

Count data

Funnel limits

I chart (Individuals chart)

Moving range (MR)

P chart

Process capability

Special cause variation

Subgroup

U chart

Variables data

$\bar{X}$ and S charts

CALCULATING SHEWHART LIMITS

I CHART

The steps for developing a Shewhart chart for individuals are the following:

1. Calculate the k–1 moving ranges and the average of the moving ranges (MR_{bar})

$$MR_{bar} = \frac{\Sigma\, MR}{k-1} = \underline{\quad}$$

2. Calculate the upper limit for the moving range using:

$$UL_{MR} = 3.27 * MR_{bar} = UL_{MR} = 3.27 \times \underline{\quad} = \underline{\quad}$$

3. Remove any moving range bigger than the ULMR and recalculate the average moving range (MR_{bar}).
   (Note: This recalculation should be done only once.)

4. Calculate the average of the k measurements (I_{bar}) for the center line (CL).

$$CL\,(I_{bar}) = \frac{\Sigma\, I}{k} = \underline{\qquad} = \underline{\qquad}$$

5. Calculate the limits for the I chart using:

$$UL = (I_{bar}) + (2.66 * MR_{bar}) \qquad\qquad LL = (I_{bar}) - (2.66 * MR_{bar})$$

$$UL = \underline{\quad} + (2.66 * \underline{\quad}) \qquad\qquad LL = \underline{\quad} - (2.66 * \underline{\quad})$$

$$UL = \underline{\quad} + \underline{\quad} = \qquad\qquad LL = \underline{\quad} - \underline{\quad} =$$

$$UL = \underline{\quad} \qquad\qquad LL = \underline{\quad}$$

6. Calculate and draw a vertical scale such that the limits "enclose" the inner 50% of the charting area and the horizontal axis covers the k time periods.

7. Plot the k measurements on the chart.

8. Draw the center line (I_{bar}) and the limits on the chart. Apply the five rules for special causes to the completed chart.

$\overline{X}$ AND S CHARTS

Symbols Associated with $\overline{X}$ and S Charts

X	Individual measurement of quality or characteristic
n	Subgroup size (number of measurements per subgroup)
k	Number of subgroups used to develop limits
Σ	Summation symbol
$\overline{X}$	Subgroup average
$\overline{\overline{X}}$	Average of the averages of all the subgroups
S	Subgroup standard deviation
S_{bar}	Weighted averages of the standard deviations of all the subgroups
A_3, B_3, B_4, c_4	Factors for computing limits and process capability
i	For that subgroup

The steps for developing $\overline{X}$ and S charts follow. All averages that are calculated should be rounded to one more decimal place (significant figure) than the values being averaged. The decimal places for the standard deviation should be the same as the averages.

1. Calculate the average, $\overline{X}$, for each subgroup:

$$\overline{X} = \Sigma\, X / n_i$$

2. Calculate S for each subgroup:

$$S = \sqrt{\Sigma\, (X - \overline{X})^2 / (n_i - 1)}$$

3. Calculate the weighted grand average, $\overline{\overline{X}}$ using:

$$\overline{\overline{X}} = \frac{\Sigma\, (n_i\, \overline{X}_i)}{\Sigma\, n_i}$$

4. Calculate S_{bar}, the center line of the standard deviation chart, using:

$$S_{bar} = \frac{\Sigma\, (n_i\, S_i)}{\Sigma\, n_i}$$

5. Calculate the control limits for the $\overline{X}$ chart using:

$$UCL = \overline{\overline{X}} + (A_3 * S_{bar})$$
$$LCL = \overline{\overline{X}} - (A_3 * S_{bar})$$

Note: A_3 is a factor that depends on the subgroup size and can be obtained from the following table.

6. Calculate the control limits for the S chart using:

$$UCL = B_4 * S_{bar}$$
$$LCL = B_3 * S_{bar}$$

Note: B_3 and B_4 are factors that depend on the size of the subgroup and can be obtained from the figure below. Note that there is no lower control limit for S when the subgroup size is less than 6.

7. Calculate a scale for the $\overline{X}$ chart so that the control limits enclose the inner 50% of the charting area. Calculate the scale for the S chart so the upper control limit is placed 25−35% below the top of the chart.

8. Plot the X bar's on the $\overline{X}$ chart and the S's on the S chart.

9. Draw the control limits and center line on the $\overline{X}$ chart. Note that the control limits for both charts are variable when the subgroup size varies.

10. Draw the control limits and center line on the S chart.

$\bar{X}$ AND S CONTROL CHART CALCULATION FORM

(This form is practical only for constant subgroup sizes.)

NAME _____ DATE _____

PROCESS _____ SAMPLE DESCRIPTION _____

NUMBER OF SUBGROUPS (K) _____ BETWEEN (DATES) _____

$$\bar{\bar{X}} = \frac{\Sigma\,(n_i\,\bar{X}_i)}{\Sigma n_i} = \text{_____} = \text{_____}$$

$$S_{bar} = \frac{\Sigma\,(n_i\,s_i)}{\Sigma n_i} = \text{_____} = \text{_____}$$

Worksheet for Calculating Limits for $\bar{X}$ Chart

$\bar{X}$ Chart	S Chart
UCL = $\bar{\bar{X}}$ + (A_3 * S_{bar})	UCL = (B_4 * S_{bar})
UCL = + (*)	UCL = *
UCL = +	UCL = _____
UCL = _____	
LCL = $\bar{\bar{X}}$ − (A_3 * S_{bar})	LCL = (B_3 * S_{bar})
LCL = − (*)	LCL = *
LCL = −	LCL = _____
LCL = _____	

Process Capability from an $\bar{X}$ and S Chart

If the process is in statistical control, the standard deviation is:
$\hat{\sigma} = S_{bar}/C_4$
$\hat{\sigma} =$ _____ / _____ = _____
The process capability is:
Practical Minimum = $\bar{\bar{X}} - 3\hat{\sigma}$
_____   −   _____   =   _____
Practical Maximum = $\bar{\bar{X}} + 3\hat{\sigma}$
_____   +   _____   =   _____
Practical Minimum = _____
Practical Maximum = _____

Table A.4   Factors for X̄ and S Charts (S_{bar} from Average of Ss)

n	A_3	B_3	B_4	C_4
2	2.66	–	3.27	0.798
3	1.95	–	2.57	0.886
4	1.63	–	2.27	0.921
5	1.43	–	2.09	0.940
6	1.29	0.03	1.97	0.952
7	1.18	0.12	1.88	0.959
8	1.10	0.18	1.82	0.965
9	1.03	0.24	1.76	0.969
10	0.98	0.28	1.72	0.973
11	0.93	0.32	1.68	0.975
12	0.89	0.35	1.65	0.978
13	0.85	0.38	1.62	0.979
14	0.82	0.41	1.59	0.981
15	0.79	0.43	1.57	0.982
16	0.76	0.45	1.55	0.984
17	0.74	0.47	1.53	0.984
18	0.72	0.48	1.52	0.985
19	0.70	0.50	1.50	0.986
20	0.68	0.51	1.49	0.987
21	0.66	0.52	1.48	0.988
22	0.65	0.53	1.47	0.988
23	0.63	0.54	1.46	0.989
24	0.62	0.56	1.44	0.989
25	0.61	0.56	1.44	0.990
30	0.55	0.62	1.38	0.992
35	0.51	0.64	1.36	0.993
40	0.48	0.67	1.33	0.994
45	0.45	0.67	1.33	0.994
50	0.43	0.70	1.30	0.995
100	0.30	0.81	1.19	0.998

For n > 25 the following formulas can be used:

$$A_3 = \frac{3}{C_4 \sqrt{n}} \qquad B_3 = 1 - \frac{3\sqrt{1-(C_4)^2}}{C_4}$$

$$B_4 = 1 - \frac{3\sqrt{1-(C_4)^2}}{C_4}$$

$$C_4 = \text{gamma function of } n^1$$

[1]Wheeler, D. J., *Advanced Topics in Statistical Process Control*, Knoxville, TN: SPC Press, 1994, Table 20.

P Chart

Once a subgrouping strategy has been determined, the following steps should be followed when constructing a P chart:

1. Calculate p {p = (number in a certain category / number in subgroup) * 100} for each subgroup.
2. Calculate Pbar = average of Ps
3. Determine the limits for the P chart.
4. Figure and draw a scale on appropriate graph paper. Plot the p points on the chart and draw in the limits and center line.

P Chart Calculation Form: Constant Subgroup Size

d = Nonconforming Sample Units per Subgroup

n = Number of Sample Units per Subgroup

k = Number of Subgroups

p = Percent Nonconforming Units = 100 * d/n

Control Limits When Subgroup Size (N) Is Constant

$$P_{bar} = \frac{\sum p}{k} = \underline{\hspace{2cm}} = \underline{\hspace{3cm}}$$

$$\sigma_p = \sqrt{\frac{P_{bar} * (100 - P_{bar})}{n}} = \sqrt{\frac{* (100 -)}{n}} = \underline{\hspace{2cm}}$$

$UL = P_{bar} + (3 * \sigma_p)$ $LL = P_{bar} - (3 * \sigma_p) =$

$UL = \underline{\hspace{1.5cm}} + (3 * \underline{\hspace{1.5cm}})$ $LL = \underline{\hspace{1.5cm}} - (3 * \underline{\hspace{1.5cm}})$

$UL = \underline{\hspace{1.5cm}} + \underline{\hspace{1.5cm}}$ $LL = \underline{\hspace{1.5cm}} - \underline{\hspace{1.5cm}}$

$UL = \underline{\hspace{3cm}}$ $LL = \underline{\hspace{3cm}}$

P Chart Calculation Form: Variable Subgroup Size

d = Nonconforming Sample Units per Subgroup

n = Number of Sample Units per Subgroup

k = Number of Subgroups

p = Percent Nonconforming Units = 100 * d/n

Control Limits When Subgroup Size (N) Is Variable

$$p_{bar} = \frac{\sum d * 100}{n} = \underline{\hspace{1cm}} * 100 = \underline{\hspace{3cm}} \text{ (center line)}$$

$$\sigma_p = \frac{\sqrt{p_{bar} * (100 - p_{bar})}}{\sqrt{n}} = \sqrt{\frac{\underline{\hspace{0.5cm}} * (100 - \underline{\hspace{0.5cm}})}{\sqrt{n}}} = \frac{\underline{\hspace{1cm}}}{\sqrt{n}} = \underline{\hspace{1cm}}$$

$$UL = \frac{p_{bar} + (3 * \sigma_p)}{\sqrt{n}} \qquad\qquad LL = \frac{p_{bar} - (3 * \sigma_p)}{\sqrt{n}} =$$

$$UL = \underline{\hspace{1cm}} + (3 * \underline{\hspace{1cm}} / \sqrt{n}) \qquad\qquad LL = \underline{\hspace{1cm}} - (3 * \underline{\hspace{1cm}} / \sqrt{n})$$

$$UL = \underline{\hspace{1cm}} + (\underline{\hspace{0.5cm}} / \sqrt{n}) \qquad\qquad LL = \underline{\hspace{1cm}} - (\underline{\hspace{1cm}} / \sqrt{n})$$

$$UL = \underline{\hspace{1cm}} + \underline{\hspace{2cm}} \qquad\qquad LL = \underline{\hspace{1cm}} - \underline{\hspace{2cm}}$$

$$UL = \underline{\hspace{3cm}} \qquad\qquad LL = \underline{\hspace{3cm}}$$

n: _____

√n: _____

3 * sigma p: _____

UL: _____

LL: _____

C Chart

Once it has been determined that the area of opportunity will be constant for each sub-group, the following steps should be followed to construct a C chart:

1. Record the count c for 20 to 30 subgroups.
2. Compute Cbar, the center line for the C chart.
3. Compute the limits for the C chart.
4. Calculate and draw a scale on the charting form. Plot the individual c points, the center line, and the limits.

C Chart Limits (Area of Opportunity Constant)

c = number of incidences per subgroup

k = number of subgroups

Note: The subgroup size is defined by the "area of opportunity" and must remain constant. Constant is defined as each subgroup +/− 25% of average subgroup size.

$$c_{bar} = \frac{\Sigma c}{k} = $$

$$UL = c_{bar} + (3 * \sqrt{c_{bar}})$$

$UL = \underline{\hspace{1cm}} + (3 * \underline{\hspace{1cm}})$ $LL = c_{bar} - (3 * \sqrt{c_{bar}})$

$UL = \underline{\hspace{1cm}} + \underline{\hspace{1cm}}$ $LL = \underline{\hspace{1cm}} - (3 * \underline{\hspace{1cm}})$

$\mathbf{UL} = \underline{\hspace{1cm}}$ $LL = \underline{\hspace{1cm}} - \underline{\hspace{1cm}}$

$\mathbf{LL} = \underline{\hspace{1cm}}$

U Chart

Once it has been determined that the area of opportunity will vary between subgroups, the following steps should be followed to construct a U chart:

1. Record the count and the size of the area of opportunity for each subgroup.
2. Determine the standard area of opportunity.
3. Compute n (area of opportunity for the subgroup divided by the standard area of opportunity) for each subgroup.
4. Compute the u statistic (count/ n) for each subgroup.
5. Compute u_{bar}, the center line of the U chart.
6. Compute the control limits for the U chart. Refer to calculation form.
7. Calculate and draw a scale on the charting form. Plot the individual u points, the center line, and the limits.

U Chart Limits (area of opportunity varies)

c = number of incidences per subgroup

n = number of standard "areas of opportunity" in a subgroup (n may vary)

u = incidences per standard area of opportunity = c/n

k = number of subgroups

Note: The standard area of opportunity will be defined by the people planning the Shewhart chart in units such as invoices, medical records, centimeters or surface area, and so on.

$$u_{bar} = \frac{\sum c}{\sum n} = $$

$$UL = u_{bar} + (3 * \sqrt{u_{bar}}) / \sqrt{n}$$
$$UL = \rule{1cm}{0.4pt} + (3 * \rule{1cm}{0.4pt}) / \sqrt{n})$$
$$UL = \rule{1cm}{0.4pt} + (\rule{1cm}{0.4pt} / \sqrt{n})$$
$$UL = \rule{1cm}{0.4pt} + (\rule{1cm}{0.4pt} / \rule{1cm}{0.4pt})$$
$$UL = \rule{1cm}{0.4pt}$$

$$LL = u_{bar} - (3 * \sqrt{u_{bar}}) / \sqrt{n}$$
$$LL = \rule{1cm}{0.4pt} - (3 * \rule{1cm}{0.4pt}) / \sqrt{n})$$
$$LL = \rule{1cm}{0.4pt} - (\rule{1cm}{0.4pt} / \sqrt{n})$$
$$LL = \rule{1cm}{0.4pt} - (\rule{1cm}{0.4pt} / \rule{1cm}{0.4pt})$$
$$LL = \rule{1cm}{0.4pt}$$

n: _____

√n: _____

UL: _____

LL: _____

## CHAPTER 6

SHEWHART CHART SAVVY: DEALING WITH SOME ISSUES

This chapter presents some issues often encountered when beginning to use Shewhart charts in improvement work. By studying this chapter the reader will learn key graphical guidelines for creating and presenting more effective charts, some typical software-created problems to avoid, and some issues and options to consider when using the I chart.

DESIGNING EFFECTIVE SHEWHART CHARTS

Chapters Three through Five contain many different types and examples of run charts, Shewhart charts, and other useful graphs. Chapter Thirteen includes seven additional case studies that use run and Shewhart charts to learn from variation in data. Although a time series chart is a fairly simple concept, the development of an effective chart for a specific situation can be very confusing. Some tips to develop additional skills related to constructing, interpreting, and using Shewhart charts follow.

Tip 1: Type of Data and Subgroup Size

When a Shewhart chart for attribute data is developed with subgroup sizes that are too small, it results in too many zeros on the graph or in a lack of a lower limit on the graph. For highly reliable process measures, the same situation occurs with data reported as 100% and no upper limit. Both of these issues make it difficult to learn about the variation in the data presented on the Shewhart chart. Guidelines for identifying an adequate subgroup size for P chart and U charts were presented in Chapter Five. G or T charts, alternative Shewhart-type charts for working with very rare events, are presented in Chapter Seven.

Continuous data (measurement) is preferable to attribute data when developing a measurement strategy for improvement projects. Continuous data enables teams to learn if changes tested are improvements more rapidly than they can learn from attribute data. Whenever it is possible to develop measures on a continuous scale it is wise to do so. For example, in learning about length of stay (LOS), subgroups of 3 to 10 measures of LOS will allow for more rapid learning about the impact of changes tested as well as causes of process variation than subgroups of 30 to 300 attribute measures of LOS (such as percentage of times > 3 days). Figures 2.2 and 2.21 illustrated the value of using continuous data rather than attribute data when available.

Tip 2: Rounding Data

It is advisable to think about the number of decimal places used when recording and using data for improvement. The average length of stay in the emergency department yesterday was calculated to be 186.37258 minutes. What should the team record? When doing calculations using a computer, always err on the side of maintaining many decimal places. Rounding the data is not necessary, nor desirable, given the computer's ability to effectively deal with many decimal places when manipulating data. Rounding upon data entry could lead to less useful limits. There are a number of guidelines about recording data when it will be used for compliance purposes that result in rounding, but those should not be applied when using data for learning. For example, many hospitals are realizing that for learning, the LOS data needs to be in minutes, rather than rounded to hours or days as typically reported in compliance data.

In thinking about how to report data, people sometimes forget that the precision of averages of multiple data points is more than that of the original data. The standard error of an average is equal to the standard deviation of the data used to calculate the average divided by the square root of the number of values averaged (subgroup or sample size). Thus, averages should usually be reported with more precision (for example, with one more decimal place) than the data used to calculate the average.

A good guideline for rounding of center lines and limits on Shewhart charts is to keep one more decimal than the statistic plotted on the chart. It is then easy to determine whether a point is above or below a line when applying the rules for detecting special cause. When presenting the data as a data grid on the chart one must often round the data to make the display usable for those analyzing the graph. Presentations of capability of a process are usually rounded to the same units as the units for the original data.

Tip 3: Formatting Charts

Shewhart charts and run charts should be presented in a way that it makes it easiest for users to learn from the variation in the data. In developing graphs for presentation, it is wise to think about what a user who is not familiar with the data or chart would need to see. Creating charts that may only be shared as a full-sized page (11 × 8.5 inches) is not ideal. Most improvement projects require multiple measures as discussed in Chapter Two and seen in Figure 2.27. It is best practice to view charts of multiple measures for an improvement project at one time (for example, on the same page). Software used to create Shewhart charts and run charts should support this method of display.

The shape of Shewhart and run charts should be rectangular. For charts with time on the horizontal axis a ratio of horizontal to vertical of 5:2 has been found to be a useful guideline. Many of the charts in this book will have approximately that ratio. Some other things to keep in mind in developing the presentation of the chart are:

1. **Vertical Scale**[1]: A good starting point is to include the upper and lower limits in the middle 50% of the graph. Use the other 50% of graph space as "white space" on either side of the limits. Do not force the graph to include 0 unless that is important to the process or measure being charted. See Figures 6.1 through 6.3 for illustrations of these scaling issues.

---

[1]Mowery, R., "Scaling Control Charts: What We Forgot to Tell You," *Quality Progress*, Nov, 1991., 6–67.

FIGURE 6.1   Appropriate Vertical Scale

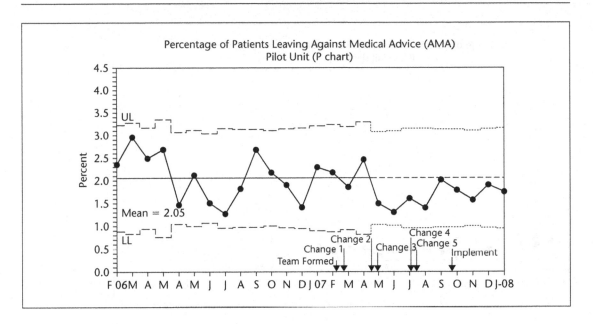

FIGURE 6.2   Vertical Scale Too Small

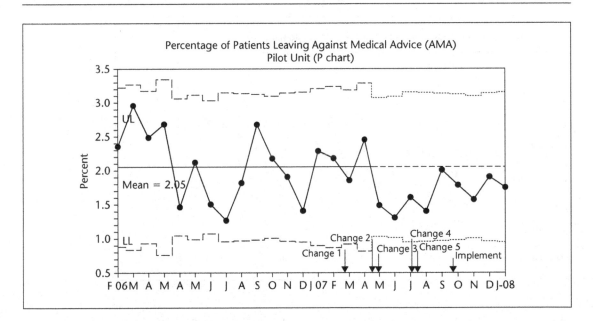

If data being graphed cannot go below 0, do not scale the graph below zero. Similarly, if the data cannot exceed 100% do not scale above 100%. Figure 6.4 illustrates a graph with a scale from −20% to 140%. While it nicely places the limits such that they utilize about 50% of the graph space, it is still an inappropriate vertical scale. It is not possible for the percentage of eligible patients who should have received angiotensin-converting enzyme inhibitors (ACEI) to exceed 100% or to be less than 0%, therefore it is not appropriate to show such a scale. Figure 6.5 shows a more appropriate scale with 100% being the maximum and 0 the minimum. In this case, the principle of using 50% of graph space as white space on either side of the limits is sacrificed for the sake of displaying an appropriate scale.

FIGURE 6.3   Vertical Scale Too Large

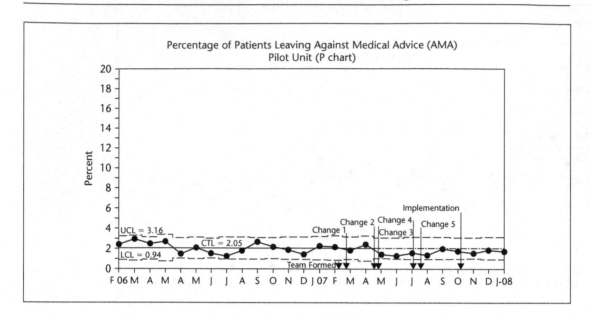

FIGURE 6.4   Inappropriate Vertical Scale Below and Above 100%

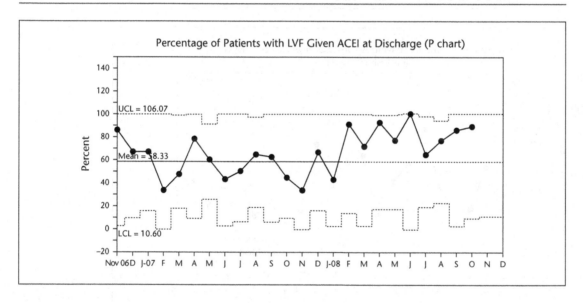

In addition, it is not always appropriate to scale all percent data from 0 to100.
If the data do not use most of this scale it may be inappropriate to scale the graph from
0 to 100% unless such a scale is necessary to include the goal on the graph. Figure 6.6 illustrates
a graph inappropriately scaled from 0 to100%. Figure 6.7 displays the graph with a more
appropriate scale.

2. **Labels**: Include user-friendly labels on vertical and horizontal axes, on centerline,
limits, and other key values (targets, baselines, requirements, and so on) on the chart.
3. **Gridlines and Data**: Keep gridlines and other lines to a minimum. At times gridlines
aid in understanding patterns in the data, however they should not be allowed to
overwhelm the graph. Figure 6.8 illustrates an overuse of gridlines. Though it may be
helpful to display the data they must be legible to be of use. Figure 6.8 also illustrates

FIGURE 6.5   Appropriate Vertical Scale Not Exceeding 100%

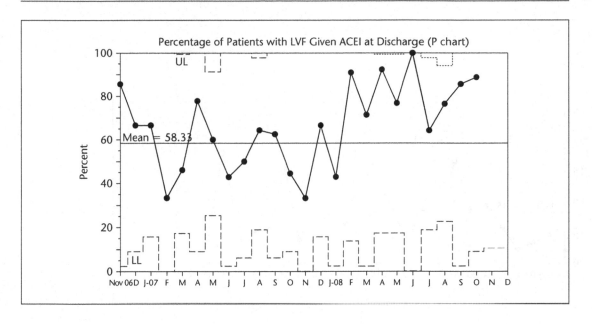

FIGURE 6.6   Inappropriate Vertical Scale Assuming Need to Scale to 100%

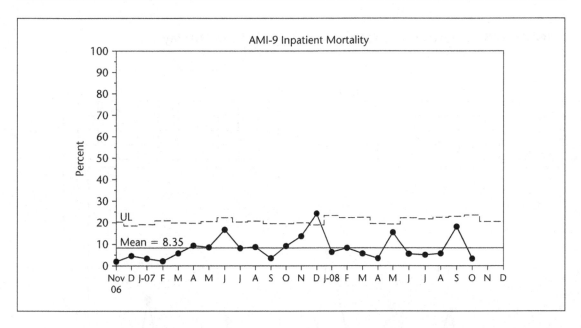

the display of illegible data. Include information such as the target or requirement on the graph but do so as a note rather than a line. In general, it is wise to avoid adding lines to a Shewhart chart that do not come from the data on that chart (the mean, upper limit, lower limit, and data line). Adding additional lines (such as a target line) may result in a chart that is subject to misinterpretation.

4. **Data Points**: Connecting the points on a run chart or Shewhart chart is optional. In Chapters Two through Five we have usually connected the plotted points when the horizontal axis is data in time order. If a line is used to connect the data points it should not overwhelm the data points, but rather help the reader in their analysis of the chart. When the data are not graphed in time order (such as in Figures 2.14, 2.15, 5.12, 5.13, 5.14, 5.18, 5.19 or Case Study Chapter Figure 13.46) it is best not to connect the data points.

FIGURE 6.7   Appropriate Vertical Scale for Range of Data

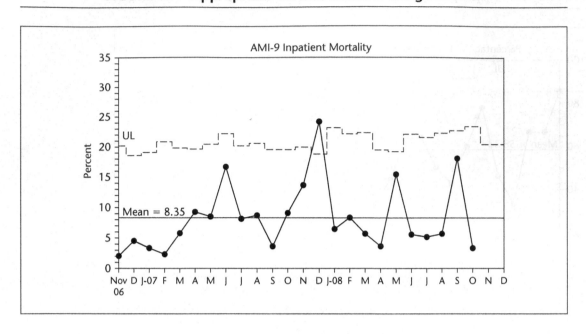

FIGURE 6.8   Overuse of Gridlines and Illegible Data Display

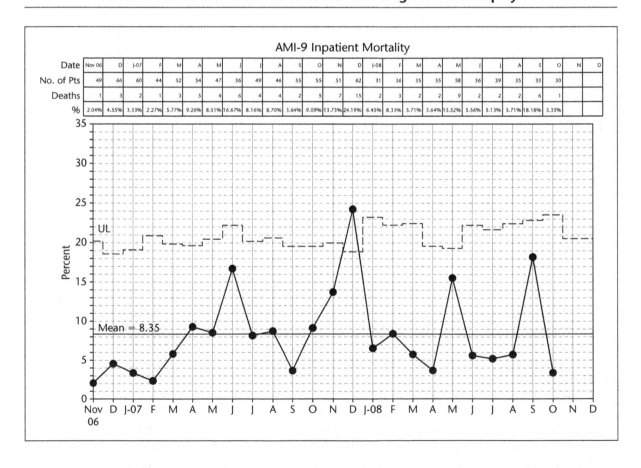

Typical Problems with Software for Calculating Shewhart Charts

When Walter Shewhart developed the control chart method in the 1920s, procedures to develop and maintain the charts manually were very important. Today most data of interest are already (or will soon be) in an electronic database. Electronic spreadsheet software can be used to do Shewhart chart calculations and prepare graphs to display the charts.

There are a number of special software programs available that are already programmed to do the calculation of limits and formatting of the charts. This can be very convenient for frequent users of Shewhart charts. But one should be cautious about approaches used in any standard statistical process control (SPC) software. The best method to evaluate the accuracy of a Shewhart chart software program is to analyze a data set where the limits are already known to be correct. Comparing the limits resulting from software under consideration to those known to be correct from an existing data set will go far to informing the user about adequacy of the software under consideration.

Some of the typical problems found with SPC software include:

1. **Estimating sigma to calculate limits.** Some programs have taken the concept of three-sigma limits and assumed the sigma in this concept referred to the usual calculation of the standard deviation. This assumption is incorrect. For a continuous data set, the formula for standard deviation is:

    $$\text{Standard deviation} = \text{Square Root } [(X - \overline{X})^2 / (n - 1)], \text{ where n is the total number of data points available.}$$

    The problem with using standard deviation as an estimate of sigma is that there is no distinction in the formula between data affected by common and special causes of variation. The estimate of sigma will be inflated when special causes are present and result in ineffective limits.

    Some software programs offer different options for calculating the sigma used in the control chart calculation. Use caution to select "recommended method" when presented with options for estimating sigma. For example, for the $\overline{X}$ and S chart, some software programs offer the "pooled standard deviation" as an option. Although this approach has good statistical properties when the data come from a stable process, the calculation is sensitive to special causes and will result in inflated limits when special causes are present in the data.

2. **Recalculating limits with every point as they are added**. SPC software typically defaults to updating limits with every data point added to the graph. As discussed in Chapter Four, when averages and limits are continuously recalculated it can result in limits that make it harder to detect special cause. The continuously updated limits can be pulled around by the most recent data. In addition, important information about earlier performance of the measure may be lost. The best technique regarding limits is to create useful baseline (often called initial) limits and then freeze and extend those limits. Chapter Four provides detailed guidance for establishing and revising limits. It is important that the user be able to direct software to use the preferred technique. Figures 6.9 and 6.10 illustrate the impact of using the incorrect technique. In Figure 6.9 using the incorrect technique results in no special cause signals throughout the graph. In Figure 6.10 use of the correct technique, establishing initial limits with 20–30 data points and extending them, results in a much clearer picture and a greater ability to detect special cause. The initial limits in Figure 6.10 indicate that revenue was stable. A shift became evident by February 2011 indicating special cause in an undesirable direction.

3. **Using most recent k points, drop oldest point out of k points and add new**. This default consists of the software being programmed to use a particular number of points for the limits. Software might be programmed to always use the most recent

FIGURE 6.9 Inappropriately Including Each New Data Point in Limits

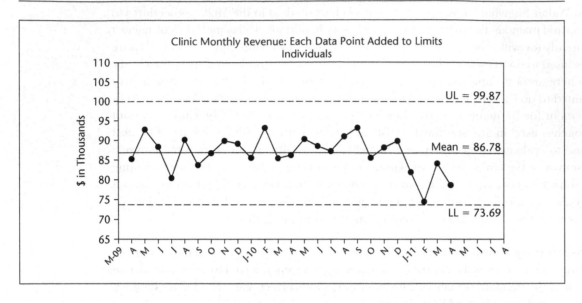

FIGURE 6.10 Impact of Appropriate Limit Technique

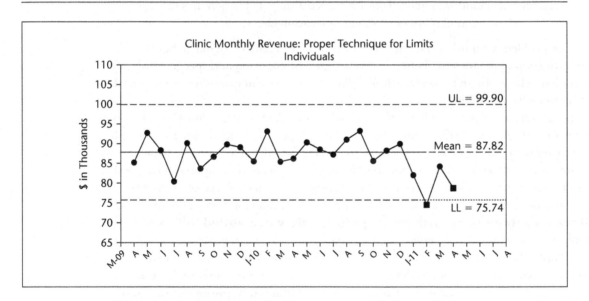

25 data points in determining the limits. When the 26th data point is added to the graph the software will exclude the first data point from the calculation of the limits. This technique can lead to a situation similar to that described in the preceding problem. The recalculation of control limits should always be done in a thoughtful, specific way rather than relying upon software defaults or options. Figure 4.14 illustrated the importance of attention to this issue.

4. **Inappropriate extension of limits with varying subgroup size.** Some SPC software improperly extends limits for data with variable subgroup size ($\overline{X}$ S, U, P charts). Options for appropriate practice when baseline data are available but no new data are yet available include:

    • Do not extend the limits but rather merely extend the center line from the baseline as seen in Chart A in Figure 6.11.

FIGURE 6.11   Proper Extension of Limits When Subgroup Sizes Are Unequal

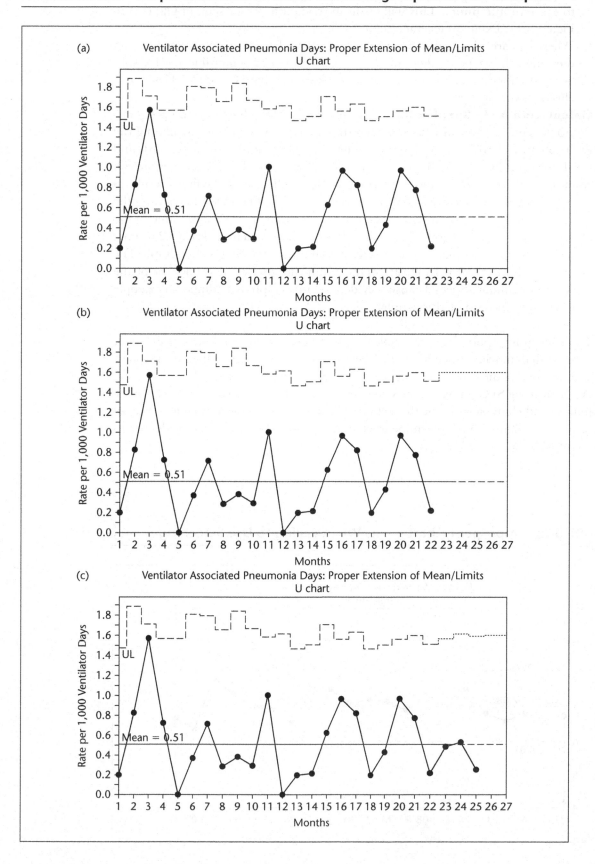

- Extend the limits by using the average subgroup size from the baseline time period to estimate the limits. This will result in straight limits as seen in Chart B in Figure 6.11. Extend the center line as usual.
- When data are added after the initial baseline limits have been constructed, extend the center line. Update the limits by using the extended center line and the subgroup size for each new data point as it is added to the chart. Chart C in Figure 6.11 illustrates this approach.

5. **Calculation of I chart limits**. Many common control chart software programs do not screen for special causes among the moving range before calculating the limits on an I chart. Failure to do this when calculating limits for the I chart (and the T chart, which uses the I chart formula for a step in the T chart calculation) can result in inflation of the I and T chart limits. Such inflation of the limits results in a reduced ability to detect special cause with the graph. Figure 6.12 illustrates the impact on an I chart when there is failure to screen for special causes among the moving ranges. The first graph shows the infectious waste data from Table 5.2 without screening the moving ranges. Note that no special cause is evident on this graph. The second graph in Figure 6.13 illustrates the graph with use of the proper use of the screening technique. Special cause is evident on this graph. An additional example is provided at the end of this chapter.

If the screening option is not available with the software being used, we suggest either using the median moving range instead of the average moving range in the calculation of the limits, or performing the screening manually as illustrated in Table 5.2.

Again, if using SPC software to develop Shewhart charts, it is prudent to check out the capabilities and characteristics of the software. This can be done by analyzing a data set that you are familiar with to determine whether the software being tested provides results consistent with the known data set.

FIGURE 6.12   Improper I Chart Limits When Failing to Use Screening

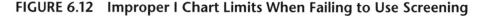

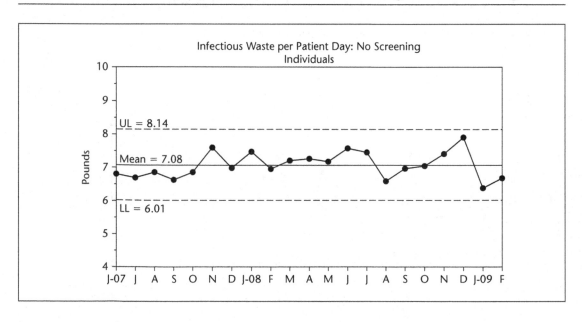

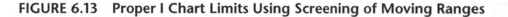

FIGURE 6.13   Proper I Chart Limits Using Screening of Moving Ranges

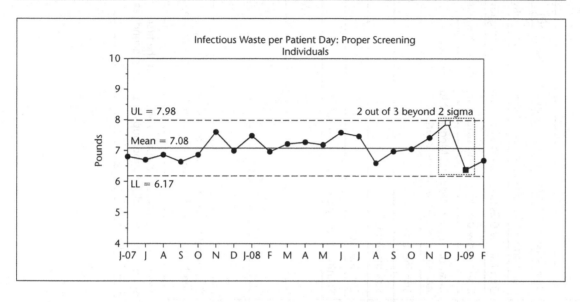

Characteristics to Consider When Purchasing SPC Software

It's wise to invest some time in reviewing a list such as that provided in Table 6.1 carefully to use it when selecting SPC software. From the authors' experience, the items listed as "must have" are essential for good software performance. Recommended features make life easier but can be worked around.

SOME CAUTIONS WHEN USING I CHARTS

Chapter Five introduced I charts as one of the basic types of Shewhart charts for studying continuous data. Examples of situations and data where a Shewhart chart for individuals can be useful include patient-specific clinical measures, monthly accounting data, laboratory test data, forecasts, and budget variances. Often the frequency of data collection cannot be controlled for these situations and types of data. Because of their simplicity, universal applicability, and the minimal amount of data required, some authors recommend that the I chart be used in almost all situations.

As discussed in Chapter Five, the I chart is less sensitive than other Shewhart charts with larger subgroup sizes in its ability to detect the presence of a special cause. Sometimes, data analyzed with an I chart will indicate a stable process, but the same data analyzed with a more appropriate chart ($\overline{X}$ and S, P chart, C chart, or U chart) will indicate the presence of special causes.

Figure 6.14 compares an I chart with a C chart for data consisting of errors made each reporting period. Note that both charts have similar limits and show the process to be stable. The fact that both of these charts have similar limits is used by some to say that an I chart can be used in place of a C chart.

Contrast the charts in Figure 6.14 to the charts in Figure 6.15. This pair of charts is for errors from the same process, but with special causes present. Note that the C chart identifies the special causes, but the I chart limits are wider and do not pick up the special causes. This is because, as was previously discussed, the order of the data affects the width of the control limits in a variables data chart such as the I chart. This is not true for an attributes chart such as the C chart. This is why it is important not to arbitrarily use an I chart when one of the other Shewhart charts is more appropriate: this can cause decision error.

Table 6.1 Characteristics to Consider When Selecting SPC Software

Category	Feature or Attribute	Must Haves	Recommended
Shewhart Control Charts	Individuals chart (also called XmR or I chart)	Standard approach should remove out-of-control **moving ranges** prior to determining average moving range for use in calculation of I chart limits).	Option to display or not display the moving range chart.
	X bar and S chart	Accommodate fixed or variable subgroup size.	Handle large subgroup sizes in each subgroup (>50).
	P chart	Accommodate fixed or variable subgroup size.	Don't show 0 as lower limit when calculation is negative.
	U chart	Accommodate fixed or variable subgroup size.	Don't show 0 as lower limit when calculation is negative.
	C chart		Don't show 0 as lower limit when calculation is negative.
	Other Times Series Charts	T and G charts.	Cusum, Moving Average, Median, Multivariate, standardized charts, prime charts.
Other Tools	Frequency plot		Stratification.
	Scatter plot		Stratification.
	Pareto chart	Can organize text data into chart.	Stratification.
	Run chart	Able place a median on the run chart.	Stratification, apply run chart rules.
	Multi-line chart	Run plot able to place more than one data line on the graph.	
Other Key Features	Uses Shewhart control chart formulas	See formulas provided in Chapter Five.	
	Update graph without having to re-build it	Must be able to save graph, reopen it, and reformat in some other way and save again.	
	Select data to include in establishing limits on the Shewhart control chart	Able to direct software to use specific points for creating baseline limits.	Document which data used to calculate the limits on the chart. Option to label values on limits and center line.
	Display two or more sets of control limits on a Shewhart chart	Ability to identify which subgroups.	As an example, must be able to arrange for the first set of limits to include subgroups 1–27, the second set subgroups 28–44.

Other Key Features	Remove data points from use in calculating the limits	Ability to designate specific data points not to be used in calculation of limits. Be able to "cause" or "ghost" a data point out (e.g., tell software to use points 1–15 and then 17–26 to create the set of limits). The point that is caused out remains on the chart but is visibly evident that it has not been used to calculate the limits.
	Display multiple charts on the same page	Support multiple charts on the same page for display purposes (multi-charting, small multiples).
	Annotate charts	Make notes on the graph.	Notes stay with a particular subgroup when the chart is updated.
	Able to use data from multiple sources (e.g., Excel, Access, others)	Suggest that it provide a "seamless" import.
	Flexible fonts on axis	Be able to control fonts for titles, labels, notes, and so on.
	Export graphs in a variety of image formats		Formats such as png, metafile, and so on.
	Markers on X axis for future data points	Be able to format graph to show format for future data points.
	Can import graphs to a report		Ability to import graphs to a report or document and link such that when graphs are updated in SPC software they will update in your report.
	Updating graphs		Ability to copy existing graph, rename it, alter title and data to create new graph with minimal additional work.

FIGURE 6.14   C Chart and I Chart for Count Data (Errors) from Stable Process

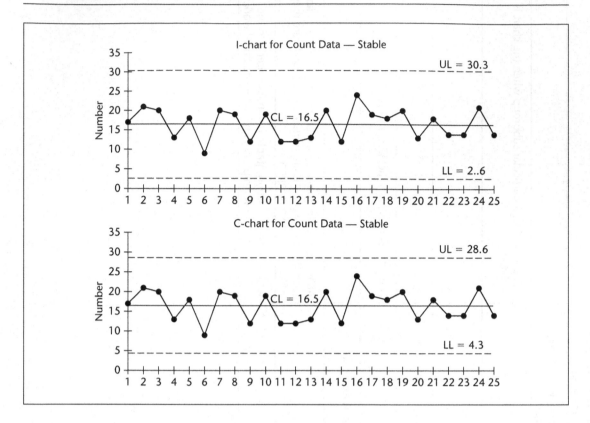

FIGURE 6.15   C Chart and I Chart for Count Data (Errors) from Unstable Process

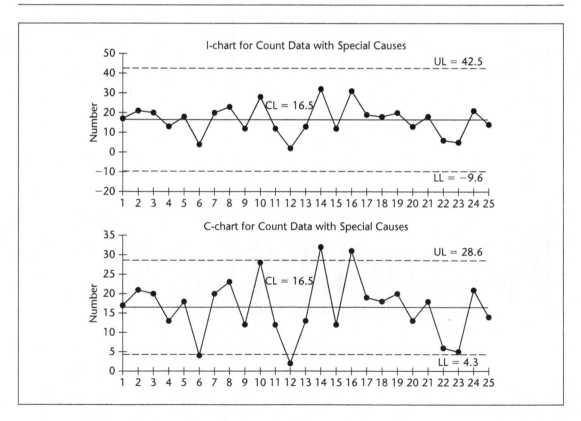

The steps for calculating limits for I charts described in Chapter Five include screening for extreme moving ranges prior to calculating the limits.[2] Some authors and software packages do not include this screening step. To execute the screening step, remove any data points above the ULMR, and then recalculate the MR using the remaining data points. This avoids inappropriate inflation of the limits on the I chart, and reduces the risk of decision errors such as missing a special cause. Figure 6.16 compares limits calculated with and without the screening for three cases. In the first case, the limits are the same (because there are no special causes). In Case 2, the wider limits without the screening step still detect the special causes. In Case 3, the wider limits pick up one of the special causes, but miss the other one. The conclusion is that the step to screen moving ranges should always be part of the I chart calculation.

FIGURE 6.16   Three Cases of I Charts with Limits Also Calculated Without MR Screening

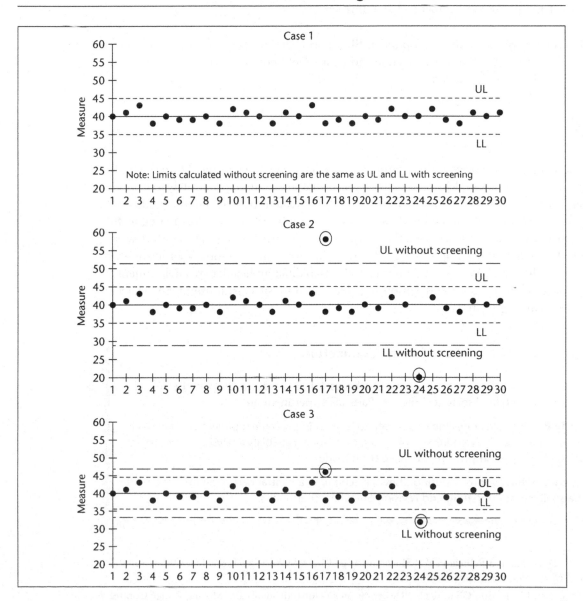

---

[2]Nelson, L. S., "Control Charts for Individual Measurements." *Journal of Quality Technology*, 1982, *14*(34).

A number of authors have published methods to improve the performance of the I chart.[3] Most of the articles deal with different approaches to estimating sigma (common cause variation) for the I chart. The key conclusion is that the moving range is the most robust approach when initially developing the limits. But once the process is stable, a more precise estimate of the common cause variation can be obtained by calculating the standard deviation of the data and dividing by the C_4 factor (see $\overline{X}$, S charts in Chapter Five for the C_4 factor). Thus, to do a capability analysis or to extend limits into the future, it may be useful to do this additional calculation, especially if less than 20 data points are available.

The article by Cryer and Ryan (1990) suggests that calculating sigma both ways (MRbar/d_2 and S/c_4) can provide important diagnostic information for interpreting an I chart:

- If both estimates are similar—stable process, use S/c_4 to estimate sigma
- If the S-based estimate is greater than the MR estimate—special causes are present
- If the S-based estimate is less than the MR estimate—autocorrelation may be present Chapter Eight discusses autocorrelation further.

The I chart is one of the most popular Shewhart charts because of its general applicability and simplicity. But as this section shows, it should not be routinely used without considering the issues discussed.

SUMMARY

This chapter presented some rather common issues that occur when using Shewhart charts in improvement work. Guidelines were given for formatting charts appropriately to include scaling, labeling, the use of additional gridlines, proper data display within the graph, and the proper approach to connecting data points on a graph. All of these formatting techniques affect the ability to learn from the chart. Some issues when using SPC software were discussed and alternative approaches offered. Some issues and options when using the I chart were discussed. When using Shewhart charts in different health care environments, being aware of these issues and options can lead to more successful use of Shewhart's method of learning from data.

Case Study Connection

Any of the seven case studies in this book would be useful as a way to deepen the reader's awareness of Shewhart chart display techniques. Particularly pertinent are:

Case Study B, which illustrates the use of data to support improvement project in a Radiology Department. This case study addresses using rare event data, capability analysis, and examples of updating charts after improvements have been made.

Case Study F, which addresses using Shewhart charts as a central part of an improvement effort. It also illustrates updating and revising Shewhart chart limits.

[3]Boes, K., Does, R., and Schurink, Y., "Shewhart-Type Control Charts for Individual Observations," *Journal of Quality Technology*, 1994, *26*(6), 188–198.

Rigdon, S., Cruthis, E., and Champ, C., "Design Strategies for Individuals and Moving Range Control Charts," *Journal of Quality Technology*, 1993, *25*(3), 274–287.

Cryer, J. and Ryan, T., "The Estimation of Sigma for an X Chart: MRbar/d2 or S/c4," *Journal of Quality Technology*, 1990, *22*(3), 187–192.

ADVANCED THEORY AND METHODS WITH DATA

## CHAPTER 7

MORE SHEWHART-TYPE CHARTS

In previous chapters, we discussed the use of run charts and Shewhart charts to learn from variation in data. The Shewhart chart applies Shewhart's theory of variation to time-series data and provides an operational definition of common and special causes of variation in a measure. This chapter presents some additional types of Shewhart charts that are useful in health care applications and some advanced methods to learn from data collected over time.

The objective of this chapter is for the reader to learn when they might apply the following types of Shewhart and other time series charts:

1. APPLY Other Shewhart Charts:
   - NP chart
   - $\bar{X}$ and Range charts
   - Median chart
   - G chart (number of opportunities between rare events)
   - T chart (time between rare events)
2. APPLY Some Alternatives to Shewhart Charts
   - Moving average
   - Cumulative sum (CUSUM)
   - Exponentially weighted moving average (EWMA)
3. USE Standardized Shewhart Chart
4. USE Multivariate Shewhart-type Charts

These specific charts were selected because all of them have been successfully used to learn from variation in health care data. Figure 7.1 shows these alternatives to the standard Shewhart charts on the chart selection diagram introduced in Chapter Five. The figure shows which of the advanced charts could be used in place of the basic Shewhart chats. Some of the reasons to consider these special charts include:

1. The desire to have more sensitivity in detecting small, persistent changes in a measure (moving average, cumulative sum, and exponentially weighted moving average charts)
2. The need for simpler calculations to be used ($\bar{X}$ and R chart, Median chart, NP chart)
3. Too many zeros on an attribute chart (G chart or T chart)
4. Different target values on the same chart (standardized charts)
5. A preference to have multiple measures analyzed together (multivariate charts)

Although we will not go into as much detail here as we did in discussing the basic Shewhart charts in Chapter Five, we will provide the background, formula to construct, and one or more examples of each type of chart.

OTHER SHEWHART-TYPE CHARTS

The expanded chart selection guide below details alternative Shewhart-type charts for each of the basic Shewhart charts.

FIGURE 7.1   Expanded Chart Selection Guide to Include Alternative Charts

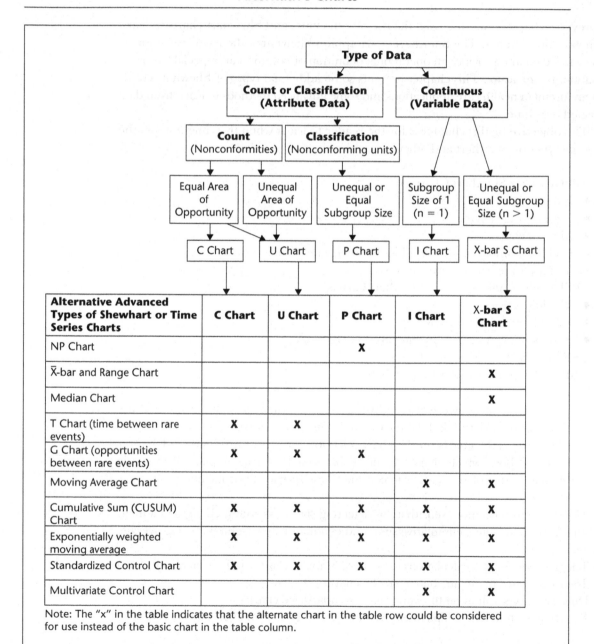

Alternative Advanced Types of Shewhart or Time Series Charts	C Chart	U Chart	P Chart	I Chart	X-bar S Chart
NP Chart			X		
X̄-bar and Range Chart					X
Median Chart					X
T Chart (time between rare events)	X	X			
G Chart (opportunities between rare events)	X	X	X		
Moving Average Chart				X	X
Cumulative Sum (CUSUM) Chart	X	X	X	X	X
Exponentially weighted moving average	X	X	X	X	X
Standardized Control Chart	X	X	X	X	X
Multivariate Control Chart				X	X

Note: The "x" in the table indicates that the alternate chart in the table row could be considered for use instead of the basic chart in the table column.

NP Chart

Chapter Five discussed two types of attribute control charts:

- Charts for classification data: P chart
- Charts for count data: C chart or U charts

The **NP Chart**[1] can be used with classification data for the special case when the subgroups are of equal size. Though people usually describe classification data with percentages, there may be some occasions where it is more convenient and useful just to plot the number of units in one of the classifications. When the subgroups are of equal size it is not necessary to convert nonconforming counts into percentages. Rather, just directly plot the count of nonconforming units (called d) for each subgroup.

Steps in Constructing an NP Chart

1. Determine the size of the subgroups (n) and collect the nonconforming units for k subgroups. The subgroup size, n, has to be sufficiently large to have nonconforming units present in the subgroup most of the time. If we have some idea as to what the historical proportion of nonconformance (p_{bar}), is we can use the following formula to estimate a recommended minimum subgroup size (see Table 5.5 in Chapter Five for more on selecting the subgroup size):

   $n = 300/p_{bar}$ (e.g., if p_{bar} is estimated to be 5%, then $n = 300/5 = 60$)

2. Calculate p_{bar}: $p_{bar} = \sum d_i / (k * n)$

3. Calculate the Center Line: $CL = n* p_{bar}/100$ or $\sum d_i / k$

4. Calculate the UL and LL:

$$UCL = np_{bar} + 3 \sqrt{np_{bar} (1 - p_{bar})}$$

$$LCL = np_{bar} - 3 \sqrt{np_{bar} (1 - p_{bar})}$$

5. Plot the center line npbar, the LL and UL, and the number of process nonconforming units, the d's.

Figure 7.2 shows an example of a completed NP chart. Each week, 20 medical records are obtained and examined for patient harm using a trigger tool. One of the measures used to monitor harm is "the number of charts with 1 or more Adverse Events in category A–D." This value is plotted each week and the NP chart used to monitor the improvement work going on in the hospital.

$\overline{X}$ and Range (R) Chart

When continuous data are obtained from a process, it is sometimes useful to learn about both the average performance of the process and the variation about the average level. For example, it may be useful to learn about the average length of stay (LOS) per month for a particular diagnosis and the variation among the cases comprising that average. In these cases, a set of two Shewhart charts is often used to study the process: one for the average and one for the variation. In Chapter Five, we introduced the $\overline{X}$ chart and the S chart for this purpose. An alternative chart, commonly used in manufacturing industries, is the

---

[1]Grant, E., and Leavenworth, R., *Statistical Quality Control*, 7th ed., New York: McGraw-Hill, 1996, 237–240.

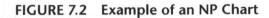

FIGURE 7.2   Example of an NP Chart

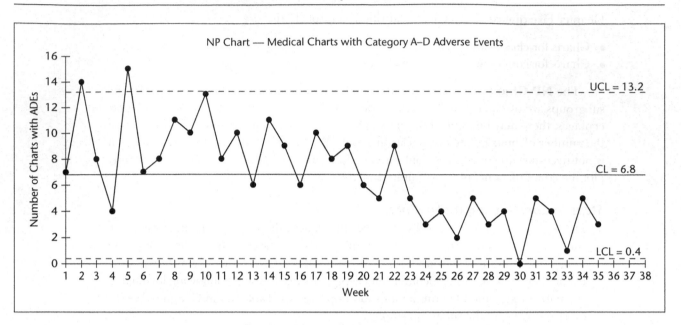

Table 7.1   Symbols Used with $\bar{X}$ and R Charts

Symbol	Description of Symbol
X	Individual measurement of quality characteristic
N	Subgroup size (number of measurements per subgroup)
K	Number of subgroups used to develop control limits
Σ	Summation symbol
$\bar{X}$ (X$_{bar}$)	Average of the individual measures within the subgroup (subgroup average)
$\bar{X}$ (X$_{doublebar}$)	Average of the averages (average of the subgroup averages)
R	Range within a subgroup (that is, subgroup range—largest minus smallest)
$\bar{R}$ (R$_{bar}$)	Average of the ranges for all subgroups
A$_2$, D$_3$, D$_4$, d$_2$	Factors for computing control limits and capability of the process
*	Multiplication symbol

$\bar{X}$ and **R chart**.[2] This set of charts requires that the subgroup size be constant and is most useful for small subgroup sizes (n = 2–10).

Table 7.1 describes the symbols and Figure 7.3 describes the formula to calculate the limits for $\bar{X}$ and R charts. An important aspect of the collection of data for the construction of $\bar{X}$ and R control charts is that the collection is done in subgroups. A subgroup for continuous data is a set (usually three to six) of measurements of some characteristic in a process, which were obtained under similar conditions or at about the same time. The $\bar{X}$ chart contains the averages of each subgroup and the R chart

[2]Ibid., Chapter 4.

FIGURE 7.3   Calculating Limits for $\overline{X}$ and R Charts

Name _____   _____ Date _____

Process _____ Sample Description _____

Number of Subgroups (k) _____ between (dates) _____ - _____

Number of Samples or Measurements per Subgroup (n) _____

$$\overline{\overline{X}} = \frac{\sum \overline{X}}{k} = \text{----------} = \underline{\quad\quad} \qquad \overline{R} = \frac{\sum R}{k} = \text{----------} = \underline{\quad\quad}$$

$\overline{X}$ Chart	$\overline{R}$ Chart
UL = $\overline{\overline{X}}$ + (A_2 * $\overline{R}$)	UL = D_4 * $\overline{R}$
UL = ___ + (___ * ___)	UL = ___ * ___
UL = ___ + _____	UL = _____
UL = _____	
LL = $\overline{\overline{X}}$ – (A_2 * $\overline{R}$)	LL = D_3 * $\overline{R}$
LL = ___ – (___ * ___)	LL = ___ * ___
LL = ___ _____	LL = _____
LL = _____	

Factors for Control Limits

n	A_2	D_3	D_4	d_2
1*	2.66		3.27	1.128
2	1.88		3.27	1.128
3	1.02		2.57	1.693
4	0.73		2.28	2.059
5	0.58		2.11	2.326
6	0.48		2.00	2.534
7	0.42	0.08	1.92	2.704
8	0.37	0.14	1.86	2.847
9	0.34	0.18	1.82	2.970
10	0.31	0.22	1.78	3.087

Note: For n = 1, use a moving range chart.

PROCESS CAPABILITY

If the process is in statistical control, the standard deviation is:

$$\hat{\sigma} = \frac{\overline{R}}{d_2} = \underline{\quad\quad} = \underline{\quad\quad}$$

Then the process capability is:

$$\overline{\overline{X}} - 3\hat{\sigma} \quad \text{to} \quad \overline{\overline{X}} + 3\hat{\sigma}$$

$$\underline{\quad} -(3 * \underline{\quad}) \quad \text{to} \quad \underline{\quad} + (3 * \underline{\quad})$$

$$\underline{\quad\quad\quad} \quad \text{to} \quad \underline{\quad\quad\quad}$$

the ranges calculated from the measurements in each subgroup. Similarly to the $\overline{X}$ and S chart, these averages and ranges are usually plotted over time, but the subgroups could also be defined in other ways.

Figure 7.4 shows an example of a completed $\overline{X}$ and R chart. Data are collected on all charges by the physician group when the principal diagnosis was pneumonia. The individual charges are organized into subgroups of five cases each by time. These charts indicate that the average charges are stable over this time period, but there is a special cause of variation among individual cases within a subgroup (the R chart). Case Study G in Chapter Thirteen shows how this $\overline{X}$ and R chart was used during an improvement project.

FIGURE 7.4 Example of an $\bar{X}$ and an R Chart

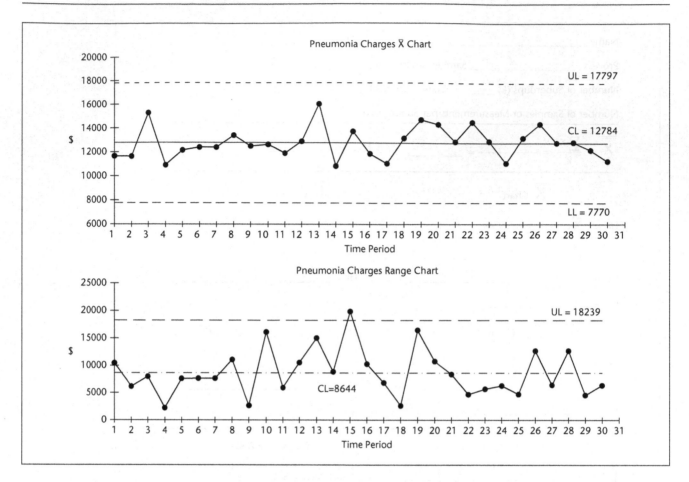

Median Chart

For continuous data, an alternative to the $\bar{X}$ chart is the median control chart.[3] The **median chart** was historically used to enable one to skip the calculation requirements of the average for $\bar{X}$ chart since the median can be determined by inspection of the data. Although the calculation of an average is rarely a barrier today, the median chart may be useful if a median is the key statistic used to monitor a process. For example, when monitoring length of stay in an emergency department, the median is often used so that one or two very long wait times do not skew the indicator of system performance. To use a median chart the subgroup must be constant and it is most convenient with an odd subgroup size (typically 3, 5, 7, or 9) where the median will be the middle value in the subgroup.

The steps to developing a median chart are similar to the $\bar{X}$ and R chart. Instead of the factor A_2, a factor A_6 is used with the median. Figure 7.5 shows the calculation sheet for a median chart including the A_6 factors for subgroup sizes from 2 to 25. A_6 is a function of the factor d_2 (see Figure 7.3) that relates the range to the standard deviation for a normal distribution.[4]

Figure 7.6 shows a median chart for office visit times. The office improvement team in the specialty clinic selected the first seven patients each day and measured their time from

---

[3]Clifford, P. C., "Control Charts Without Calculations," *Industrial Quality Control*, 1959, *15*(11), 40–44.

[4]Wheeler, D., and Chambers, D., *Understanding Statistical Process Control*, SPC Press, Knoxville, TN, 1992.

FIGURE 7.5   Calculating Limits for Median Charts

Name _____ Date _____

Process _____ Sample Description _____

Number of Subgroups (k) _____ between (dates)_____ - _____

Number of Samples or Measurements per Subgroup (n) _____

$$\overline{\overline{X}} = \frac{\sum Medians}{k} = \text{----------------} = \underline{\hspace{2cm}} \qquad \overline{R} = \frac{\sum R}{k} = \text{-------------} = \underline{\hspace{0.5cm}}.\underline{\hspace{0.5cm}}$$

Median Chart	Factors for Median Control Limits

$$UL = \overline{\overline{X}} \quad + \quad (\quad A_6 \quad * \quad \overline{R} \quad)$$

$$UL = \quad\quad + \quad (\quad\quad * \quad\quad)$$

$$UL = \underline{\hspace{5cm}}$$

$$LL = \overline{\overline{X}} \quad - \quad (\quad A_6 \quad * \quad \overline{R})$$

$$LL = \quad\quad - \quad (\quad\quad * \quad\quad)$$

$$LL = \underline{\hspace{5cm}}$$

n	A_6
2	1.881
3	1.187
4	0.795
5	0.691
6	0.549
7	0.509
8	0.432
9	0.412
10	0.363
11	0.350
12	0.316
13	0.308
14	0.282
15	0.276
16	0.255
17	0.251
18	0.235
19	0.231
20	0.218

FIGURE 7.6   Median Chart for Visit Times

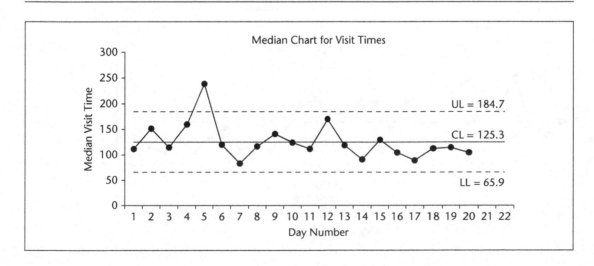

check-in to checkout. They were concerned that average visit times had recently crept up above their standard of two hours (120 minutes). The team did not want a single long visit time to affect their overall average, so they used the median chart to minimize that impact. Note that another way to deal with time data that can be skewed to long waiting times is to use a transformation of the data. This approach is discussed in Chapter Eight.

Figure 7.7 shows a second example of a median chart for daily length of stay (LOS) data in the emergency room. A judgment sample of 15 patients is selected each day to monitor performance. The median chart was selected to minimize the impact of a few individual patients with very long LOSs.

SHEWHART CHARTS FOR RARE EVENTS

Rare events are defined here as events that do not usually occur when the process is observed, so a value of 0 is often recorded. Rare events can cause the standard Shewhart charts for attribute data (P chart for Classification data; C chart or U chart for Count data) that were described in Chapter Five to become ineffective. In order to develop effective attribute Shewhart charts, two important characteristics of these charts should be considered. First, in order to better monitor improvement in the process, the chart should have a lower control limit. Second, it is desirable to have the size of the subgroup large enough so that some nonconformities or nonconforming units are found in most subgroups. Our experience has been that in order to develop a useful attribute chart, less than 25% of the subgroups should have no nonconforming units (plotting "0" on the chart). With more than 25% calculations and rules used with the chart become questionable. The size of a subgroup plays an important role in achieving these two characteristics.

Often we can design our data collection plan (design our subgroups for the Shewhart chart) so that we do not have too many zeros in our recorded data. If we are sampling, we can increase our sample size so that we expect to see the event of interest. If we are already using all available data, we can adjust the time period for defining subgroups:

- For things that don't occur every hour, we pick daily subgroups.
- For things that don't occur every day, we pick weekly or monthly subgroups.
- For things that don't occur every month, we can pick quarterly or annual subgroups,

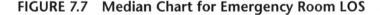

FIGURE 7.7   Median Chart for Emergency Room LOS

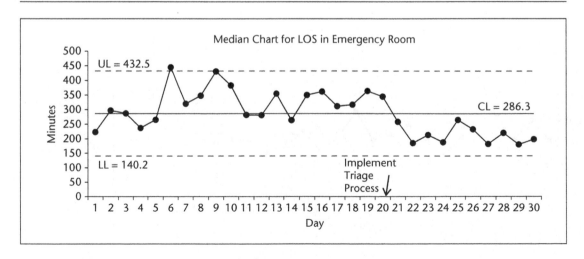

- For things that don't occur every year, we pick decades (number of Category 4 hurricanes)
- And so on

Table 5.5 described minimum subgroups size for effective P charts, which depends on the expected value of p, the average percent for the event of interest. For count data, the Poisson distribution is used to develop the control limits. On a C chart, whenever C_{bar} is less than 9, there will not be a lower control limit. C_{bar} has to be greater than 1.4 to expect $< 25\%$ of the subgroup values to be non-zero.

The problem is that for improvement work, we often want to look at our systems at least monthly. We can go only so far with subgrouping strategies before we encounter the problem of subgroups that exceed a month. So we switch to a different strategy to form subgroups that better foster learning. When the attribute we are interested in studying is a relatively rare event, the guidelines in Table 5.5 often cannot be met. In these cases, the basic Shewhart charts may not be useful to detect improvement. An alternative in these cases is to develop Shewhart charts for the time or number of opportunities between events as shown in Figure 7.8. Chapter Two introduced the concept of transforming rare event data to time or cases between events. Chapter Three (Figures 3.30 through 3.32) showed how to develop a run chart for cases between data.

FIGURE 7.8   Run Chart of Rare Event and Time Between Incident of the Event

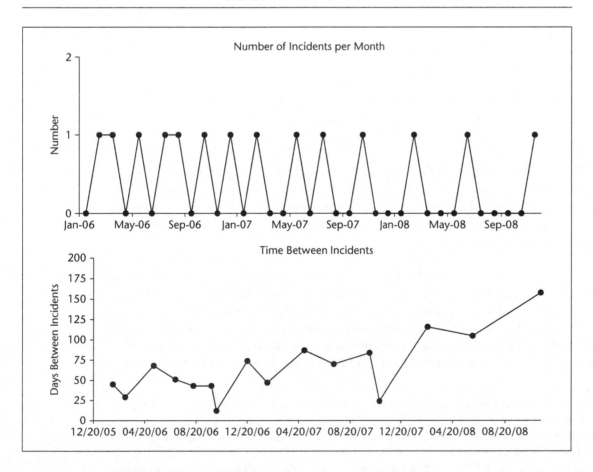

For example, in monitoring hospital infection rates, the time between infections has been used to assess improvement because of the relatively low rates of infection and the simplicity of interpretation of the chart. The current value of this statistic can be updated every day and a chart of time (or opportunities, cases, bed days, and so forth) between infections can be updated each time an infection occurs on the hospital floor, without having to determine the appropriate denominator. The desired direction on this type of chart will always be up as this will indicate more time or more cases between undesirable events. The next two sections describe G charts for opportunities between events and T charts for time between events.

G Chart for Opportunities Between Rare Events

The **G chart** (or Geometric chart) is an alternative to the P chart, C chart, or U chart when the incident of interest is relatively rare and some discrete determination of opportunity (cases, patients, admits, line insertions, and so on) can be obtained.[5] The G chart allows each occurrence to be immediately evaluated on the chart rather than having to wait to the end of a time period before the data point is plotted. The G chart is particularly useful for verifying improvements (such as reduced infections) and for processes with low rates. Improvements are indicated by higher values (more cases between incidents) on the G chart. Because of the skewed nature of the geometric distribution, there is no lower control limit for the G chart, but the standard run rules can be applied because the center line is adjusted to the theoretical median of the distribution.

The calculation of control limits is based on the geometric distribution:

Determine the incident of interest (for example, pressure ulcer) and the unit that determines the opportunity for the incident (for example, occupied bed days).

$$g = \text{number opportunities or units between incidents}$$
$$g_{bar} = \text{average of g's}$$
$$CL = 0.693 * g_{bar}$$
$$UL = g_{bar} + 3 * \text{square root } [g_{bar} * (g_{bar} + 1)]$$
$$LL = \text{there is no lower control limit}$$

Notes:

1. The UL is approximately 4 times g_{bar} (or 5.7 times the CL) for quick visual analysis.
2. Since the count data on a g chart are usually highly skewed, the plotted data will not be symmetric around the average (g_{bar}). The theoretical median = 0.693 * mean for the geometric distribution should be used for the center line when it is desirable to apply the shift rule (8 consecutive points above or below center line).

Figure 7.9 is an example of a G chart developed for a specific type of infection in an intensive care unit (ICU). The bottom graph in the figure is a U chart with the number of infections per 100 admissions plotted each month. Although the infection rate appeared to have improved, there was still not a special cause signal on the chart. The top chart is a G chart calculated for the same data. The median is used as the center line (CL = 10.4; the mean value was 15.0). The next to the last point is above the UL. The admissions between

[5]Benneyan J.C.: Number-between g-type statistical quality control charts for monitoring adverse events. *Health Care Management Science* 2001, 4, 305-318.

Benneyan J.C.: Performance of number-between g-type statistical control charts for monitoring adverse events. *Health Care Management Science*, 2001, 4, 319-336.

Kaminsky FC, Benneyan JC, Davis RB, and Burke RJ, "Statistical Control Charts Based on a Geometric Distribution", *Journal of Quality Technology*, 1992, 24(2), 63-69.

Wall, R., et al., "Using Real Time Process Measurements to Reduce Catheter Related Bloodstream Infections in the ICU," *BMJ Journal of Quality and Safety in Health Care*, 2005, 14, 295–302.

FIGURE 7.9   G Chart for Number of ICU Admissions Between Infections

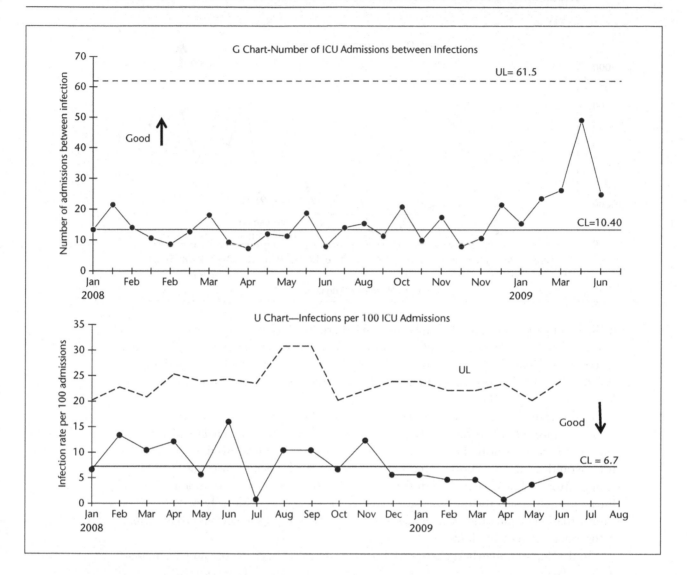

infections have increased to the point that special cause is detected. This special cause for the next to the last point on the G chart provides the evidence that the infection rate has decreased. This signal confirms the visual pattern for the last six occurrences.

Figure 7.10 shows a second example of the G chart. A hospital tracks Adverse Drug Events (ADEs) using their automated system. When they find an ADE, they count the number of doses dispensed since the previous occurrence. An improvement team was formed in July and they collected data on the last 20 ADEs from the automated system and developed a G chart. Since the chart indicated a stable process with a center line of 7,657 doses, they extended the limits and began their improvement work. The ADE that occurred on February 18, 2011 signaled a special cause indicating a reduction in the rate of adverse drug events. Because all the ADE events after the team formed were above the extended center line, they planned to update the limits to reflect the new process.

T Chart for Time Between Rare Events

The **T chart** (or time-between chart) is an alternative to a standard attribute chart when the incident of interest is relatively rare and a measurement of time between each occurrence of

FIGURE 7.10   G Chart for Doses Dispensed Between ADEs

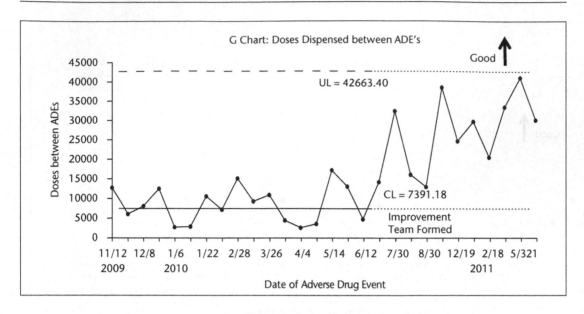

the incident can be obtained.[6] Similar to the G chart, the T chart allows the evaluation of each incident (called nonconformity for count data or nonconfirming unit for classification data) to be evaluated as it occurs rather than having to wait to the end of a standard time period before the data point is plotted. The T chart builds on the "time-between" run chart described in Chapter Three.

If the rate of occurrence can be modeled by the Poisson distribution (the usual assumption for a C chart or U chart), then the times between occurrences will follow an exponential distribution. The exponential distribution is highly skewed, so plotting the times would result in a control chart where the standard special cause rules would not be appropriate. The exponential distribution can be transformed to a symmetric Weibull distribution by raising the time measure to the $1/3.6 = 0.2777$ power or $[y = t^{0.2777}]$. This transformation of the time (days, hours, minutes, and so on) between events is done as part of the calculation of the limits.

To develop this Shewhart chart, first determine the incident of interest and the measure of time (days, hours, minutes, and so on) between each incident. The easiest way to collect the data is to record the exact time that an incident occurs and subtract the time that the previous incident occurred. Often the time can be recorded to the nearest days, but if two or more events can occur on the same day, the hours should also be recorded. Because the construction of the chart is based on an I chart calculation, the chart limits can be sensitive to a few data points. Try to get at least 20 incidents to establish limits. Once you have an estimate of the time between events, you can determine how far back in time you need to go to collect data. For example, if the event has historically occurred about once a week, go back at least 20 weeks to collect data. For an event that is expected to occur about once per quarter, collect historic dates for the previous five years.

The limits for the T chart are calculated by transforming the time data, then using the formulas used for the I chart (Chapter Five) to calculate limits for the transformed data. These limits are then transformed back to the original scale for display with the original data.

$$t = \text{time between incidents}$$
$$y = \text{transformed time } [y = t^{0.2777}].$$

[6]Nelson, L., "A Control Chart for Parts-Per-Million Nonconforming Items," *Journal of Quality Technology*, July 1994, *26*(3), 239–240.

MR_{bar} = average moving range of y's

remove any MRs > 3.27*MR_{bar} and recalculate the average MR_{bar}' (MR_{bar}')

Y_{bar} = average of y's (center line)

$$UL = Ybar + 2.66 * MR_{bar}'$$
$$LL = Ybar - 2.66 * MR_{bar}'$$

Transform the center line and the limits back to time scale before plotting chart by raising them to the 3.6 power:

$$Limit = (transformed\ limit)^{3.6}$$

Notes:

1. Conduct the usual screening of MRs to calculate the average moving range.
2. Be careful to not have any zeros in the data (for example, two rare events occurring at exactly the same time). Increase precision (hours vs. days, minutes vs. hours, and so forth) when any data values will be recorded as zero (or add 0.5 units to the calculated time for the second data point recorded as the same time).
3. As the upper limit transformed back to the original scale can appear to be very large (people view it as "not reasonable"), sometimes the T chart is displayed on a logarithm scale so that the limits appear more symmetrical. This also creates more visual sensitivity around the lower limit of the chart.

Figure 7.11 shows an example of a T chart for sentinel events (death or serious injury) in a health system. The number of days between each event is the focus of the chart. The top chart is the I chart based on the transformed data. The middle chart shows the T chart (limits transformed back to time scale) with the original days between plotted. The bottom chart is the same information as the middle T chart, but the y-axis uses a logarithm (log_{10}) scale. The run of 9 consecutive points above the center line is a signal of improvement. Note that all three of the charts tell exactly the same story, with different visual emphasis, so that the users can determine which chart they prefer for presentation or decision making. The default should be to present the chart on the original time scale.

Figure 7.12 shows a second example of a T chart. A hospital requires documentation any time a foreign object is retained during a procedure. An improvement team was formed to reduce the number of incidents of "retained foreign objects." Historical data indicated that an incident occurred only about once per month. Because data had only been collected for the last year, they prepared a T chart using the last 15 incidents before their improvement work began. As they tested changes they continued to plot an additional point each time a new incident occurred. After observing eight consecutive points above the center line, they used the signal of special cause to conclude that their changes had increased the time between incidents of retained foreign objects. They continued to record events and recalculated the center line and temporary limits after they had 12 data points representing their improved process. The average days between foreign object retention improved from 21 to 85 days.

SOME ALTERNATIVES TO SHEWHART-TYPE CHARTS

All of the Shewhart charts discussed in Chapter Five, and thus far in Chapter Seven, have the feature that each plotted point contains information based only on data in that subgroup. The calculation of the plotted statistic does not use data from other subgroups. Thus, each point can be treated independently. Some of the rules for determining a special cause (such as a run of 8 consecutive points above or below the center line [also called a shift] and the trend rule) incorporate information from other points.

FIGURE 7.11 T Chart (Transformed Data, Original Time Scale, Log₁₀ Scale)

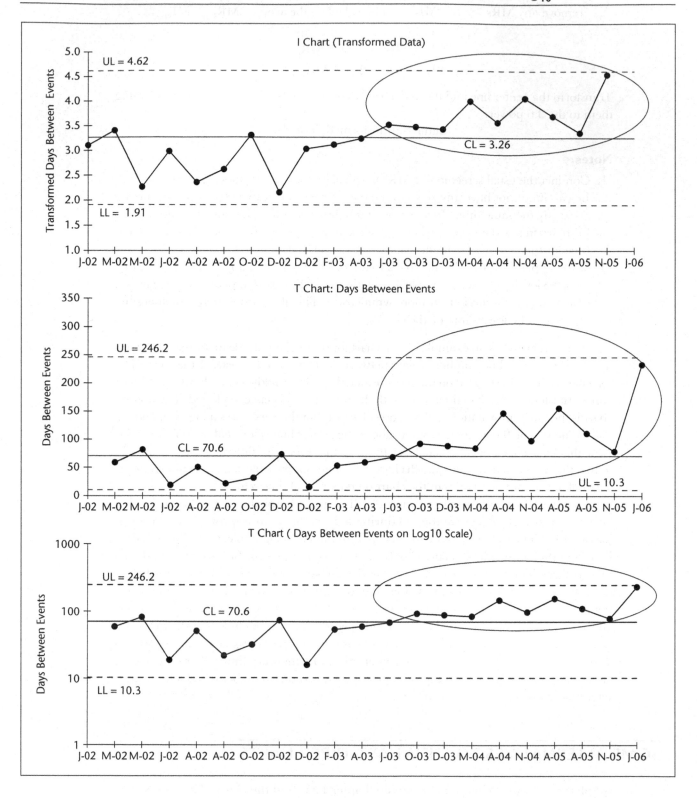

FIGURE 7.12   T Chart for Days Between Retained Foreign Objects

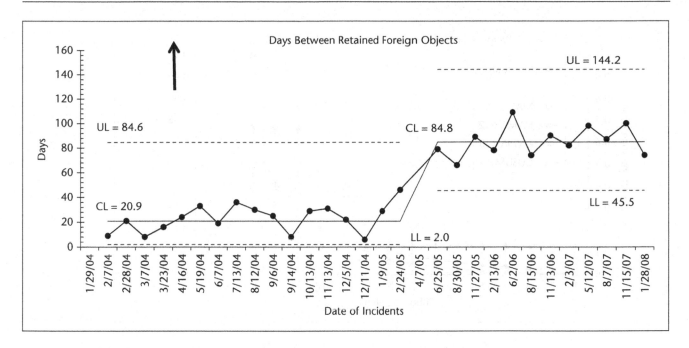

This section discusses some alternative time series charts that incorporate information from other subgroups when calculating the statistic to plot.[7] The advantage of using these time-weighted charts is the ability to detect small changes in the measure on the chart. An important disadvantage is that the plotted statistics are not independent from subgroup to subgroup and thus the Shewhart rules for runs and trends cannot be used. Only Rule 1 from Chapter Five (points outside the limits) can be used to detect special causes. Often users of these alternative charts forget about this lack of independence and improperly interpret the chart.

These weighted charts should not be considered to be replacements for the universal use of Shewhart charts. They are best used in specific situations where the process stability has been obtained and it is desirable to detect small changes in a process measure or to maintain a measure at its target value. Three types of time series charts will be discussed here: moving average (MA); cumulative sum (CUSUM); and exponentially weighted moving average (EWMA). Figure 7.13 shows the weights used for different versions of these three charts.

Moving Average Chart

A **moving average** (MA) chart uses averages calculated from consecutive subgroups created from consecutive observations. The MA chart is a common alternative to an individual chart when it is important to detect small, persistent shifts in the process average. Typically moving averages of 2–12 are used. A moving average of 12 is sometimes used with monthly data to plot an annual value and average out any seasonal effects (such as for asthma health measures). A moving average of 7 is often used with daily data to get a whole week in each subgroup. A moving average of 3 months is often used each month since board reports are based on quarterly data. As an example, Figure 7.13 showed the weighting scheme for moving averages of three and of five and the calculated moving averages are shown in Table 7.2:

[7]Roberts, S. W., "A Comparison of Some Control Chart Procedures," *Technometrics*, *8*(3), August 1966, 411–430.

FIGURE 7.13 Weighting Schemes for Alternative Charts

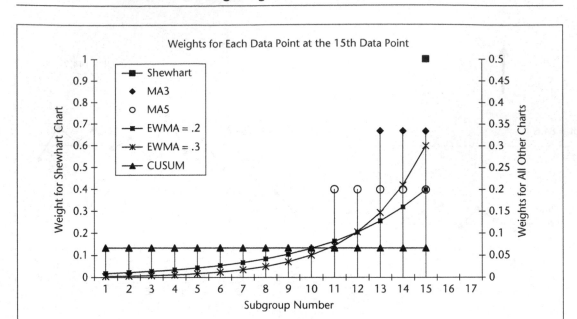

Table 7.2 Calculated Moving Averages of Three and Five

Subgroup	1	2	3	4	5	6	7	8	9
Measure	10	8	7	8	6	10	9	8	16
MA$_3$	10.0	9.0	8.3	7.7	7.0	8.0	8.3	9.0	11.0
MA$_5$	10.0	9.0	8.3	8.3	7.8	7.8	8.0	8.2	9.8

The moving average of three is constructed by averaging the last three subgroup values and plotting this average as a point. Several points in the moving average will be impacted by a single point that is affected by a special cause. The example in Table 7.2 shows the measure for nine subgroups with a moving average (MA) of length three (MA3) and five (MA5) calculated for each subgroup.

For both of these MA statistics, the calculated value for the first subgroup is 10.0, the first subgroup value and the moving average for the second subgroup is the average of the first two values. Note that in a moving average chart, the first few subgroups are special since there is not yet enough data to average three or more values. Thus, the UL and LL will be wider for the first few subgroups until the full number for the moving average are available. In general, the MA3 for subgroup i is the average of the means from subgroups i-2, i-1, and i.

Figure 7.14 shows four charts to illustrate the use of moving averages. The top chart shows run charts of quarterly HbA1c values for a diabetic patient. The individual values as well as moving averages of three and five are shown on the graph. The moving averages (plotted points), are averages calculated from artificial subgroups created from consecutive observations. Because each moving average incorporates historical data, the moving averages are not independent (this lack of independence over time is called **autocorrelation**). Note that none of the standard Shewhart chart special rules can be used, and be cautious when visually interpreting any trends or cycles in the moving average chart.

FIGURE 7.14   Moving Average Charts

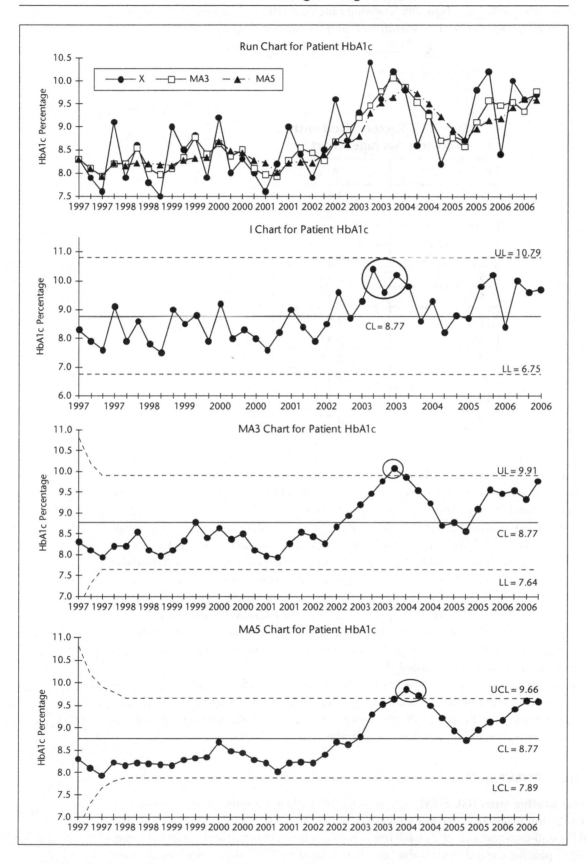

The control limits for a moving average chart use the same formula and factors as the and $\overline{X}$ chart (see Table 7.3). Typically a moving range with the same length as the moving average is used to determine the measure of common cause variation.

$$CL = \overline{X} = \text{average of subgroup values}$$
$$UCL = \overline{X} + (A_2 * \overline{R})$$
$$LCL = \overline{X} - (A_2 * \overline{R})$$

Table 7.3   Factors Used with Moving Average Chart

n	A_2
1	2.66
2	1.88
3	1.02
4	0.73
5	0.58
6	0.48
7	0.42
8	0.37
9	0.34
10	0.31
11	0.29
12	0.27

The bottom two charts in Figure 7.14 show moving average charts (MA3 and MA5) for the HbA1c. Because the moving averages are not independent, detecting runs or other trends is complex. Several points located near the control limits (2 out of 3 consecutive points in the outer third of the limits or beyond) on an MA chart do not have the significance they would on a traditional Shewhart control chart. Therefore the only rule that can be used to detect special causes on a moving average chart is a point(s) outside the control limits. Note that both of the MA charts detect special causes that were detected in the I chart (second from top) using the "2 out of 3 points in the outer third" rule.

As discussed above, moving average statistics are often misinterpreted when they are used to communicate performance. Exhibit 7.1 is a simple example that shows reviewers interpreting a three-month moving average statistic. This example illustrates the complexity on interpretation of this statistic. The comments for June and July are not consistent with the basic data, and will probably lead to improper reactions, making things worse, or frustrating process owners. So the complexity of interpreting the visual patterns in the charts is a big disadvantage of a moving average chart. Only consider using a moving average chart instead of an I chart when it is important to detect small, persistent changes or when there are seasonal patterns that it is desirable to average out of the data.

Cumulative Sum (CUSUM) Chart

The **cumulative sum (CUSUM)** statistic was introduced in Chapter Three as an alternative statistic for a run chart (see last section in Chapter Three on CUSUM run charts). The CUSUM statistic is the sum of the differences between the data points and a selected target. Instead of plotting the individual value, the chart using the CUSUM technique displays the cumulative evidence of change. The chart gives a clear presentation of changes in average

EXHIBIT 7.1   INTERPRETING MOVING AVERAGE STATISTIC OF INFECTION RATES

Month	Infections	Moving Average	Comments After Looking at Moving Average Statistic
March	7		
April	0		
May	2	3.0	
June	4	2.0	"Nice to see a 50% improvement this month from last month; please send a congratulatory note to the ICU manager"
July	2	2.7	"Oops, looks like things are getting worse this month, get Infection Control to visit the ICU"

levels and provides a visual indication of when the change began to occur. Figure 7.13 showed that each previous data point on the chart is given equal weight in the CUSUM statistic. So as the number of data points accumulates, the CUSUM is based on an increasing amount of data.

The cumulative sum statistic (S_i) is the sum of the deviations of the individual measurements from a target value:

$$S_i = S_{i-1} + (X_i - T), \text{ where}$$

S_i is the ith cumulative sum,

X_i = the ith observation,

T = Target (often the historical average)

An example of these calculations was shown in Chapter Three for patient satisfaction data (Table 3.7). Sometimes, when plotting the CUSUM statistic, the target value is added to S_i to make the plotted value more familiar. A stable process would thus appear in runs up and down around the target. Figure 7.15 shows the CUSUM run chart from Figure 3.44 in Chapter Three. The average of all the available data points is used as the target so the chart is forced to begin and end at the same value (the target of 88.3, as this value is added to each point before plotting).

A CUSUM control chart is designed to quickly detect change in performance associated with a small persistent change in the plotted statistic.[8] When the process is stable at the target level, the CUSUM statistic runs randomly at or above a horizontal axis (no slope). When a special cause occurs, the CUSUM slopes upward or downward and will eventually cross a control limit. The CUSUM chart will more quickly detect an average shift of one-half to two standard deviations than the I chart. Since the calculation of the control limits for a CUSUM chart are rather complex, applications are done with special software or a programmed spreadsheet calculation.

[8]Banard, G. A., "Control Charts and Stochastic Processes," *Journal of the Royal Statistical Society B21*, 1959, 230–271.

Evans, W. D., "When and How to Use Cu-Sum Charts," *Technometrics*, 1963, *5*, 1–22.

FIGURE 7.15   CUSUM Run Chart of Patient Satisfaction Data from Figure

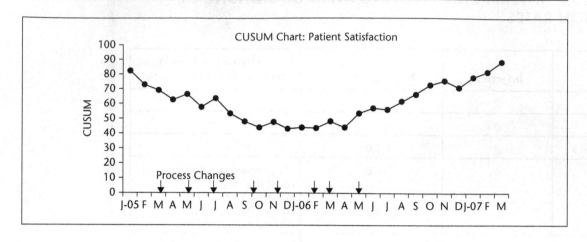

FIGURE 7.16   CUSUM Charts for Patient Satisfaction

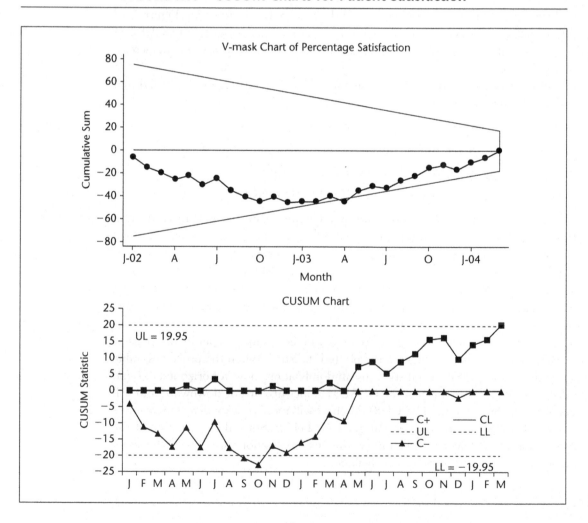

The CUSUM chart should be considered whenever data points are infrequent, difficult to obtain, or expensive, and it is desirable to quickly detect small changes in the process operating level. Figure 7.16, using the patient satisfaction data from Table 3.4, shows two different ways to develop control limits for this CUSUM chart:

1. Traditional V-mask (top chart in Figure 7.16). A "mask" in the shape of a V is laid over the CUSUM run chart with the origin over the last plotted point. Previous points (to the left of the current value of interest) outside the mask indicate the process has shifted.
2. An alternative form of limits (bottom chart in Figure 7.16) that required two CUSUM statistics to monitor increases (CUSUM value > 0) or decreases (CUSUM < 0) in the series.

The V-mask was used in the past when CUSUM charts were manually plotted for real time monitoring of processes. Today these calculations will be done using a computer. The CUSUM chart with more standard control chart limits is preferred, even though it requires the complexity of plotting and interpreting two series. Only the formula for this form of CUSUM charts is presented here. To calculate the control limits, a target and a measure of common cause variation (sigma) are first determined:

T = the average of the data series, a reference value, or a target (goal).

σ = an estimate of the common cause variation of the plotted points (this could come from the screened moving ranges of the data points, a pooled estimate of the within subgroup variation, or a theoretical value).

k = an allowance or slack value used in the CUSUM calculation. The value k can range from 0.2 to 1.0, but it is usually selected as 0.5 to best match the risks of a Shewhart chart for a stable process. Tables are available to select optimum values of k for different assumptions.[9]

Next, two cumulative series have to be calculated:

1. Accumulate derivations **above the target** with one statistic, $C+$
2. Accumulate derivations **below the target** with another statistic, $C-$

$C+$ and $C-$ are called upper and lower CUSUMS, respectively. The statistics are computed as follows:

$$C_i+ = \max [0, x_i - (T + k\sigma) + C_{i-1}+]$$
$$C_i- = \min [0, (k\sigma - T) + x_i + C_{i-1}-]$$

where T, k, and σ are defined above and x_i is the current data value. The control limits are set at plus or minus $h*\sigma$ from 0 (target). The value of h is usually set at 4 (when $k = 0.5$) to match the performance of the traditional Shewhart chart, but other combinations of k and h can be selected to meet specific objectives for the chart. See earlier reference by Lucas (1976) for a detailed discussion of these strategies. In analyzing a CUSUM chart the only rule for detecting special cause used is a point(s) beyond the limits. Either of the plotted series (C_i+ or C_i- going outside the control limit is an indication of a special cause. The slope of the plotted series can provide an indication of when the shift in the process average began. The bottom chart in Figure 7.16 shows the computational form

---

[9]Lucas, J., "The Design and Use of V-mask Control Schemes," *Journal of Quality Technology*, January 1976, *8*(1), 1–12. Evans, W. D., "When and How to Use Cu-Sum Charts."

Table 7.4 Calculation of CUSUM Statistic and Limits

Month	% Sat (X)	Average	X-Average (Si)	CUSUM	Screened MRs	C +	C −	CL	Upper Limit	Lower Limit
J-02	82	88.30	−6.30	−6.30		0.00	−4.08	0	17.73	−17.73
F	79	88.30	−9.30	−15.59	3	0.00	−11.16	0	17.73	−17.73
M	84	88.30	−4.30	−19.89	5	0.00	−13.24	0	17.73	−17.73
A	82	88.30	−6.30	−26.19	2	0.00	−17.32	0	17.73	−17.73
M	92	88.30	3.70	−22.48	10	1.49	−11.40	0	17.73	−17.73
J	80	88.30	−8.30	−30.78	12	0.00	−17.48	0	17.73	−17.73
J	94	88.30	5.70	−25.07	14	3.49	−9.56	0	17.73	−17.73
A	78	88.30	−10.30	−35.37	16	0.00	−17.64	0	17.73	−17.73
S	83	88.30	−5.30	−40.67	5	0.00	−20.72	0	17.73	−17.73
O	84	88.30	−4.30	−44.96	1	0.00	−22.80	0	17.73	−17.73
N	92	88.30	3.70	−41.26	8	1.49	−16.88	0	17.73	−17.73
D	84	88.30	−4.30	−45.56	8	0.00	−18.96	0	17.73	−17.73
J-03	89	88.30	0.70	−44.85	5	0.00	−16.04	0	17.73	−17.73
F	88	88.30	−0.30	−45.15	1	0.00	−14.12	0	17.73	−17.73
M	93	88.30	4.70	−40.44	5	2.49	−7.20	0	17.73	−17.73
A	84	88.30	−4.30	−44.74	9	0.00	−9.28	0	17.73	−17.73
M	98	88.30	9.70	−35.04	14	7.49	0.00	0	17.73	−17.73
J	92	88.30	3.70	−31.33	6	8.97	0.00	0	17.73	−17.73
J	87	88.30	−1.30	−32.63	5	5.46	0.00	0	17.73	−17.73
A	94	88.30	5.70	−26.93	7	8.95	0.00	0	17.73	−17.73
S	93	88.30	4.70	−22.22	1	11.44	0.00	0	17.73	−17.73
O	95	88.30	6.70	−15.52	2	15.92	0.00	0	17.73	−17.73
N	91	88.30	2.70	−12.81	4	16.41	0.00	0	17.73	−17.73
D	84	88.30	−4.30	−17.11	7	9.90	−2.08	0	17.73	−17.73
J-04	95	88.30	6.70	−10.41	11	14.39	0.00	0	17.73	−17.73
F	92	88.30	3.70	−6.70	3	15.87	0.00	0	17.73	−17.73
M	95	88.30	6.70	0.00	3	20.36	0.00	0	17.73	−17.73

of the CUSUM for the patient satisfaction data. Table 7.4 shows the calculations of the CUSUM statistics and the limits for the chart in Figure 7.16.

When a special cause is indicated on a CUSUM chart, the plot of the CUSUM statistic can be useful in determining the specific time period when the impact of the special cause first occurred. For example, in Figure 7.16, the special cause on the high side shows up after data point 27(M), but the CUSUM had a change in slope at point 16(A) (the C_i+ value started increasing after point 16). So the time period between points 16 and 17 would be a productive time period to look to identify circumstances associated with the special cause.[10]

Another issue when using a CUSUM chart is when to "restart" the CUSUM value. As the statistic is cumulative, all of the information in previous data values continues to be included in the CUSUM value plotted. After a special cause is detected and an appropriate reaction is taken, it is recommended to restart the CUSUM statistic at 0. Otherwise, the statistic would continue to indicate the special cause situation. Another option when restarting the CUSUM series is to use a "fast initial response" feature, restarting the CUSUM statistic to a fixed value rather than 0.[11]

Figure 7.17 shows a second example of a CUSUM chart. This example was introduced earlier in this chapter and evaluates quarterly HbA1c values for a diabetic patient. The chart is based on a target value of 8.77 = the average of the series. The chart shows the upper CUSUM staying near zero for the first half of the chart, meaning the measure is trending below the average HbA1c for this time period. This is verified by the lower CUSUM of the data trending downward with a special cause indicated with the 8th data point in 2001. It appears that the measure was running slightly below the average

FIGURE 7.17   CUSUM Chart of HbA1c Values

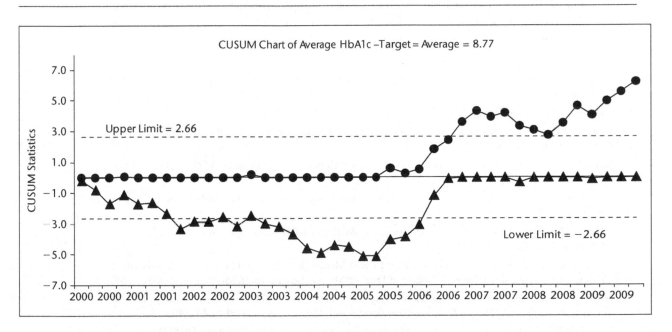

[10]Khoo, M., "Determining the Time of a Permanent Shift in the Process Mean of CUSUM Control Charts," *Quality Engineering*, 2005, *17*, 87–93.

[11]Lucas, J., and Crosier, R., "Fast Initial Response for CUSUM Quality-Control Schemes: Give Your CUSUM a Head Start," *Technometrics*, 1982, *24*(3), 199–205;.

Elder, R., Provost L., and Ecker, O., "USDA CUSUM Acceptance Sampling Procedures," *Journal of Quality Technology*, 1980, *13*, 59–64.

(downward slope) until the 17th point, when it became equal to the average (flat series). Starting with the 25th point, the series appears to be above the average until the end. A special cause for the upper CUSUM occurs on the 28th point (2006) indicating that the average HbA1c is now higher than the target. The point where the upper CUSUM becomes positive (point 25, 2005) should be investigated to understand the special cause.

Because of the complexity in both construction and interpretation of a CUSUM chart, some improvement teams are reluctant to use it. One option in these situations is to use a run chart or conventional Shewhart chart to present the data and annotate changes, but also do a behind the scene analysis of the data using a CUSUM chart to signal special causes.[12] The discussion of CUSUM here has focused on measures based on continuous data. CUSUM charts can also be used with attribute data and risk-adjusted data. See references for further discussion.[13]

The CUSUM chart has been discussed in the health care literature for more than thirty years.[14] In the past ten years, there have been numerous applications of CUSUM charts in health care systems described in the literature.[15] A study of these references may make improvers more comfortable with CUSUM charts.

Exponentially Weighted Moving Average (EWMA)

The **Exponentially Weighted Moving Average (EWMA)** control chart was introduced by Roberts.[16] The data series is the same as a geometric moving average, which is often used in economic models. The EWMA provides a formal way to use historical data which is intuitive to users. Morton et al. illustrate use of the EWMA chart in monitoring infections.[17] Figure 7.18 shows an EWMA for the same patient satisfaction data used in the CUSUM section. This chart does not show any clear special causes in the data.

The CUSUM chart gave the same weight to each previous data value. The logic of the EWMA is that the more recent data are likely to represent the current process more than very old data. More weight therefore is given to the most current data, less to the

[12]Lucas, J., "Combined Shewhart-Cusum Quality Control Schemes," *Journal of Quality Technology*, 1982 *14*(2), 51–59.

[13]Lucas, J., "Counted Data CUSUMs," *Technometrics*, 1985, *27*(2), 129–134.

Elder, R., Provost L., and Ecker, O., "USDA CUSUM Acceptance Sampling Procedures," *Journal of Quality Technology*, January 1981.

Reynolds M., and Stoumbos, Z., "A CUSUM Chart for Monitoring a Proportion When Inspecting Continuously," *Journal of Quality Technology*, 1999, *31*(1), 87–108.

Steiner, S., and et al., "Monitoring Surgical Performance Using Risk-Adjusted Cumulative Sum Charts," *Biostatistics*, 2000, *1*(4), 441–452.

[14]Wold, H., "The CUSUM Plot: Its Utility in the Analysis of Clinical Data," *New England Journal of Medicine*, 1977, *296*, 1044–1045.

[15]Sibanda, T., and Sibanda N., "The CUSUM Chart Method as a Tool for Continuous Monitoring of Clinical Outcomes Using Routinely Collected Data," BMC Medical Research Methodology, 2007, *7*(46).

Noyez, L., "A Review of Methods for Monitoring Performance in Healthcare Control Charts, CUSUM Techniques and Funnel Plots," *Interactive Cardiovascular* and *Thoracic Surgery*, 2009, *9*, 494–499.

Biau, D., "Quality Control of Surgical and Interventional Procedures: A Review of the CUSUM," *Quality and Safety in Health Care*, 2007, *16*, 203–207.

Chang, W. R., and McLean, O. P., "CUSUM: A Tool for Early Feedback About Performance?" *BMC Medical Research Methodology*, 2006, *6*(8).

[16]Roberts, S. W., "A Comparison of Some Control Chart Procedures."

[17]Morton, A. P., et al., "The Application of Statistical Process Control Charts to the Detection and Monitoring of Hospital-Acquired Infections," *Journal of Quality in Clinical Practice*, 2001, *21*(4), 112–117.

FIGURE 7.18   EWMA Data for Patient Satisfaction Data

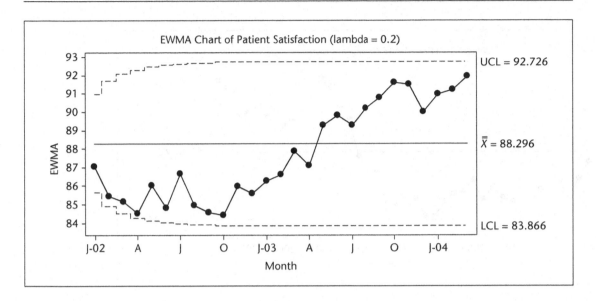

immediately past data, even less to data from two periods ago, and so on. These weights decrease exponentially: if 50% (.50) of the weight is given to the most recent data point, 50% of 50% (.25) would be given to the prior point, and $0.50^3 = .0625$ to the point before that. The exponentially weighted moving average (EWMA) statistic (z_i) is defined as:

$$z_i = \lambda x_i + (1 - \lambda)z_{i-1}$$

where z, is the data point, and $0 < 1\lambda < 1$ is a constant selected for the chart (note: usually set z_0 = the average of the series). The calculation of the statistic and the control limits would be done using a spreadsheet or appropriate software.

The control limits for the EWMA control chart are:

$$UCL = \mu_0 + 3\sigma\sqrt{\frac{\lambda}{(2 - \lambda)}\left[1 - (1 - \lambda)^{2i}\right]}$$

$$CL = \mu_0$$

$$LCL = \mu_0 - 3\sigma\sqrt{\frac{\lambda}{(2 - \lambda)}\left[1 - (1 - \lambda)^{2i}\right]}$$

The average (μ_0) of the data is usually used for the center line and σ is usually calculated using the screened moving range. As i gets larger, the term $[1 - (1 - 1)^{2i}]$ approaches infinity and the control limits reach a steady state value:

$$UCL = \mu_0 + 3\sigma\sqrt{\frac{\lambda}{2 - \lambda}}$$

$$CL = \mu_0$$

$$LCL = \mu_0 - 3\sigma\sqrt{\frac{\lambda}{2 - \lambda}}$$

Experience with EWMA charts suggests that a λ value between 0.1 and 0.3 gives the best performance. There are formal ways to estimate an optimum value for a particular

FIGURE 7.19   EWMA Data for HbA1c Values for Diabetic Patient

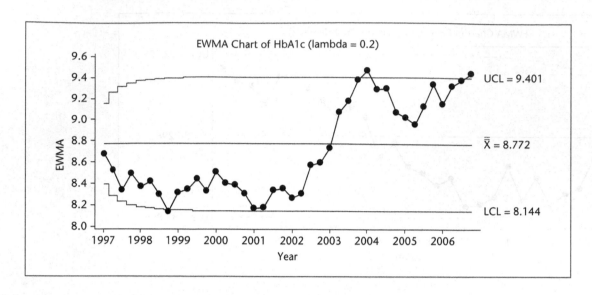

measure.[18] A large value of λ close to 1 approaches an I chart, whereas a small λ puts more weight on the previous data values. The two previous references give some rational for picking a value for λ.

Figure 7.19 shows a second example of an EWMA chart for the HbA1c values for a diabetic patient introduced earlier in the chapter. The low values detected in the CUSUM chart are also outside the control limit here. The high values starting after sample number 25 go above the upper limit at point 29.

Standardized Shewhart Charts

Shewhart charts with variable subgroup sizes ($\overline{X}$ and S chart, P chart, U chart) result in variable control limits. Sometimes this complexity in the appearance of the chart results in them not being used. An alternative is to create constant limits using the **standardized Shewhart chart**.[19] The statistics for any of the types of Shewhart charts can be transformed so that the resulting Shewhart chart has a mean (center line) of 0 and standard deviation of 1 (thus limits of ± 3.0). All the rules for special causes can be used with standardized Shewhart charts.

The transformation for standardization is:

$$S = (X - \mu) / \sigma,$$

where S is the standardized value, X is the original data value; μ is the mean, and σ the standard deviation of the original data. Using this transformation, data for all the types of Shewhart charts can be transformed so that the resulting chart has limits that are always:

$$CL = 0$$
$$UL = 3$$
$$LL = -3$$

---

[18]Hunter, J. S., "The Exponentially Weighted Moving Average," *Journal of Quality Technology*, October 1986, *18*(4), 203–210; Crowder, S. V., "Design of Exponentially Weighted Moving Average Schemes," *Journal of Quality Technology*, July 1989, *21*(3), 155–162.

[19]Nelson, L. S., "Standardization of Shewhart Control Charts," *Journal of Quality Technology*, October 1989, *21*(4), 287–289.

Table 7.5 shows the procedure to transform data from three different types of Shewhart charts to standardized charts. Figures 7.20, 7.21, and 7.22 show standardized charts for some of the examples from Chapter Five of the three types of charts with variable limits. Note that the general pattern of the plotted points on these charts and the interpretation of the chart is the same are the original charts in Chapter Five.

In addition to these three preceding standardized charts, Table 7.5 shows the formula for an I chart where there are different targets for various groups of the data points. In Chapter Five, an example of this type of chart for monitoring budgets was included (see Figure 5.5). This chart could be used in monitoring patient health when there are different expectations from time period to time period. Standardized control charts can also be used when some of the subgroups have different expected variation.

Multivariate Shewhart-Type Charts

A key concept discussed in Chapter Two on the use of data in improvement projects was that multiple measures (for example, a family of measures) were usually required to successfully document an improvement in health care systems. But all of the Shewhart charts discussed in Chapters Five and Six, and thus far in Seven, have been charts for one

Table 7.5   Creating Standardized Statistics for Shewhart Charts with Variable Limits

Shewhart Chart Type	Statistic Plotted	Mean of Statistic	Sigma of Statistic	Standardized Value to Plot
P chart	$P_i = 100^* d_i/n_i$	$P_{bar} = 100^* \Sigma d_i/\Sigma n_i$	$\sigma_p = \sqrt{P_{bar}^*(100-P_{bar})/n_i}$	$\dfrac{Pi-P_{bar}}{\sigma_p}$
U chart	$U_i = \Sigma c_i / \Sigma o_i$	$U_{bar} = \Sigma d_i / \Sigma n_i$	$\sigma = \sqrt{U_{bar}/O_i}$	$\dfrac{Ui-U_{bar}}{\sigma_U}$
$\bar{X}$ (with S)	$\bar{X}_i = \Sigma x_i / n_i$	$\bar{\bar{X}} = \Sigma n_i X_i / \Sigma n_i$	$\sigma\bar{x} = S_{bar} / \sqrt{n}$	$\dfrac{X_{bar}-\bar{\bar{X}}}{\sigma_{bar}}$
I chart (with variable group targets)	X_i	$\bar{X}_j = \Sigma x_i/n_i$ for each group j	$\sigma_x = MR/1.128$	$\dfrac{X_i-\bar{X}}{\sigma}$

FIGURE 7.20   Standardized $\bar{X}$ Chart from Figure 5.5, Chapter 5

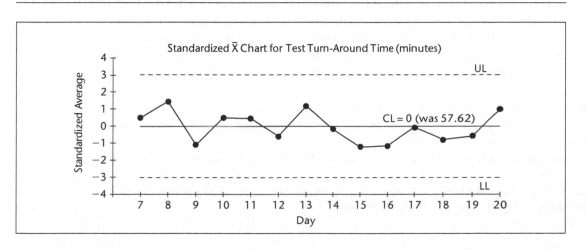

FIGURE 7.21   Standardized P Chart (Data Chapter 5, Fig. 5.11, P Chart with Variable Limits)

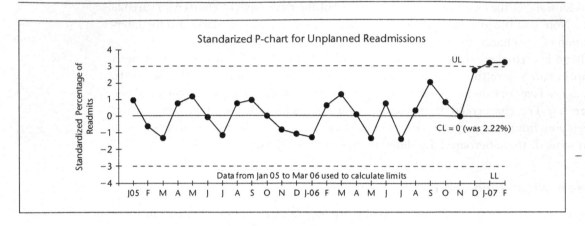

FIGURE 7.22   Standardized U Chart (Data from Figure 5.24, U Chart with Variable Limits)

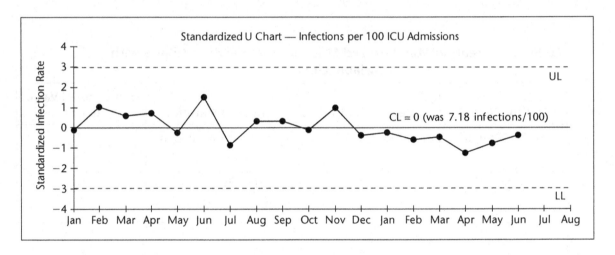

measure (an outcome or process measure). This is usually appropriate because we are interested in how each of the individual measures is affected by changes and often special causes that are specific to a particular measure. But there are times where it would be useful to jointly consider the performance of multiple measures at the same time (in one Shewhart-type chart). That is the objective of multivariate control charts.[20]

A multivariate control chart analyzes how multiple measures jointly influence a process or system. For example, you might use multivariate control charts to investigate how blood pressure, cholesterol levels, and blood sugars are varying for a diabetes patient. When the measures of interest are related to each other, the use of a multivariate chart has the ability to evaluate changes in the correlation structure as well as changes in the levels

---

[20]Jackson, J. E., "Quality Control Methods for Two Related Variables," *Technometrics*, 1959, *1*(4), 359–376.

Kourti, T., and MacGregor, J. F., "Multivariate SPC Methods for Process and Product Monitoring," *Journal of Quality Technology*, 1966, *28*(4), 409–428.

Elder, R. S., and Provost L. P., "Efficient Control Charts for Wastewater Laboratories," *American Laboratory*, July 1983.

Sullivan, J. H., and Woodall, W. H., "A Comparison of Multivariate Control Charts for Individual Observations," *Journal of Quality Technology*, 1966, *28*, 398–408.

FIGURE 7.23   General Form of Multivariate Control Chart
(T² Chart for Three Measures)

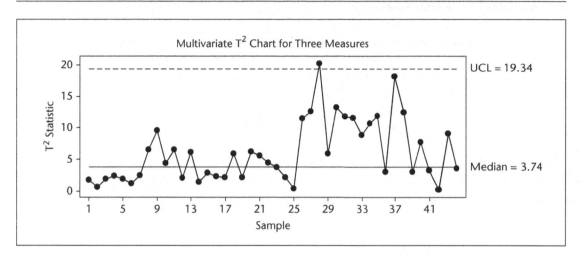

of the measures. Figure 7.23 shows the general form of a multivariate control chart. All of the rules for detecting special cause may be used with the multivariate control chart.

The primary advantage of a multivariate control chart is that a single control limit is used to determine whether the process is stable. However, multivariate charts can be more difficult to interpret than classic Shewhart control charts. For example, the scale on multivariate charts is unrelated to the scale of any of the measures, and special cause signals do not reveal which measure (or combination of measures) caused the signal. Another reason for the slow adoption of multivariate charts is the complexity of the calculation of the statistics and limits which require some knowledge of matrix algebra. The charts should begin to see more use as options for these multivariate charts appear in standard software for control chart calculations.

The multivariate equivalent to the Shewhart I chart or $\bar{X}$ chart for continuous data (see Chapter Five) is called the T^2 chart (often called Hotelling's T^2 chart[21]). To develop limits affected by only common cause variation, the construction of a T^2 chart is typically divided into two phases:

- Phase I: The analysis of a preliminary set of data that is assumed to be in a state of statistical control to develop control limits. This phase of data collection should include at least twenty subgroups of data so that the center line and limits are estimated with good precision. The subgroups associated with any signals of special causes are removed and then recalculated before using them in Phase II. One approach is to develop I charts for each of the measures that will be used in developing the T^2 chart and make sure they are all stable.
- Phase II: Use the limits (and summary statistics) estimated in Phase I to analyze data collected in the future. This distinction of phases is important with multivariate charts

---

[21]Hotelling, H. H., "Multivariate Quality Control Illustrated by the Air Testing of Sample Bombsights," *Techniques of Statistical Analysis*, 1947, 111–184.

Tracy, N., Young, J., and Mason, R., "Multivariate Control Charts for Individual Observations," *Journal of Quality Technology*, 1992, *24*(2), 88–95.

Sullivan, J. H., and Woodall, W. H., "A Comparison of Multivariate Control Charts for Individual Observations," *Journal of Quality Technology*, 1996, *28*(4), 398–408.

because the standard formulas are not robust to the presence of special causes in the Phase I data. For an I chart, there are some alternative methods to calculate the limits that are more robust to special causes.[22]

The Hotelling T^2 distance was proposed by Harold Hotelling in 1947. The statistic accounts for the covariance structure of the multiple measures of interest. The T^2 distance is a constant multiplied by a quadratic form obtained by multiplying the following three quantities:

$$T^2 = n(\bar{X} - \bar{\bar{X}}_0)s^{-1}(\bar{X} - \bar{\bar{X}}_0)$$

where n is the size of the subgroup, is the vector of the p sample means of the subgroup means, is the vector of the p sample subgroup means, and is the inverse of the pooled covariance matrix:

$$S = \frac{1}{n-1}\sum_{i-1}^{n} X_i - \bar{X}_i(X_i - \bar{X}_i)$$

Changes in the average, variation, or correlation structure all result in larger values of T^2, so there is no lower control limit. The upper control limit is:

$$UCL = \frac{knp - kn - np + p}{kn - k - p + 1}F_{\alpha, p, kn-k-p+1}$$

with n denoting the subgroup size, k the number of subgroups, and p the number of variables. The value of α for the F statistic is chosen so that $\alpha/(2p) = 0.00135$. This approximates the three-sigma limits for a Shewhart chart (assuming a normal distribution for the measures). The F-statistic can be found in a table in most statistics books or as a function in Excel.

When the T^2 statistic exceeds the control limit, additional analysis is required to determine the source of the special cause. One way to do that is to examine the individual Shewhart chart for each measure. A number of other alternatives have also been proposed.[23] Note: all the control chart rules for special causes can also be used with the T^2 chart.

Table 7.6 shows data from a hospital's financial system. The chief financial officer was interested in determining whether the financial situation had changed during the last two years as a number of new ideas were implemented in the charge and cost systems in the hospital. Because she knew that there were correlations among the measures, she chose to use a T^2 chart to study the variation in the measures.

Figure 7.24 shows initial T^2 (Phase I) chart calculated using the baseline data from 2004 and 2005. The T^2 chart indicates a stable process, so the limits (and estimated means and covariance matrix) were used to extend the chart for 2006 and nine months in 2007 (Phase II use of T^2 chart in Figure 7.24). The extended chart in Figure 7.25 shows special causes starting in February 2006. The financial measures seemed to return to the 2004–2005 levels after February 2007. The T^2 chart does not provide any information on which measures are contributing to the special causes, thus I charts for each measure can be used to understand the special cause.

[22]Williams, J., Woodall, W., and Birch, J., "Distribution of Hotelling's T^2 Statistic Based on the Successive Differences Estimator," *Journal of Quality Technology*, July 2006, *38*(3), 217–229.

[23]Hayter, A. J., and Tsui, K., "Identification and Quantification in Multivariate Quality Control Problems," *Journal of Quality Technology*, 1994, *26*(3), 197–208.

Table 7.6   Monthly Hospital Financial Data (Units 5 Millions of Dollars) over Four Years

Month	Costs	Charges	Profit
J-04	161	289	102
F	169	311	105
M	155	282	109
A	172	305	110
M	180	327	115
J	163	296	97
J	175	312	98
A	153	268	96
S	171	289	87
O	180	316	116
N	161	279	83
D	152	294	110
J-05	182	316	93
F	173	316	129
M	170	328	130
A	179	321	106
M	172	309	124
J	168	299	74
J	158	284	105
A	180	322	83
S	162	284	79
O	188	339	113
N	172	311	137
D	168	299	98
J-06	157	296	119
F	148	308	137
M	161	328	167
A	164	335	190
M	170	332	153
J	140	280	162
J	163	330	166
A	168	324	176
S	141	285	147
O	144	295	106
N	136	268	76
D	150	295	126
J-07	131	276	94
F	133	279	127
M	180	338	132
A	191	332	114
M	185	338	124
J	167	309	109
J	152	268	65
A	169	301	85
S	160	270	78

FIGURE 7.24   T² Chart for First Two Years' Financial Data

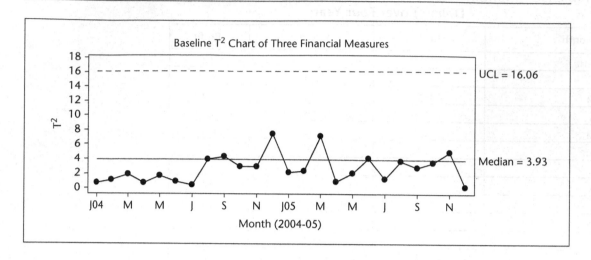

FIGURE 7.25   T² Chart for Three Financial Measures—Baseline Limits Extended

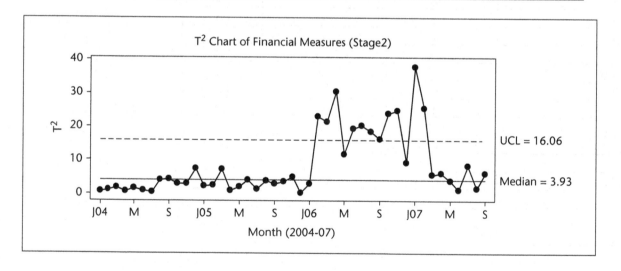

Figure 7.26 shows the three I charts for the three financial measures. The limits are based on the first two years of data (same as the T² chart). The chart for charges is stable, while both the costs and profit I charts show special causes beginning early in 2005. Thus the indicators of special causes can be attributed to the lower costs and increased profits in 2005. Both of these charts appear to have returned to the 2004–2005 levels in 2006.

Multivariate charts can also be developed using CUSUM and EWMA statistics. Specialty software is required for these charts.

FIGURE 7.26   I Charts for Three Financial Measures (Limits Based on 2004–2005 Data)

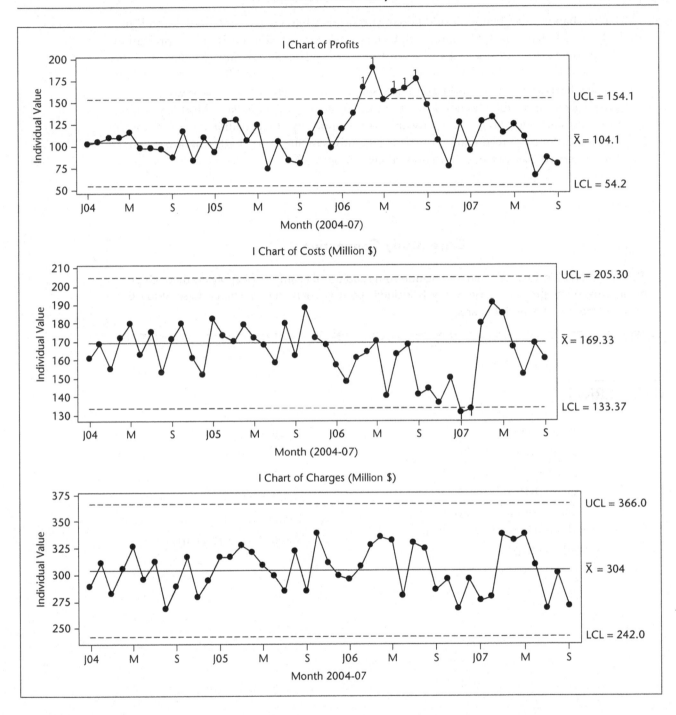

SUMMARY

This chapter described some additional types of Shewhart charts (NP Chart, $\bar{X}$ and Range charts, Median chart, G chart, and T chart) that are useful in health care applications and some advanced methods to learn from data collected over time (Moving Average, CUSUM, and EWMA). The Standardized Shewhart Chart and Multivariate Shewhart-type Charts were also introduced. These specific charts were selected because all of them have been successfully used to learn from variation in health care data. Most applications of these charts are done using software so the complexity of calculation and display is not an issue. But the interpretation of these alternatives to Shewhart charts can be tricky since the standard special cause rules do not always apply.

Case Study Connection

The case studies in Chapter Thirteen include some additional examples of applying these charts on improvement projects. Case Study B includes both G charts and T charts. Case Study G includes the use of X and R charts.

KEY TERMS

Autocorrelation

Cumulative sum (CUSUM)

Exponentially weighted moving average (EWMA)

G chart [number of events, items, and so on between rare events]

Median chart

Moving average

Multivariate Shewhart-type charts

NP chart

Standardized Shewhart chart

T chart (time between rare events)

$\bar{X}$ and Range (R) charts

## CHAPTER 8

SPECIAL USES FOR SHEWHART CHARTS

This chapter describes a number of modifications to Shewhart charts that may be useful in special situations. When applying Shewhart charts to measures from health care processes, some situations arise where the basic methods need to be modified. This chapter addresses some of these common situations. The objective is to make the reader aware of these complexities and learn how to deal with them when they show up in improvement work.

The following situations are discussed in this chapter: Shewhart charts with a changing center line; Shewhart charts with seasonal effects; transformation of data with Shewhart charts; Shewhart charts for autocorrelated data; Shewhart charts for attribute data with large subgroup sizes (over-dispersion); comparison charts; confidence intervals and confidence limits; and Shewhart charts for case-mix adjusted data.

SHEWHART CHARTS WITH A CHANGING CENTER LINE

All of the charts presented thus far in this book have a constant, horizontal center line. There are some circumstances when it may be appropriate to include a center line that varies:

1. When there are consistent seasonal or day-of-the-week effects that are expected to repeat from period to period.
2. When there is an expected increase (growth) or decrease (decline) in the center line.
3. When other factors would lead to an expectation that the center line will be different at certain time periods in the chart.

In all these cases, an approach similar to the standardized charts described in Chapter Seven could be used to adjust the data so that the center line is a constant value. But it may be useful to the users of the chart to maintain the nonconstant center line for ease of interpretation and for using the chart for prediction.

Shewhart Charts with a Sloping Center Line[1]

Figure 8.1 shows an example of an I chart for the U.S. median percentage of obesity since 1989. The center line is based on a linear regression analysis (Y = median, X = year, with 1989 = year 1). The analysis shows a system increasing at a stable rate of about 0.9% per year.

---

[1]Grant, E. L., and Leavenworth, R. S., *Statistical Quality Control*, 7th ed., New York: McGraw-Hill, 1980, 298–302.

FIGURE 8.1 **Chart with Slanted Center Line for Obesity Data**

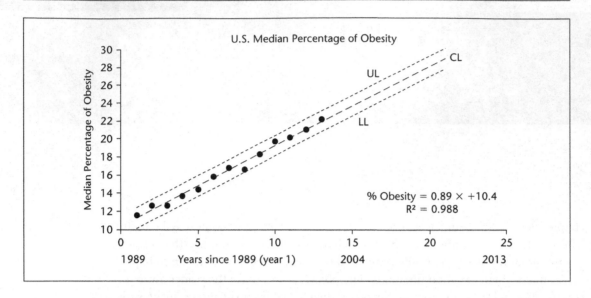

U.S. Median Percentage of Obesity

% Obesity = 0.89 × +10.4
R² = 0.988

Median Percentage of Obesity

Years since 1989 (year 1)

1989   5   10   2004   20   2013

CL, UL, LL

The steps to construct a Shewhart chart with a trend are outlined below for individual measurements. Regression analysis is used to develop the center line. Note that the moving range cannot be used directly as before, but rather the moving range is based on the residuals from the regression line. Using the moving range directly will result in an inflated estimate of the common cause variation due to the trend.

1. Develop a regression line for the data versus time.
2. Calculate the residual for each data value (R_i = Expected Value from Regression − X_i).
3. Calculate k–1 moving ranges (MR_R), using the residuals. Calculate:

$$\overline{MR}_R \ (\Sigma MR_R)/ \ (k-1)$$

4. Use the $\overline{MR}_R$ with the usual control chart constants to screen the $\overline{MR}_R$ and to calculate the location of the limits on chart:

$$\pm \ 2.66 * \overline{MR}_R$$

5. Draw in the center line for the chart using the values estimated from the regression line. Use the first and last subgroups in the data set, and then connect these points with a straight line.
6. Draw in the control limits using the values calculated in step 4 to determine how far above and below the center line the limits should be placed. It is easiest to measure from the center line values from step 5 at the ends of the data set, and then connect these points to obtain each limit.

    (Note: all these steps can be done using a spreadsheet and graphics package such as Excel).

Although interpretation of the control chart with a trend is essentially the same as for conventional control charts, the special cause rule of six points trending up or down should not be used, due to difficulties in interpreting the trend relative to the sloping data points. In addition to special causes associated with specific circumstances, the slanted control chart may show signals of special causes if the trend is not linear.

FIGURE 8.2   Shewhart Chart for Delay for an Appointment

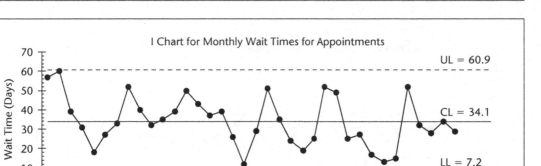

Shewhart Charts with Seasonal Effects

A second example is based on a measure with suspected **seasonal effects**, one that is expected to change during different seasons of the year. A group of pediatricians monitor key measures for their asthma patients. Figure 8.2 shows an I chart for one of their monthly measures: wait time for an appointment. Some of their Shewhart charts showed special causes (in both positive and unfavorable directions), but the doctors were concerned that maybe these were just simply seasonal variations rather than evidence of improvement or problems. Some of their theories for seasonal effects were associated with flu season, asthma seasons, and back-to-school appointments.

There are a number of ways to study seasonal effects. For continuous data (wait times here), one way is to fit a time series model to the data that includes seasonal effects.[2] Then use the model to adjust the data to remove these effects. The residuals from the model can then be studied on a Shewhart chart to see if there are other special causes (for example, from improvement efforts). A simpler, alternative approach is to compute the average for each month, calculate the average deviation from the center line, and use an $\overline{X}$ and S chart to determine if any of the months are special. At least two years of historical data are needed to do this, and it is useful to have three or more years.

Figure 8.3 shows the $\overline{X}$ chart for the average deviations from the center line of each of the 12 months (in time order on the chart). The S chart was also constructed and was stable. The $\overline{X}$ chart shows three months special high (January, February, and August) and three months special low (May, June, and July).

Based on this analysis these seasonal effects were determined to be important:

High Months	Average Deviation	Low Months	Average Deviation
January	18.9	May	−13.7
February	16.6	June	−16.7
August	17.6	July	−8.4
Average	17.7	Average	−12.9

[2]Nelson, C. R., *Applied Time Series Analysis for Managerial Forecasting*, San Francisco: Holden-Day, 1973.

FIGURE 8.3   Study of Average Deviations (from Overall Average) for Wait Times

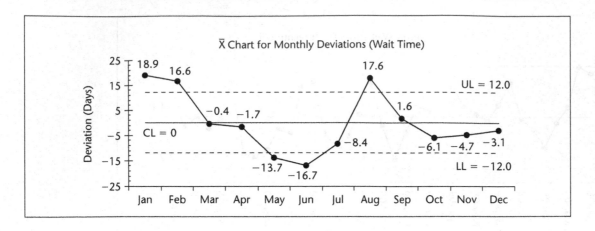

FIGURE 8.4   Individual Chart for Adjusted Wait Times

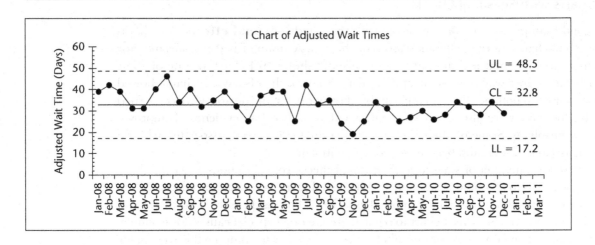

Having determined the monthly effects, the monthly data could be adjusted by adding and subtracting these effects. This approach is a modification to the standardized charts discussed in Chapter Seven with the average deviation as the target for the high and low months. Figure 8.4 shows this I chart for the adjusted wait time data. The common cause variation in this chart is much less than the initial chart in Figure 8.2; thus, with the seasonal effects removed, the I chart is more sensitive to detect special causes. Some users of a chart like this would be uncomfortable with the adjusted data and the fact that the chart is not useful for prediction of the actual wait times for future months.

Another choice is to use the monthly effects to adjust the center line to display a different expectation for each of the months with an important effect. Then the limits are calculated from the appropriate center line each period. Figure 8.5 shows this format for the wait time chart from Figure 8.2. An advantage of this presentation is that when using the chart for prediction, the expectation for future months is clear (for example, this January and February are coming up, so we can expect a longer wait time for an appointment).

Figure 8.6 shows a P chart for another of the team's monthly measures: the percentage of their asthma patients who had emergency visits in the last month. For attribute data like this, the use of rational subgroups defined by each month can be used to test for

FIGURE 8.5 Wait Time Chart with Adjusted Center Line

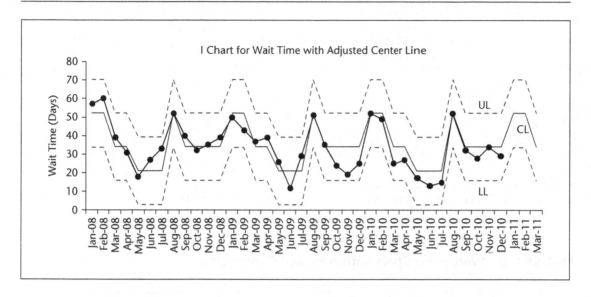

FIGURE 8.6 Shewhart Charts for Emergency Asthma Visits

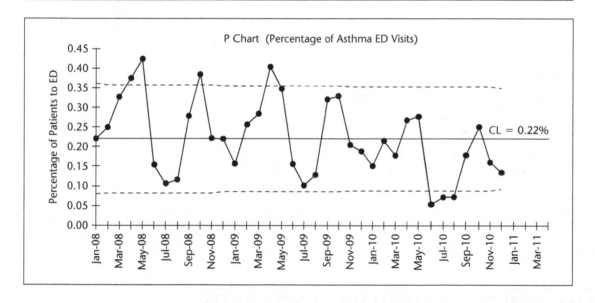

the importance of seasonal effects. Figure 8.7 shows a P chart for this measure using the same data as in Figure 8.6, but with the 12 subgroups defined by each month of the year. April, May, and October are special on the high side, whereas June, July, and August are special with fewer emergency visits for asthma patients. Figure 8.8 shows the P chart from Figure 8.6 with the center lines adjusted for these special months. After accounting for the seasonal effects, there is a run of more than eight points below the adjusted center line in the last year (starting in November 2009). This is a signal that there has been a consistent reduction in emergency room visits. This trend was not clear in the original chart in Figure 8.6 because of the special monthly effects. Although this chart with the adjusted center line is more complex visually than the standardized chart, users may prefer it for predicting outcomes in future months.

FIGURE 8.7   P Chart to Study Monthly Effects

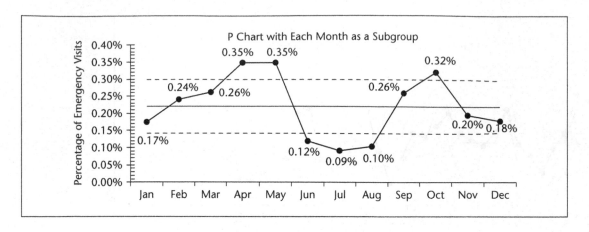

FIGURE 8.8   Wait Time Chart with Adjusted Center Line

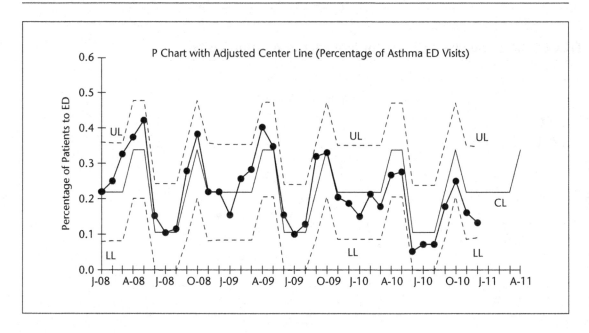

TRANSFORMATION OF DATA WITH SHEWHART CHARTS

Chapter Two discussed the use of transformations to enhance learning from data. Shewhart charts are very robust to a variety of distributions of data. Some authors have mistakenly assumed that a Shewhart chart is based on a normal distribution and suggest testing data for fit to a normal distribution prior to developing a Shewhart chart. As discussed in Chapter Four, this approach is the opposite of Dr. Shewhart's intention to first establish the stability of data using the Shewhart Chart, and then consider statistical inferences of interest (such as a capability analysis as described in Chapter Five). So the complexity in this chapter of introducing transformations is not to achieve a normal distribution. But sometimes a transformation is useful when Shewhart's methods lead to a chart that is not helpful for learning.

Chapters Five and Six warned about the effect of the distribution of data on an I chart. The limits for an I chart will be more sensitive than an $\bar{X}$ chart to the shape of the distribution of the measurements, but in most cases the limits still provide a good economic balance between overreacting and underreacting to variation in the process (Chapter Four details the costs of these two mistakes). However, when the data range over more than an order of magnitude (10, 100, 1,000, and so on) or when the data are highly skewed in one direction (for example, measurements of time) the limits on the I chart will benefit from transformation of the data.

In these extreme cases, it was suggested that the measurements be transformed prior to developing the Shewhart chart to alleviate these situations. Common transformations are the logarithm for multiple orders of magnitudes and the square root for skewed data. What are indications on an I chart that we might have an extreme case?

1. If the lower limit is below zero for a measure that has to be greater than or equal to zero (for example, time to complete a service)
2. If significantly more than half of the data are below the average (obvious by visual inspection)

The options in these extreme cases are:

Option 1: Put the data in subgroups and create an $\bar{X}$S (or R) chart. The Central Limit Theorem states that the averages for any distribution will approach a symmetric distribution (specifically a normal distribution) as the number of values averaged increases. But the S chart may still be affected by the skewness. If there are numerous special causes on the S chart, a transformation may still be useful.

Option 2: Transform the data into a more symmetric distribution.

Typical transformations for data (X) that are highly skewed are:

- Square Root $\sqrt{X}$
- Logarithmic: $\log_{10} X$ or $\ln X$ (no 0 values possible for the measure)
- Reciprocal of data: $1/X$ (no 0 values possible for the measure)

When an initial I chart indicates that the data may be highly skewed, the following steps should be considered:

1. Create a frequency plot of data.
2. If the frequency plot is not symmetric, and you don't think that special causes are the dominating issue, try transformations to get data symmetric.
3. Deal with 0 values in order to use the logarithm or reciprocal transformation. A common default is to add a small value to all the data points or to set 0 value at half the lowest value in the data set.
4. Look at frequency plots of the transformed data to see if it is symmetric.
5. Once a transformation is found where the distribution is somewhat symmetric, calculate I chart limits using transformed data.
6. Do reverse transformation of the center line and limits in order to plot the data in its original units.
7. Plot the chart using the original data and the limits that have been transformed back into the original units.

8. Sometimes it is more appropriate to present the data on a logarithm scale so it is easier to visually see points below the center line.

9. Note that the estimates of the mean (and other statistics) in the original scale for the reverse transformed values will be biased. Adjustments to these estimates should be made, depending on the transformation used.

An example of using a transformation with an I chart, is the presentation of the T chart (time between incidents) illustrated in Chapter Seven. A power transformation was used to get the data symmetric ($y = x^{0.2777}$) and then after the center line and limits were calculated, they were transformed back into the original scale using $t = y^{3.6}$.

As another example of using a transformation, Figure 8.9 shows an I chart for the time required to complete a report after close of business at the end of each week. The system was originally designed to produce a report within two hours of close of business. In March, some reports were not available until the following day. An investigation completed in July produced the data used to develop the I chart. The chart shows special causes in March but a run of 11 points below the center line in the most recent weeks. However, the lower limit for the chart was less than 0 (for time data) and more than half the points were below the center line. Both of these are sign of a Shewhart chart that may not be useful for learning. A transformation of the data should be considered in situations like this.

Figure 8.10 shows frequency plots for the original data (in minutes), and also a square root and log base 10 transformation of the data. The skewness of the original data appears clear from this picture. The square-root transformation still shows a skewed distribution, whereas the data from the logarithm transformation looks symmetrical with a spike at the grouping with the value 2.7. The logarithm was selected as an appropriate transformation and the I chart in Figure 8.11 calculated from these data.

The I chart in Figure 8.11 can be easily interpreted and special causes identified. The pattern of special causes is much clearer when using the limits calculated from the transformed data. A disturbing pattern not obvious in the original chart is the steady increase in completion time during the last month. Although this presentation of the chart is fine for understanding the patterns of variation, many users are more comfortable analyzing

FIGURE 8.9   Ineffective I Chart for Time to Complete Administrative Task

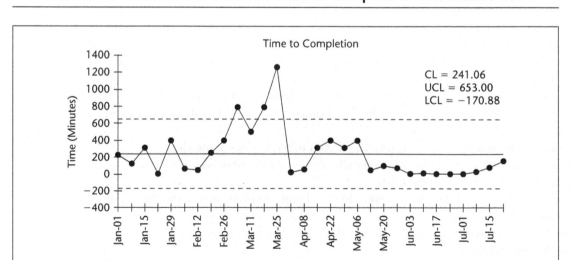

data in the units to which they are accustomed (minutes in this case). Figures 8.12 and 8.13 show steps 6, 7, and 8 (from previous list) for developing Shewhart charts for transformed data. The center line and limits are transformed back to the original scale (minutes) and plotted with the original data (Figure 8.10). Note that the center line and lower limit are compressed near the bottom of the chart, making it difficult to see whether points are above or below the limit. Another option is to plot the exact same data on a logarithmic vertical axis (Figure 8.13). This last chart appears like Figure 8.11, but the units are in minutes. For display, pick a presentation (Figures 8.11, 8.12, or 8.13) that is most comfortable to the users. Figure 8.12 is the most common presentation.

FIGURE 8.10   Frequency Plots for Data and Transformations (Time for Weekly Task)

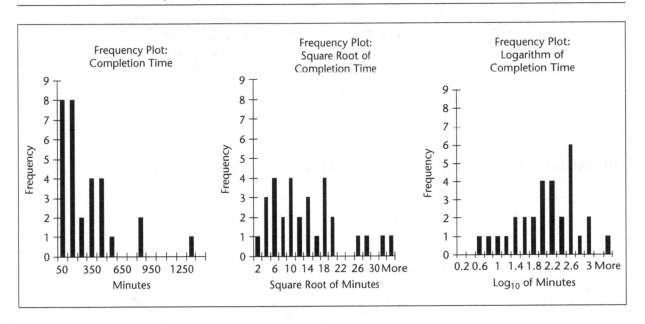

FIGURE 8.11   I Chart Developed from Transformed Data

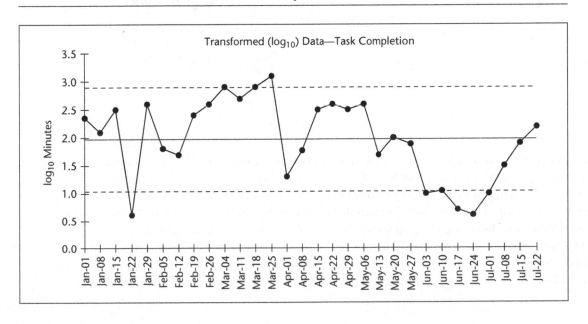

FIGURE 8.12   I Chart Transformed Back to Original Scale

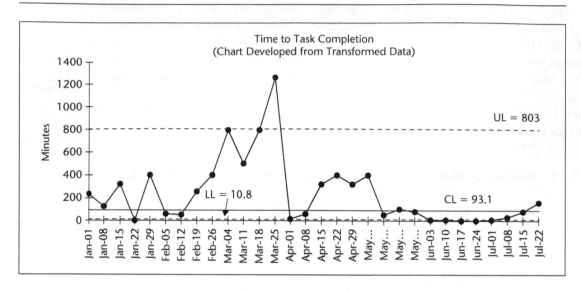

FIGURE 8.13   I Chart for Transformed Data Displayed on a Log$_{10}$ Scale

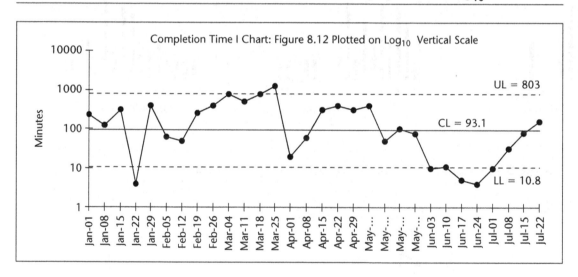

Sometimes it is also useful to transform data even when using an $\overline{X}$ and S chart. Figure 8.14 shows the initial $\overline{X}$ and S chart for a measure of time from arrival in the emergency department until initiating treatment (for a particular group of patients). A number of points on the S chart indicated special causes. Investigation of the data indicated that these subgroups all had some extreme (but not unusual) waiting times.

The frequency plots in Figure 8.15 indicated a highly skewed distribution of waiting times which became symmetric with a log$_{10}$ transformation. An $\overline{X}$ and S chart was calculated on the transformed data. Then the statistics ($\overline{X}$, S), center line, and limits were

FIGURE 8.14 X̄ and S Chart for ED Times from Arrival to Treatment

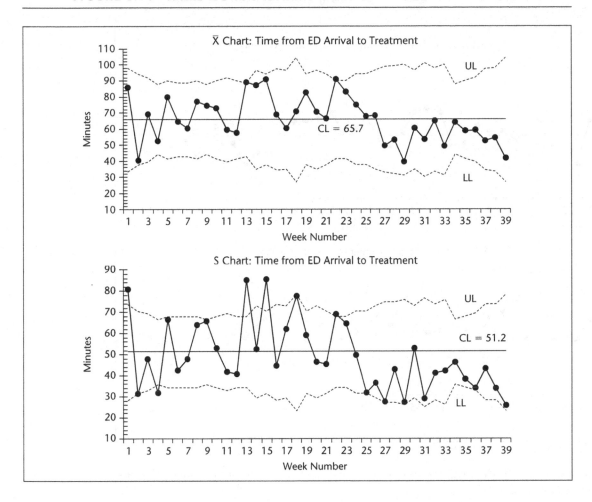

FIGURE 8.15 Frequency Plots for Original and Log$_{10}$ Transformed Data

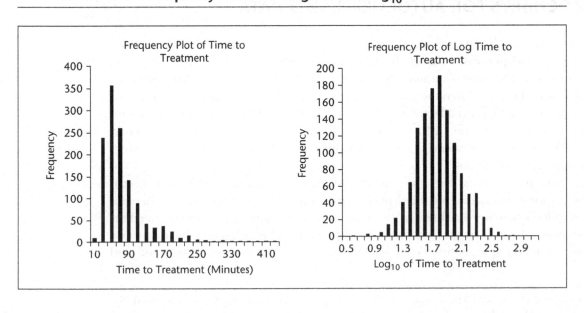

FIGURE 8.16 $\bar{X}$ and S Chart Based on Log$_{10}$ Transformed ED Times

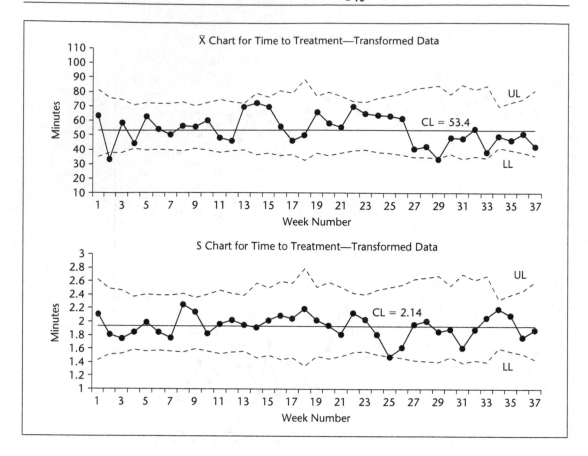

transformed back to the original time scale. The charts based on the transformation are shown in Figure 8.16.

SHEWHART CHARTS FOR AUTOCORRELATED DATA

A basic assumption in determining the limits for Shewhart charts is that the data for each subgroup are independent—that is, the data from one subgroup does not help us predict another period. The most common way this assumption is violated is when special causes are present in the data. Then the subgroups associated with the special causes tend to be more alike than subgroups affected only by common causes. The result is that these subgroups show up as "special," which is exactly what the chart was designed to do. Thus, most of the time when someone is concerned with autocorrelation, there are special causes to uncover and learn about.

But sometimes process operations or data collection procedures result in data affected only by common causes that is not independent from subgroup to subgroup. This phenomenon is called **autocorrelation**.[3] With a positive autocorrelation, successive data points will be similar. For time-ordered data, subgroups close together will tend to be more alike than subgroups far apart in time. With negative autocorrelation, successive points will tend

---

[3]Montgomery, D. C., and Mastrangelo, C. M., "Some Statistical Process Control Methods for Autocorrelated Data," *Journal of Quality Technology*, 1991, *23*, 179–193.

to be dissimilar, resulting in a sawtooth pattern. Shewhart charts with autocorrelated data may be analyzed for evidence of special cause using Rule 1 only (a point outside the limits). The autocorrelated relationship between the plotted points would make all the additional rules used with Shewhart charts invalid. With continuous data (I chart and the $\overline{X}$ and S chart and the other advanced charts for continuous data discussed in Chapter Seven), the usual limits might not be accurate expressions of the common cause variation, and the autocorrelation will result in an increase in false signals of special causes. Limits for charts made for continuous autocorrelated data may require adjustment before the limits are usable. For attribute data, the limits are useful for analysis and require no adjustment to be made.

A common example of autocorrelation in clinical operations is analyzing data that is managed in a computerized registry for patients with chronic diseases such as diabetes, asthma, or cardiovascular disease. Typically these patients visit the clinic every two to four months and clinical tests and observations are done to monitor their health status. In some clinics, the average value or overall percentage of the various measures in the registry are summarized each month and used to monitor the performance of the clinic for that particular population of patients (see case study at the end of Chapter One for an example of this practice). The autocorrelation problem occurs because the data for most patients is not updated each month; this is done only for patients who come in for a visit. If one-third of the patients come in during the current month and have their data updated, the monthly summary will use the same data as the previous month for two-thirds of the patients. This creates a statistical relationship—that is, autocorrelation—between the monthly measures.

When analyzing autocorrelated data, the difficulty is in separating the effect of special causes from false signals created by the autocorrelation. Figure 8.17 shows an I chart for the average glycated hemoglobin test (HbA1c value) from a registry of about 130 adult patients with diabetes. Patients are scheduled to visit the clinic every three months, so about one-third visit each month and their registry values are updated.

The chart indicates numerous special causes: 10 points outside limits, runs below the center line, and numerous points near the limits. Are these special causes or the impact of autocorrelation due to the use of the registry values? Because of the way the data are collected for this chart, autocorrelation was expected.

One way to examine the autocorrelation is to create a scatter diagram by plotting each point versus the point after it (data point i and data point I + 1). Figure 8.18 shows the scatter diagram for the HbA1c data in Figure 8.17. The current subgroup value is plotted on the x-axis with the point immediately after it on the y-axis. A regression analysis and

FIGURE 8.17   Chart for Average HbA1c Values from Registry

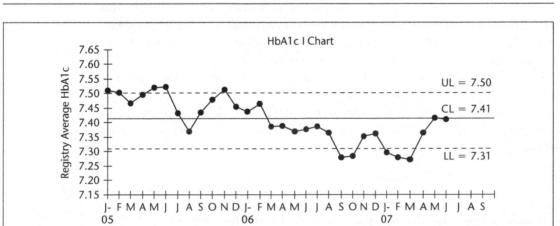

FIGURE 8.18   Scatter Plot to Evaluate Autocorrelation of Registry Data

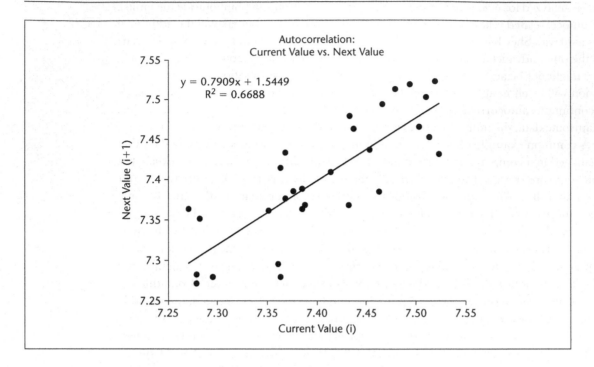

the R^2 value (R^2 is the correlation squared and represents the percentage of the variation in the next month's value that can be explained by the current subgroup value). The square root of this value, r, is the correlation coefficient and represents the autocorrelation (r = 0.82 here). Shewhart charts are robust to low levels of autocorrelation. If the autocorrelation coefficient is less than 0.50, the autocorrelation issue can be ignored, but if it is greater than 0.80, some alternative should be considered.[4] If the autocorrelation is between 0.50 and 0.8, addressing it is at the discretion of the user.

The following are some of the approaches to deal with autocorrelation detected on a Shewhart chart:

1. Identify the source of the autocorrelation and take appropriate actions to learn from it and incorporate it into improvement strategies.
2. If the autocorrelation is due to the sampling or measurement strategy, modify the data collection to reduce its impact.
3. Continue to learn from and monitor the process as a run chart (using only visual analysis, not using run chart rules). When the autocorrelation coefficient is greater than 0.8, the patterns on the run chart cannot be interpreted directly. Sudden changes or unusual data points will be readily apparent on the chart.
4. Use time series analysis to model the data series and analyze the residuals from the time series using a Shewhart chart.[5]
5. For continuous data, make adjustment to the control limits to compensate for the autocorrelation (see footnote 2). The recommended adjustment is to increase the limits by multiplying by the factor:

$$1/\sqrt{1 - r^2} \text{ or sigma} = \overline{MR} / [d_2 * \text{sqrt } (1 - r^2)]$$

---

[4]Wheeler, D., *Advanced Topics in Statistical Process Control*, Knoxville, TN: SPC Press, 1995, Chapter 12.

[5]Nelson, *Applied Time Series Analysis for Managerial Forecasting*.

FIGURE 8.19 I Chart with Limits Adjusted to Compensate for Autocorrelation

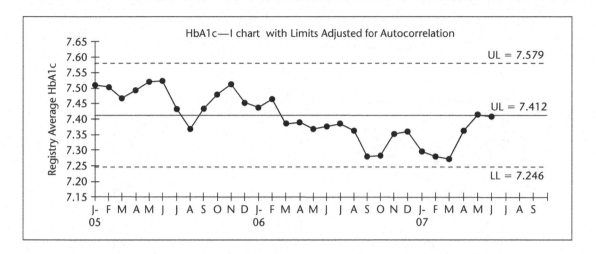

FIGURE 8.20 I Chart for Visit Cycle Time in a Specialty Clinic

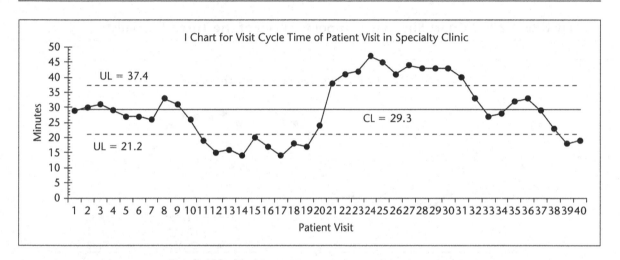

Figure 8.19 shows the I chart in Figure 8.17 with the adjustment in option 5. Note that all of the data points are inside the limits on the I chart. Because of the autocorrelation, none of the alternative rules for special causes can be used to identify special causes.

Because the limits for attribute charts are calculated from theoretical formula based on a statistical distribution, autocorrelation does not affect the limits. So even with autocorrelation, the limits can be used to detect special causes using Rule 1 (a point outside the limits), but none of the other four rules for special causes can be used to identify special causes.

As noted at the beginning of this section, a process measure that contains many special causes will often exhibit patterns that look like autocorrelation. For example, the I chart in Figure 8.20 was prepared by the team to study the visit cycle time for consecutive patients in a specialty clinic where three different doctors practice.

After viewing the chart, one of the team members expected problems with autocorrelation, so the team prepared the scatter plot in Figure 8.21. The high value of r^2 (autocorrelation = .905) could indicate autocorrelation that must be dealt with in order to use the limits on the chart. But, when reviewing the chart, the clinic receptionist noted that "it was pretty clear which of the specialists were in the office each day." From her experiences, she was aware of different average cycle times for each of the doctors. Based on the receptionist's

FIGURE 8.21 **Scatter Plot for Autocorrelation**

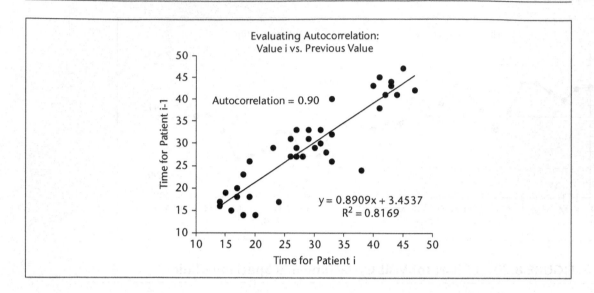

FIGURE 8.22 **I Chart Showing Symbol for Each of the Three Specialists**

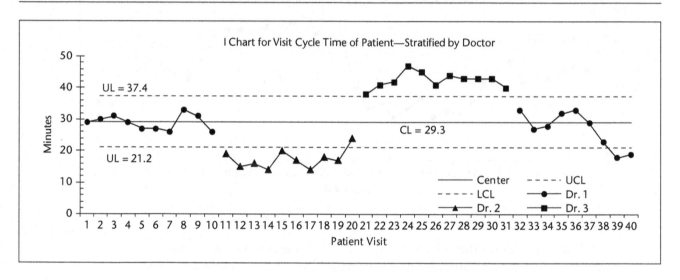

comments, the QI team prepared the chart in Figure 8.22, with a different symbol for each of the three specialists. The patterns associated with the doctors are very clear. So it is critical to do a thorough analysis of special causes before thinking about autocorrelation.

In summary, the effect of autocorrelation on time-ordered charts can create some complications in interpreting data. Some useful guidance includes:

- When learning from data using a run chart, don't use the three probability-based rules for detecting a signal (shift, trend, number of runs) as they are based on an assumption of independence of the data. When using run charts with autocorrelated data rely only on visual analysis of the graph.
- When using a Shewhart Chart, the only rule useful for detecting special cause is Rule 1, a point outside the limits. Rules 2–5 should not be applied with any Shewhart chart that contains autocorrelated data.
- When working with autocorrelated continuous data, the limits will be affected by the autocorrelation. You can adjust the limits to account for this prior to analyzing the chart.

- When working with autocorrelated attribute data, the calculation of the limits is not affected by the autocorrelation; the limits do not require any adjustment.
- If your autocorrelated data are from a registry, another approach may be useful for learning with Shewhart charts. Consider obtaining data each month from only the tests or visits conducted in that last month. Using this approach a particular patient's data will only be used when new tests or evaluations are done. The summary from these data will be independent and thus will not be autocorrelated. Using this approach, standard Shewhart and run charts can be used and analyzed with all the usual rules for detection of special cause on a Shewhart chart or signals on a run chart.

SHEWHART CHARTS FOR ATTRIBUTE DATA WITH LARGE SUBGROUP SIZES (OVER-DISPERSION)

Chapter Five described the calculations to develop Shewhart charts for attribute data (P, C, and U charts). Sometimes, applying these formulas with very large subgroup sizes can result in charts that are not very useful. The plotted data points have much more variation than that expected from the theoretical calculation of limits based on the Binomial or Poisson distribution. This problem has been called "**over-dispersion**" in health care applications.[6] This phenomenon can occur quite often when using measures from administrative databases to develop the charts.

Figure 8.23 shows an example of a P chart from the call center of a health care organization. From the call center database, it is easy to determine the number of current eligible members of the health plan who communicated with the organization each month. The subgroup size each month is the total active membership (from 8,755 members in January 2007 up to 22,300 members in August 2007). The result is a P chart where the limits appear to be "very tight" and most of the points are outside the control limits.

The question then becomes: Are all these points outside the limits due to special causes, or is something else going on here? The sigma in the formula for the P chart is:

$$\sigma_p = \sqrt{P_{bar}(100 - P_{bar})/n}$$

so the variation in the limits is affected by the average percentage and the subgroup size (n). This method to estimate sigma is often called the sampling variation because the subgroup size is some type of sample from the process of interest. As discussed in Chapter Five, the limits are not affected by the variation in the plotted points. For any given value of p, the limits will thus get tighter and tighter as the subgroup size increases. For very large subgroup sizes (such as average subgroup size greater than 5,000), the sampling variation becomes very small and thus the limits appear to be tight. Unless the process is perfectly stable, eventually points will be outside the limits.

Prime Charts (p′ and U′)

A number of authors have made suggestions to deal with this over-dispersion situation.[7] The difficulty is that the adjustments recommended do not differentiate cases when special

---

[6]Spiegelhalter, D., "Handling Overdispersion of Performance Indicators," *Journal of Quality and Safety in HealthCare*, BMJ, 2005, *14*, 347–351.

[7]Heimann, P. A., "Attributes Control Charts with Large Sample Sizes," *Journal of Quality Technology*, ASQ, 1996, *28*, 451–459.

FIGURE 8.23   P Chart with Control Limits That Appear "Very Tight"

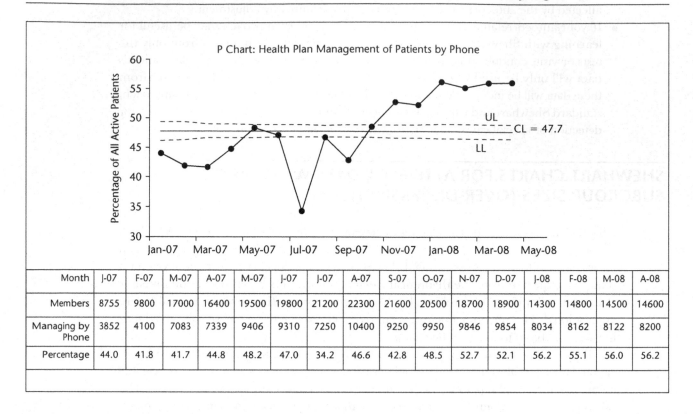

P Chart: Health Plan Management of Patients by Phone

Month	J-07	F-07	M-07	A-07	M-07	J-07	J-07	A-07	S-07	O-07	N-07	D-07	J-08	F-08	M-08	A-08
Members	8755	9800	17000	16400	19500	19800	21200	22300	21600	20500	18700	18900	14300	14800	14500	14600
Managing by Phone	3852	4100	7083	7339	9406	9310	7250	10400	9250	9950	9846	9854	8034	8162	8122	8200
Percentage	44.0	41.8	41.7	44.8	48.2	47.0	34.2	46.6	42.8	48.5	52.7	52.1	56.2	55.1	56.0	56.2

FIGURE 8.24   Data from Figure 8.23 on a P′ Chart

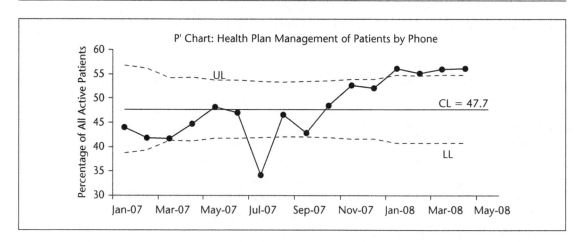

P′ Chart: Health Plan Management of Patients by Phone

causes really are dominating the variation in the measure. Interpretation by subject matter experts is required. The most useful method, called a P prime (P′) chart, presented here was developed by Laney.[8] Figure 8.24 shows a P′ chart for the data in Figure 8.23. Note that the limits in this case appear more reasonable or useful and that important special causes are still detected on the chart.

First develop the appropriate attribute chart (P or U chart). If the limits appear "too tight" and very large subgroup sizes are involved, look for ways to further stratify the data

---

[8]Laney, D. B., "Improved Control Charts for Attribute Data," *Quality Engineering*, 2002, *14*, 531–537.

(monthly into daily subgroups, organization data into department subgroups, and so forth). If you still end up with large subgroup sizes and a chart that is full of special causes, spend time with the subject matter expert trying to identify and understand the special causes. If you are not able to learn from the special causes, then use the following method to develop a modified attribute chart.

The method developed by Laney and presented here uses the attribute chart calculation of sigma to get the sampling variation and then uses the standardized chart (from Chapter Seven) to calculate a sigma that is based on the process variation (between subgroup variation). The I chart of the standardized values is used to develop the process sigma. Then the total variation is transformed back to the original scale by multiplying the two estimated sigmas (sampling and process). The following example is for the P′ chart (U′ charts are similar):

Step 1: Calculate the P chart (getting p_i and σ_{pi} for each subgroup).

Step 2: Convert the individual p values to z-values using

$$z_i = [p_i - p_{bar}] / \sigma_{pi}.$$

The use the I chart calculation (Chapter Five) of moving ranges to determine the sigma for z-values:

$$\sigma_{zi} = \text{screened } \overline{MR} \text{ divided by } 1.128.$$

(Note: as with any I chart, it is very important to screen the moving ranges for special causes prior to calculating the average moving range).

This sigma value will be greater than 1.0 if there is over-dispersion (more variation than expected from the theoretical calculation based on the binomial variation).

Step 3: Transpose the z chart calculations back to p values to get the limits for the P′ chart:

$$CL = p_{bar} \text{ (same as original p chart)}$$
$$UCL = p_{bar} + 3\,\sigma_{pi}\,\sigma_{zi}$$
$$LCL = p_{bar} - 3\,\sigma_{pi}\,\sigma_{zi}$$

that is multiplying the theoretical sampling sigma (σ_{pi}) by the between-subgroup sigma (σ_{zi}).

The P′ chart in Figure 8.24 is based on these three steps. The U charts follow the same three steps with:

$$\sigma_c = \sqrt{u_{bar} / n}$$

Figure 8.25 is a second example of applying this method to a U chart for medication errors from different hospitals in a system. The data are obtained from a screening of computer order entry of prescriptions in the hospitals for one month. The screening system picks up the possible errors and they are then reviewed by the pharmacist and corrected if necessary. Subgroup sizes (number of prescription entries for the month) ranges from 4,467 to 27,203 per hospital.

The quality analyst sequenced the hospitals on the U chart from the smallest to largest denominator (for example, see funnel plot format, see Chapter Five). The points for one-half of the hospitals were outside the U chart limits (seven low and five on the high side). The U chart was reviewed with the improvement team working on reducing medication

FIGURE 8.25 U Chart and U′ Chart for Medication Errors

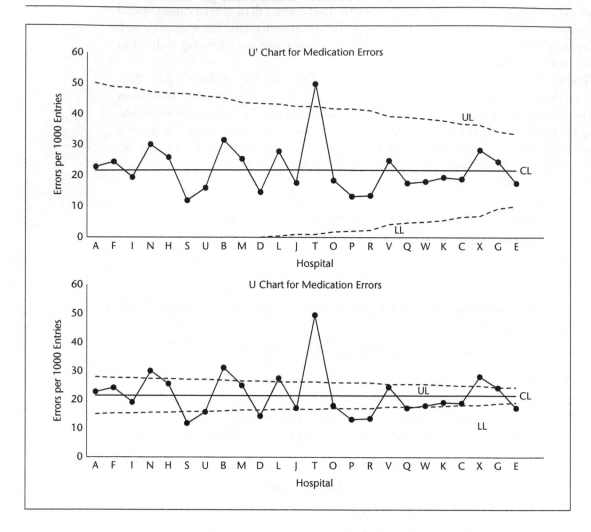

errors. After reflecting on the hospitals below the lower limit, the team (especially the system lead pharmacist) did not feel it was worthwhile to spend time further investigating these hospitals because many them had the same systems and experience as others inside the limits. The team also questioned whether the hospitals on the high side were "special" and pushed back on the methods to determine the limits.

Based on this conversation with the subject matter experts (and the very large subgroup sizes), the quality analyst created the U′ chart shown at the top of Figure 8.25. This chart indicated that only hospital T (with 50 errors per 1,000 entries) was special. The team quickly shifted their focus to the specific circumstances associated with that hospital and the common cause variation from the rest of the hospitals.

It is very important not to just automatically switch to a these modified charts until the source of the over-dispersion has been thoroughly investigated.[9] Only when subgroup sizes are above 1,000 should the adjustment be even considered. The purpose of Shewhart's method is to optimize learning, not to eliminate special causes. The example in Figure 8.26 shows the problem of jumping to the modified chart without thorough investigation of the special causes in the initial Shewhart chart.

---

[9]Mohammed, M. A., and Laney, D., "Overdispersion in Health Care Performance Data: Laney's Approach," *Journal of Quality and Safety in Health Care*, 2006, *15*, 383–384.

FIGURE 8.26   P Chart and P′ Chart for Self-Management Goals in 14 Clinics

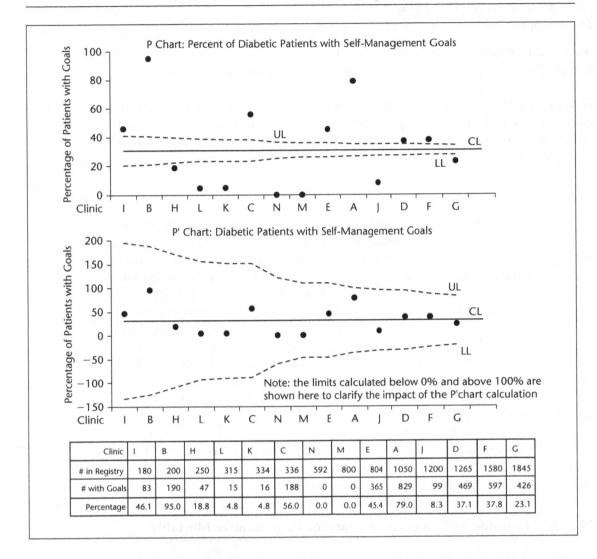

Clinic	I	B	H	L	K	C	N	M	E	A	J	D	F	G
# in Registry	180	200	250	315	334	336	592	800	804	1050	1200	1265	1580	1845
# with Goals	83	190	47	15	16	188	0	0	365	829	99	469	597	426
Percentage	46.1	95.0	18.8	4.8	4.8	56.0	0.0	0.0	45.4	79.0	8.3	37.1	37.8	23.1

The charts in Figure 8.26 are based on the evaluation of a process measure used in an improvement project to take better care of patients with diabetes. The health care providers in each of the system's 14 clinics were trained and coached to encourage their patients to set their own goals for better managing their disease. After six months, the measure of "percentage of patients with self-management goals" was extracted from each clinic's registry and used to create the top chart in Figure 8.26. When the analyst saw that all of the plotted points were outside the P chart limits, she quickly recalculated the limits using the P′ chart method. The P′ chart showed all of the clinics inside the control limits.

After her initial positive reaction that "the P′ chart limits looked better," the analyst realized that the limits for most of the clinics were below 0 and above 100% (thus, essentially no useful limits). She decided to spend more time understanding what was happening in the clinics based on the initial P chart. She found that the two clinics with 0 goals set did not have this field installed in their registry, so 0 values were recorded for these two clinics by default. From interviews with the five other clinics below the lower limit she learned that because of turnover, short staffing, and other priorities, they had not been able to make self-management a priority in their clinics. The clinic with 95% of patients with goals offered some great tips for getting all of a clinic's patients involved in self-management.

The other clinics above the upper limit all felt they were making progress and would attain the goal of 85% by the end of the year.

This example emphasizes the cautions in using the modification to P and U charts:

1. Don't consider the adjustment unless the subgroup sizes are very large (in this last example they ranged from 180 to 1,845, not enough to make the P chart limits ineffective). In cases where average subgroup sizes are very large (>3,000), first try using different subgrouping strategies to the stratify the data into smaller rational subgroups.

2. Spend time with subject matter experts trying to understand and learn from the initial indications of special causes on the attribute chart before considering the modification to these charts.

Comparison Charts

Another type of analysis sometimes confused with a Shewhart chart is called a comparison chart. Comparison charts are primarily useful for classifying performance measures into exemplary performance, average performance, or substandard performance. **Comparison charts** compare an organization's outcomes to its comparison group or to its risk-adjusted data. A comparison chart consists of observed rates, expected rates, and expected ranges (upper and lower limits) for a given time frame. The expected range is similar to a confidence interval (discussed in the next section) and describes the degree of certainty with which a given point could be different from the average population value. The organization used a 99% expected range to calculate the limits. An outlier is a data point that fails the hypothesis test that the observed value is not different from the expected value. Figure 8.27 shows the format for a comparison chart. In the recent past the Joint Commission used comparison charts.

Some organizations use Shewhart and comparison charts to complement each other, offering two different views of data. Using both charts together, leaders can determine whether they are comfortable with their organization's level of performance or whether a performance improvement initiative should be undertaken.[10]

FIGURE 8.27   Example of Comparison Chart for Perioperative Mortality

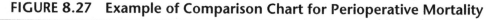

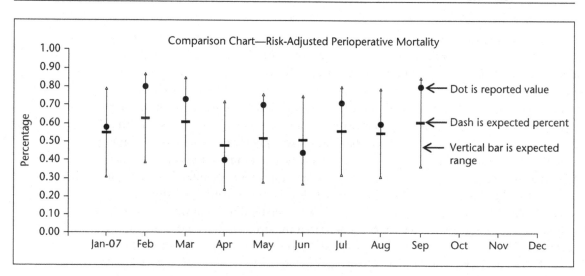

[10]Lee K., and McGreevey, C., "Using Comparison Charts to Assess Performance Measurement Data," *Joint Commission Journal of Quality Improvement*, 2002, *28*(3), 90–101.

We recommend that comparison charts never be used without a Shewhart control chart for two reasons:

1. Before valid comparisons can be made, the process under investigation should be stable, that is, predictable within limits (in statistical control). This follows the same logic as capability analysis addressed in Chapter Five.

2. Comparison charts are examples of using measures for judgment rather than for improvement. If a comparison chart leads to the conclusion that improvement is appropriate, the organization still needs to determine the appropriate improvement strategy based on analysis of a Shewhart chart. Should they adopt a strategy for common cause or for special cause? Only a Shewhart chart can aid in their determination of an appropriate improvement strategy. This is discussed further in Chapter Four. In addition, those working in the improvement effort need measures displayed in a way that will help them tell whether changes are improvements. A run chart or Shewhart chart is necessary for this. A comparison chart is not capable of helping a team discern whether a change is an improvement. Chapter Two addresses the difference between data used for judgment and data used for improvement.

Confidence Intervals and Confidence Limits

When people who have studied statistics are first exposed to Shewhart charts, they sometimes confuse the calculation of the limits with confidence intervals. A **confidence interval**, or an interval estimate, is a range of values with an associated probability or confidence level. *Confidence limits* are the lower and upper boundaries of a confidence interval, that is, the values that define the range of a confidence interval. The probability quantifies the chance that a calculated interval is expected to contain the population parameter of interest. If independent samples are taken repeatedly from the same population, and a confidence interval calculated for each sample, then a certain percentage (confidence level) of the intervals are expected to include the unknown population parameter.

The correct interpretation of a confidence interval is based on repeated sampling. For example, if samples of the same size are drawn repeatedly from a population, and a 95% confidence interval for the means is calculated from each sample, then 95% of these intervals should contain the population mean.

The usefulness of confidence intervals in quality improvement studies is limited because of the analytic nature of improvement work (see Chapter Two on analytic and enumerative studies). Deming emphasized the appropriate role of confidence intervals: "A confidence interval has operational meaning and is very useful for summarization of results of an enumerative study. I use confidence intervals in legal evidence in enumerative studies. But a confidence interval has no operational meaning for prediction, hence provides no degree of belief for planning."[11]

A confidence interval:

- Provides a range of values based on observations from a sample
- Gives information about closeness of estimates from the sample to an unknown population parameter
- Is stated in terms of probability, usually 90%, 95%, or 99%

The width of the confidence interval gives us some idea about how uncertain we are about the unknown parameter (average, standard deviation, percent, rate, and so on). A very wide interval may indicate that more data should be collected before anything very

---

[11]Deming, W. E., *Out of the Crisis*, Cambridge, MA, MIT Press, 1982, 132.

definite can be said about the parameter. The width of the confidence interval is determined by the variation of the measure in the population of interest and the sample size used to develop the estimate.

As example of a confidence interval, Chad Crumly, of the University of Georgia Department of Mathematics, produced this explanation:

> The 90% confidence interval for the number of people, of all ages, in poverty in the United States in 1995 (based on the March 1996 Current Population Survey) is "35,534,124 to 37,315,094." A confidence interval is also itself an estimate. It is made using a model of how sampling, interviewing, measuring, and modeling contribute to uncertainty about the relation between the true value of the quantity we are estimating and our estimate of that value.[12]

The procedures used to calculate confidence intervals make some important assumptions:

1. The data used to develop the interval is from a random sample from a known population of interest.
2. The data are identically and independently distributed.
3. Assumptions about the form of the distribution of the data in the population lead to specific formula to calculate the interval.

The second assumption implies that the data come from a stable distribution—the exact issue that a Shewhart chart is designed to evaluate. The first assumption results in confidence intervals not being useful in improvement work because the population of interest is usually in the future, and it is not possible to get a random sample.

To illustrate the form of a confidence interval, Figure 8.28 shows an $\bar{X}$ and S chart for length of stay for a particular type of admission. If the measures of length of stay (LOS) were based on a random sample from all patients discharged during the month, then the confidence interval could be used as an indicator of how precisely we have estimated the mean LOS for the month.

Figure 8.29 shows 95% confidence intervals calculated for each month. The average for the 20-month period is also shown on the plot as a reference point.

Confidence intervals for the mean are based on the following formula:

> where u is the population average that we are interested in estimating and t is from a table of student's t distribution with a is selected at 0.025 to obtain a 95% confidence interval.

Most statistical software programs include an option to calculate confidence intervals when statistical tests are done.

For months when the confidence intervals overlap, one could assume that there is no difference in the population average length of stay for those months. The confidence interval for March 2004 indicates that the average length of stay during that month is significantly higher than most of the other months. Note that this was also identified as a special cause on the $\bar{X}$ chart.

Following similar procedure confidence intervals can be established for other parameters of interest like percents, differences, rates, standard deviations, and so forth. The formulas are included in most basic statistics books.[13]

---

[12]Crumly, C. *Confidence Intervals*. The University of Georgia Department of Mathematics and Science Education. http://jwilson.coe.uga.edu/EMAT6680Fa06/Crumley/Normal/Normal7.html.

[13]Rickmers, A., and Todd, H., *Statistics, an Introduction*, New York: McGraw-Hill, 1967.

FIGURE 8.28   X̄ and S Chart for Length of Stay

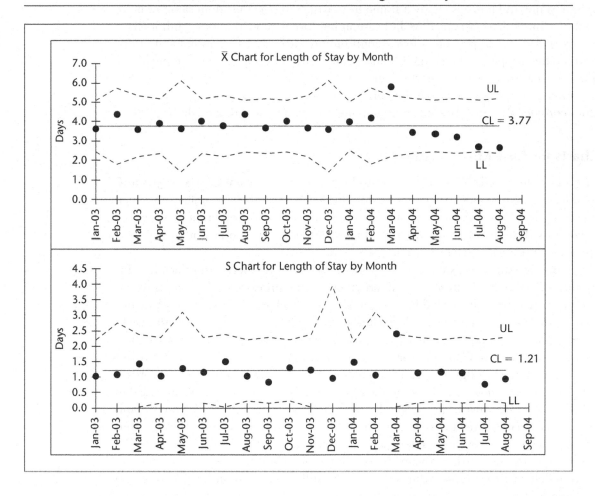

FIGURE 8.29   95% Confidence Intervals for Average Monthly Length of Stays

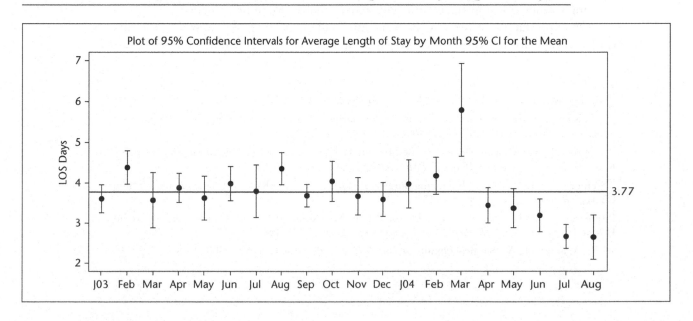

Because most improvement work uses judgment or convenience samples (see Chapter Two, Sampling) and there is rarely a frame from which to select random samples if we wanted to, confidence intervals have little use in improvement work. Some authors have suggested that they can provide a lower bound to the variation of an estimate, but this depends on the sampling scheme used to collect the date (for example, we might purposely sample extremes to understand performance under a wide range of conditions). In addition, a confidence interval describes the range in an estimate due to sampling variation but does not consider the many possible nonsampling errors and biases that might be present.

Shewhart Charts for Case-Mix Adjustment

Chapter Two discussed the need for data to be risk, severity, or **case-mix adjusted**. These adjustments are done to account for differing levels of complexity or illness between groups of patients when making comparisons of outcomes across different providers or organizations. This is important when data are being used for comparison or accountability; it can also be important in some research projects.[14]

In improvement work, studying differences between providers can offer ideas for improving the system of interest for all providers. Some improvement projects would benefit from taking into account differences in severity of subjects when studying practice patterns or the effect of changes made to clinical processes.[15] Our ability in health care to risk/severity adjust our data is evolving as we continue to understand the factors that affect various health outcomes. Computer programs are available to do risk/severity adjustment using complex models. Logistic regression analysis based on data from patient records is one of the most common approaches to these programs. Examples of factors included in the adjustment models are age, race, gender, body size, and comorbidities. If your organization is able to risk adjust the data you are using for an improvement project without slowing down your improvement efforts, then use the risk-adjusted data.

Because data used for improvement are not intended to judge people but to learn, a Shewhart chart based on unadjusted data may still be very useful for learning and improvement in many cases. A number of authors have studied the need for case-mix adjustment with control charts. In their study of mortality rates, Marshall and Mohammed concluded: "There is moderate-good agreement between signals of special cause variation between observed and risk-adjusted mortality."[16] The references below contain examples of using various risk-adjustment strategies in data analysis for improvement.[17]

One approach is to present the usual attribute chart, then also show the case-mix expected value for the statistic (C, U, or P) on the same chart. Figure 8.30 shows a P chart

[14]Kuttner, R., "The Risk-Adjustment Debate," *N England Journal of Medicine*, 1998, *339*, 1952–1956.

[15]Tekkis et al., "Mortality Control Charts for Comparing Performance of Surgical Units: Validation Study Using Hospital Mortality Data," *BMJ, 326*, 12 April, 2003.

[16]Marshall, T., and Mohammed, M., "Case-Mix and the Use of Control Charts in Monitoring Mortality Rates after Coronary Artery Bypass," *BMC Health Services Research*, 2007, *7*, 63.

[17]Steiner S., and Cook, R. "Monitoring Surgical Performance Using Risk-Adjusted Cumulative Sum Charts," *Biostatistics, 1*(4), 2000, 241–452.

Eisenstein, E., and Bethea, C., "The Use of Patient Mix-Adjusted Control Charts to Compare in-Hospital Costs of Care," *Health Care Management Science 2*, 1999, 193–198.

Webb, A. and Fink, A. "Surgical Quality of Care," *Hospital Physician*, February, 2008, 29–37.

FIGURE 8.30   Expected Values from Case-Mix Adjustment on Shewhart Chart

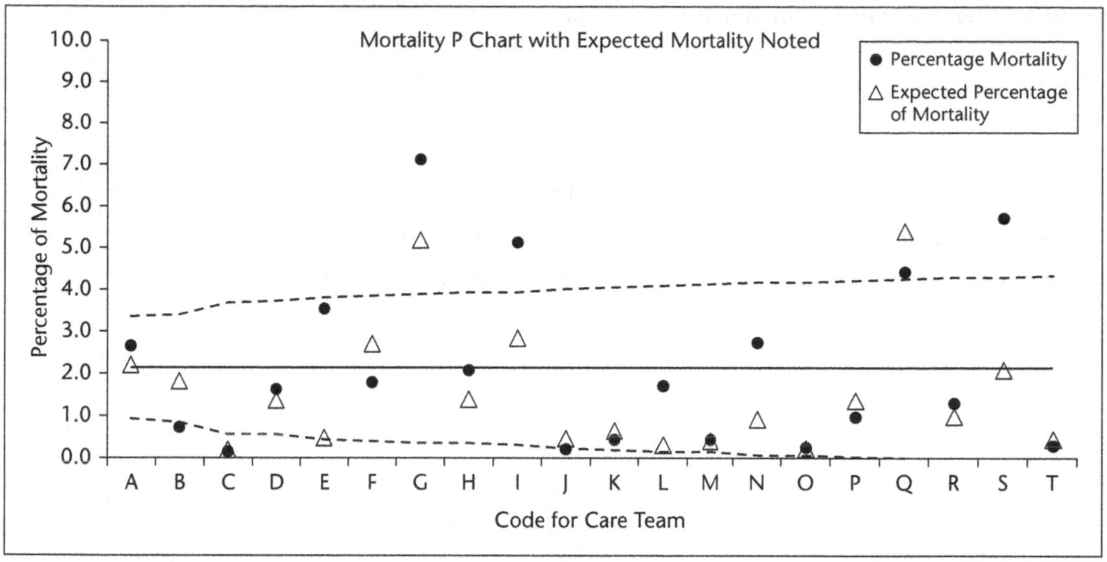

Mortality P Chart with Expected Mortality Noted

● Percentage Mortality
△ Expected Percentage of Mortality

for mortality subgrouped by the care teams in the hospital. The chart is a funnel chart (see Chapter Five for more on funnel limits) with the teams with the most eligible patients on the left of the chart. The triangle symbol represents the expected percentage of mortality based on a case-mix adjustment model. Note that teams B and C are both below the lower limit. Team B's expectation is near the center line, whereas the expectation for team C is below the lower limit. So team B appears to be a special cause, while their case-mix can explain the low value for team C.

On the high side, teams G, I, Q, and S are above the upper limit. Both teams G and Q have expected values above the upper limit; their high values are probably due to the severity of their patients. But teams I and S have expected values near the center line, so the special cause is due to something else besides the case-mix expectation.

Another option for analyzing case-mix adjusted data is to obtain the case-mix adjusted data for each case and develop an $\overline{X}$ and S chart subgrouped by care team for these adjusted data.

SUMMARY

This chapter presents some approaches to deal with common issues that can arise when SPC methods are used in health care improvement work. When using Shewhart charts in different health care environments, being aware of these issues and options can lead to more successful use of Shewhart's method of learning. Shewhart charts with changing center lines can be used to deal with measures that are expected to increase or decrease or vary by season. The uses of transformations can turn ineffective charts into charts with more useful limits. If autocorrelation is present in a measure, methods to deal with it were discussed. Special charts called "prime charts" can be used with attribute measures with very large subgroup sizes. This often occurs when analyzing administrative data.

Confidence intervals and comparison charts, both of which are sometimes confused with Shewhart charts, were described. Some additional suggestions for case-mix adjusted data were presenting, building on the discussion in Chapter Two.

KEY TERMS

Autocorrelation

Case-mix adjustment

Comparison charts

Confidence intervals

Over-dispersion

Seasonal effects

Transformation of data

## CHAPTER 9

DRILLING DOWN INTO AGGREGATE DATA FOR IMPROVEMENT

Heath care data are often reported in a highly aggregated form. Using this data for improvement can be a challenge. This chapter introduces a **Drill Down Pathway** for learning from aggregated data. The Drill Down Pathway uses the methods discussed in Chapters Four and Five. To drill down effectively into highly aggregated data requires the use of the appropriate Shewhart chart, an understanding of special and common cause improvement strategies, and the skills of disaggregation and rational subgrouping. In this chapter the reader will learn to display data at the aggregate level to determine system stability. After this, the reader will learn of an often overlooked step in data analysis. This step involves disaggregating (or stratifying) the data and displaying it with all units on a *single* Shewhart chart to determine whether a part of the system is special cause when compared to the rest of the system. The reader will learn how stratifying, rational subgrouping, and rational ordering can be used with aggregate data to better learn from this data for improvement.

WHAT ARE AGGREGATE DATA?

Aggregate data are data related to a dimension of quality that has been combined from parts of a system (such as different units, providers, services, departments, patient groups) or combined over time. Aggregating this data often provides important summary information—a big-picture view—of the level of performance related to that measure. Aggregate data are often useful for oversight, judgment, or comparison purposes. Some common examples of aggregate data in health care include:

- Quarterly percentage of patients getting angiotensin-converting enzyme inhibitors (ACEI) appropriately aggregated from monthly data
- Average post–coronary artery bypass graft (CABG) mortality for a group of 14 cardiologists
- Fall rate for an organization aggregating multiple units
- Fall rate for a system of six hospitals
- Annual percentage of patients harmed
- Overall hospital patient satisfaction score aggregated from satisfaction scores related to admitting, nursing care, housekeeping, and so on
- Average patient waiting time in a clinic with four providers
- Average supply costs per inpatient aggregated from all units
- Average STAT lab turn-around time aggregated from multiple labs
- Percentage mortality aggregated for a system of 12 hospitals

WHAT IS THE CHALLENGE PRESENTED BY AGGREGATE DATA?

Our health care environment abounds with highly aggregated data. If this data were merely being collected and reported we might not need the methods in this chapter. The fact is that we want to, and often are expected to, react to the information in the data and make things better . . . but the challenge is how? Aggregated data presents challenges as we move from using it for comparison or accountability to using it for improvement. Chapter Two addresses some of the differences between data for improvement, accountability, and clinical research. Aggregation often makes it very difficult to detect useful patterns of variation. In addition, internal scorecards or payer report cards often transform the raw data into indices. This transformation can make understanding the data even more challenging. For example, a hospital (Hospital F) was looking at a report card that compared their performance to that of seven of their peers using data from a federal payer. The report card is presented in Table 9.1.

When reviewing the report Hospital F noted that their accidental puncture and laceration (APL) score was 1.64. At a review meeting, someone asked "What does an APL score of 1.64 *mean*?" The answer was not immediately evident to anyone. The APL score of 1.64 could have been a rate or the percentage of cases with an APL. The key provided with this report card clarified that an APL score of 1.64 represented a ratio of actual-to-expected APLs. It consisted of the actual number of APLs that occurred in their organization divided by the number of APLs expected for their organization utilizing a predictive formula. The predictive formula was proprietary and not available to the group using this data. Any indexed number greater than one meant that the hospital had more APLs occur than was expected given their patient population.

Table 9.1   Clinical Quality Measures Comparative Summary

Clinical Quality Measures Comparative Summary									
Excerpt—Inpatient Care: Medicare Populations A and B from 2/2005 to 1/2006									
Dimension	Measure	Hosp. A	Hosp. B	Hosp. C	Hosp. D	Hosp. E	Hosp. F	Hosp. G	Hosp. H
Volume	Total Cases	5,206	10,997	7,328	8,251	4,721	7,421	5,883	7,247
Utilization	Cost per Case	0.81	1.28	0.89	1.21	1.07	0.95	0.99	1.19
	ALOS	0.94	1.1	0.86	1.09	0.94	0.88	0.99	1.07
Clinical Care	Mortality	0.70	0.99	1.15	1.02	1.38	0.74	1.03	1.01
	Accidental Puncture and Laceration	1.18	1.22	0.86	1.04	1.15	**1.64**	0.94	1.27
	Cardiac Complications Resulting from a Procedure	0.81	1.13	1.04	0.82	0.77	0.53	1.17	1.06
	Postoperative Infections	0.92	1.46	0.63	0.87	1.19	0.89	1.21	0.84

Note: All data indexed. Index = actual divided by expected. An index of < 1.00 is favorable. All data case-mix adjusted and grouped using grouper *******.

This measure was designed to compare hospitals and account for differences in the case mix of their patients. The resulting data can be challenging for people interested in using it for improvement in a number of ways:

- The index is not very "human-scale" for sensing the harm occurring to patients (for example, "What does an APL of 1.64 mean for our patients?").
- The data are old by the time they are viewed (typically six months to two years).
- The predictive formula for estimating expected APLs may vary each year. This adds an additional layer of complexity when working to understand the variation in this data over time.

Sometimes aggregate data are presented as a payer scorecard that scores the organization in defined areas and then totals the score for aggregate organizational score. Table 9.2 displays a small portion of one such payer report card.

Table 9.2   Excerpt From Clinical Quality Measures Comparative Summary Report Card

Excerpt: XYZ Payer Report Card		
Inpatient Care: 2/2005 to 1/2006		
Obstetrical Care (34 points possible in this section; 600 for entire report card)		

A. Hospital's Percentage of C-Sections Is:	Possible Points	Our Points
17% or less	12	
17.1–18	8	
18.1–19	6	
19.1–21	3	3
21.1–23	1	
23.1 or >	0	
Bonus: Achieve 15% or <	5	0
B. Percentage of VBACs Attempted Is:		
70% or >	10	
60–69%	5	
50–59%	3	
40–49%	2	
30–39%	1	1
25–29%	0	
C. Staff MDs Review CS and VBAC Data Quarterly	4	4
D. Percentage of C-Section Wound Infections:		
<1 %	8	
1.1–2%	3	
2.1–3 %	1	
> 3 %	0	
Section Total	34	8

In familiarizing themselves with this scorecard this organization noted that a higher score indicated better performance. They determined that their organizational total the previous year for the entire scorecard (all sections combined) was 499/600, but only 466/600 this year. They wanted to go to work to improve this score. Their first questions was "What does a score of 466 mean? How did we get it? Where do we begin?" The aggregate score didn't yield any clues as to where to focus improvement resources. In this scorecard various clinical areas are identified and rated. The total for each area is added and a grand total obtained. If the score is lower this year than last, what does that mean in terms of where to focus learning and improvement? Do we focus improvement in clinical areas in which scores were low? Areas in which the score decreased compared to last year? If the score is lower this year than last in one of these areas, does that mean things are really worse there this year or is some variation to be expected without the variation signaling a significant change in care? How do we get started with improvement now that we know we have a score of 466 this year compared to a 499 the year before? (Note: see Case Study D in Chapter Thirteen for a case study related to this scorecard.)

It's not uncommon to see an annual report aggregating data and listing the quarterly or annual average for each key measure such as the excerpt shown in Table 9.3. The organization is able to note things such as the fact that last year the organization's annual unplanned readmission rate was 5.6 per 100 discharges, and this year to date it is 4.9. The organization might conclude that it has improved.

But what if the organization had been viewing its data monthly, rather than quarterly, and displayed it using the appropriate Shewhart chart as shown in Figure 9.1? (Chapter Twelve provides additional examples of the powerful learning available to leaders by moving from static displays of data to data appropriately displayed over time.)

Here we can see that this measure appears to have improved starting in January 2010, as evidenced by special cause, but the Shewhart chart reveals that they did not hold on to that gain in subsequent months. Thus, although the average unplanned readmission rate is lower for this year to date than last year, the Shewhart chart makes it clear that any improvement gained during the year has been lost.

Aggregated data may assist an organization in judging performance as good or bad relative to desired performance. This is something organizations ought to, and want to, know. Aggregated data, however, often obscure important information related to the dynamic nature of the system. Aggregated data may lead to erroneous conclusions that a system is improving or degrading when that may not be so. Data in the aggregated form rarely provide useful information for improving performance.

Table 9.3   Excerpt from Medical Center Balanced Scorecard

Measure	Last Year	Year to Date	Target
Employee Satisfaction Score	3.5	3.6	4.0 or higher on 1–5 scale
Customer Satisfaction Press Ganey (Percentage Excellent and Very Good)	82	84	90
Labor as Percentage of Net Revenue	29	27	26
Net Revenue	26,178,400	25,869,300	26,754,250
Surgical Site Infection Rate	2.1	1.9	1.0
Unplanned Readmission Rate	5.6	4.9	5.0

FIGURE 9.1   Shewhart Chart Revealing Improvement Not Maintained

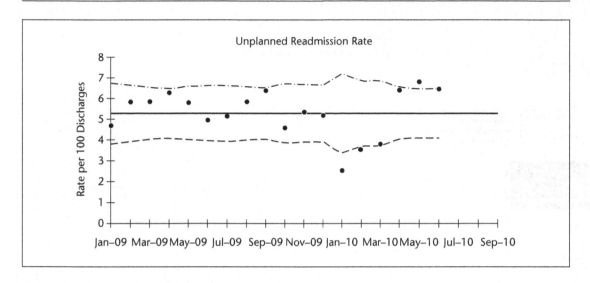

Fortunately some tools and methods exist for learning more from aggregated data. These tools and methods may aid in obtaining more useful information related to accountability and, in addition, generate ideas for improvement for clinical or organizational performance. The tools and methods for learning from aggregate data for improvement include:

- Statistical Process Control (SPC) tools
- The Drill Down Pathway
- The Model for Improvement to test changes and make improvements in the system

The SPC tools are discussed in Chapters One through Eight; the Model for Improvement is detailed in Chapter One. The remainder of this chapter will detail the Drill Down Pathway.

INTRODUCTION TO THE DRILL DOWN PATHWAY

The Drill Down Pathway, illustrated in Figure 9.2, includes the following basic steps:

- Identify the aggregate measure of interest
- Clarify the measure
- Create a Shewhart chart for the measure at the aggregate level
- Drill down into the measure:
  - By organizational unit (placing all units on the same Shewhart chart)
  - By placing each unit on its own Shewhart chart
- Use rational subgrouping with Shewhart charts to learn more about the causal system for this measure
- Use SPC tools to learn from the data and then use PDSA cycles to test ideas for improvement
- Use PDSA cycles to implement successful changes

FIGURE 9.2   The Drill Down Pathway

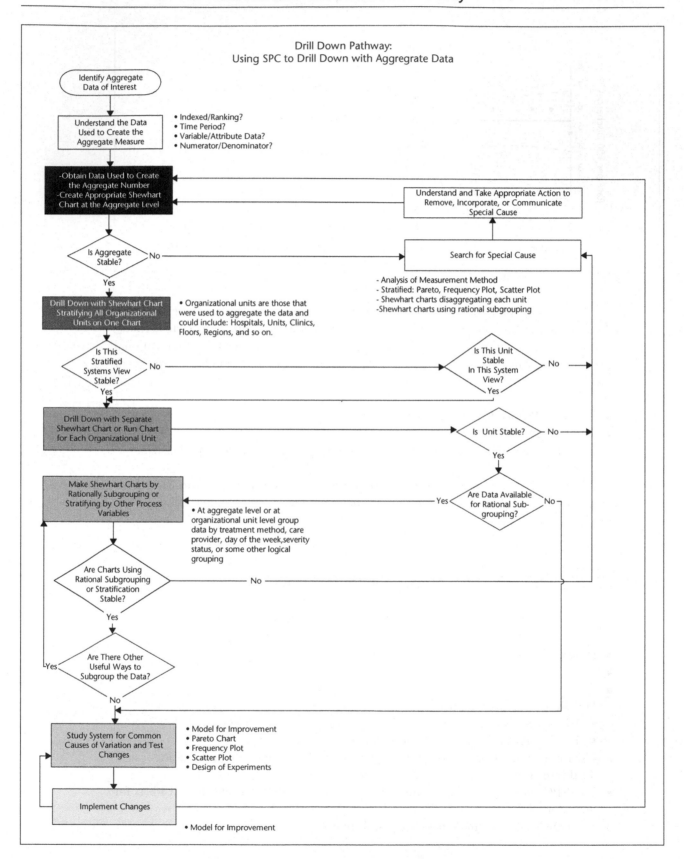

The Drill Down Pathway uses Shewhart charts and the techniques of stratification (specifically disaggregation), sequencing, and rational subgrouping. The concept of stratification was introduced in Chapter Two.

Stratification

Stratification involves the separation and classification of data according to selected variables or factors. The object is to find patterns that help in understanding the causal mechanisms in the process. In drill down stratification will refer specifically to **disaggregation**, separating data from different organizational units (departments, time periods, regions, and so forth) for presentation on a Shewhart chart

Figure 9.3 illustrates the value of stratifying aggregated data. The organization had a database containing mortality data and another with admissions data. They decided to create a U chart looking at deaths per 100 admissions each month. When viewing the mortality rates for their five-hospital system this organization did not see any evidence of special cause. Disaggregating the data and displaying all five hospitals on the same Shewhart chart revealed a special cause variation. Some hospitals were special related to mortality when compared to the other hospitals in their system. This provided the organization with an opportunity to learn more about mortality in their system.

FIGURE 9.3   Comparison of Aggregated and Disaggregated Mortality Data

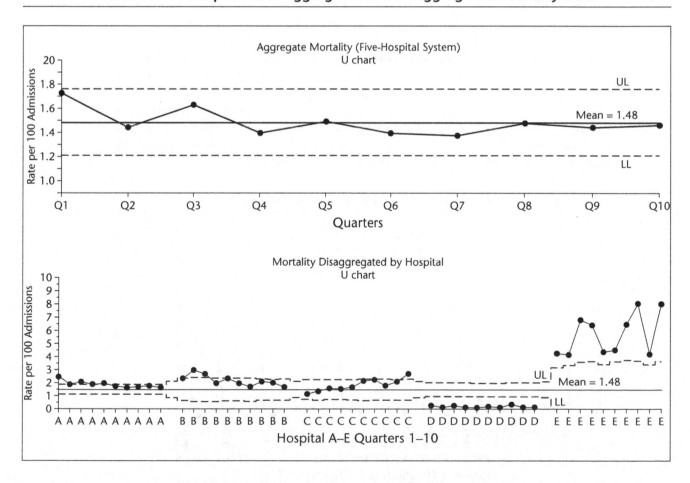

Hospitals A and B had been special cause to the rest of the system with high mortality but were within the system limits more recently. Hospital C had been within the system but had been showing an increasing mortality rate and recently became special cause to the system. Hospital D was special cause with consistently low mortality. Hospital E was special cause to the system with consistently high mortality. Some of the special cause variation was understood and related to the different types of patients cared for at the hospitals in their system. But after looking at data adjusted for patient case mix, it was clear that not all the special cause variation was attributable to the different patient populations. The leadership team felt there was much to be learned by studying the disaggregated data.

Sequencing

Sequencing is the ordering of data on a Shewhart chart. Figure 9.3 illustrates one of two sequencing strategies. Figure 9.3 displays the data sequenced by each hospital (quarters 1–10) and addresses the question "Is any hospital special cause when viewed as a system?" Figure 9.4 displays the data sequenced by quarter (hospitals A–E) and addresses the question "Did anything impact our entire system in one particular time frame?" In Figure 9.4 we don't see a time period (quarter) when all of the organizations exhibit special cause. If we had, it would indicate that something had happened in this time period to affect mortality at all five hospitals in the system. Instead what is evident from Figure 9.4 is that hospital E is consistently special cause to the rest of the system.

Rational Subgrouping

This step involves stating a theory or posing a question and then grouping data for Shewhart chart analysis in a way designed to help learn about the theory or answer that question. Shewhart's concept of **rational subgrouping** involves organizing data from the process in a way that is likely to give the greatest chance for the data in each subgroup to be alike and greatest chance for data in other subgroups to be different.

The aim of rational subgrouping is to include only common causes of variation within a subgroup, with all special causes of variation occurring between subgroups. Examples of rational subgrouping include forming subgroups of the data by shift, by location, by provider, or by diagnosis. Chapter Four discusses rational subgrouping further.

FIGURE 9.4   Comparison of Sequencing Strategies

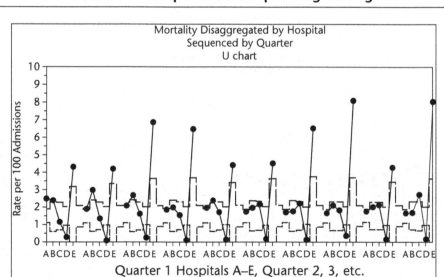

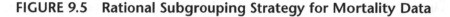

FIGURE 9.5   Rational Subgrouping Strategy for Mortality Data

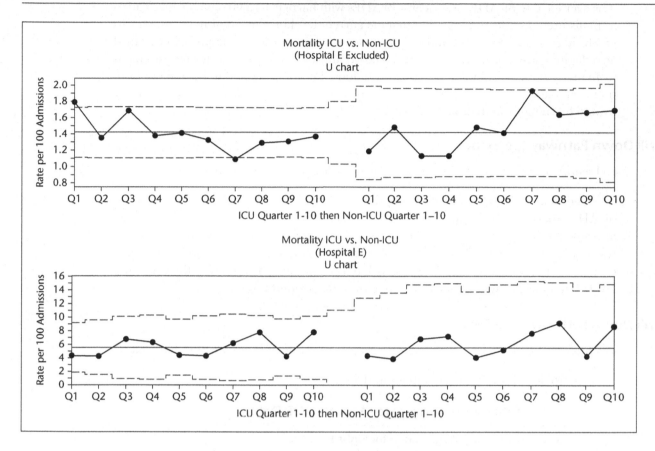

Figure 9.5 illustrates rationally subgrouping the mortality data for hospitals A–D by ICU deaths versus non-ICU deaths each month. The top Shewhart chart in this figure reveals that ICU mortality shows special cause and is improving. The first three quarters are special cause high (two out of three consecutive points two sigma or beyond). After this the data decreases and special cause in the desired direction is evident by Quarter 7. Non-ICU mortality is highly variable but stable (Quarter 7 is not outside the upper limit). Hospital E was special cause to the system and their data was viewed separately. The bottom graph in Figure 9.5 shows that ICU deaths are not improving at Hospital E. There are many other possible ways to rationally subgroup this mortality data: by unit, by DRG, by provider, by ethnic group, and so on.

AN ILLUSTRATION OF THE DRILL DOWN PATHWAY: ADVERSE DRUG EVENTS (ADES)

This section will illustrate the use of the Drill Down Pathway with a case study involving adverse drug events (ADEs). An eight-hospital system routinely collected and aggregated data on ADEs which caused harm to patients (NCC MERP Index for Categorizing Errors, categories E through I).[1] They used a combination of self-reporting and computerized triggers for ADEs with follow-on chart review to identify ADEs per 1,000 doses. The data

---

[1]National Coordinating Council for Medical Errors Reporting and Prevention, http://www .nccmerp.org.

from all eight hospitals was aggregated and reviewed quarterly at the corporate level. The average rate of ADEs was nearly 15 ADEs with harm per 1,000 doses of medication administered. Leadership decided that the current level of harm that their system was producing was unacceptable and decided to focus their resources on improvement aimed at reducing patient harm from ADEs. The organization sought ideas for improvement from many sources including other organizations. They also wanted to learn more from their own data. Using the Drill Down Pathway (Figure 9.2) they took the following journey toward learning from their aggregated data:

Drill Down Pathway Step One

● Identify aggregate data of interest and gain understanding of that data

The quarterly ADE rate was comprised of a numerator consisting of the number of ADEs that result in harm (detected by both computerized triggers and self reporting) and a denominator consisting of the number of doses of medication dispensed. The rate was adjusted to a rate/1,000 doses dispensed. Data were submitted monthly from each of the eight organizations and aggregated to a single rate per quarter at the corporate level. The hospitals were readily able to retrieve their monthly data.

Drill Down Pathway Step Two

● Obtain data used to create the aggregate and display on appropriate Shewhart chart

See Table 9.4 for aggregated monthly data.

Table 9.4   Aggregate Monthly ADE Data

Systemwide Data Aggregated for Eight Hospitals		
Month	Total ADEs	Doses Dispensed/1,000
J/05	1129	70.80
F	1194	80.14
M	1158	75.35
A	1199	76.06
M	1077	74.98
J	1135	75.96
J	1150	70.80
A	1206	80.47
S	1169	76.68
O	1193	81.88
N	1224	75.29
D	1155	78.54
J/06	1181	79.73
F	1119	80.65
M	1192	81.85
A	1112	77.29
M	1088	71.21
J	1060	75.85

To organize their analysis, the team used a simple form, illustrated in Table 9.5, to record their theories about the aggregated data and describe the way they would display the data.

Using the Shewhart Chart Selection Guide (provided at the back of this book), the team selected a U chart. which is appropriate for count data where the area of opportunity (subgroup size) varies. Their first U chart of the aggregate data displayed monthly is shown in Figure 9.6.

The team summarized what they had learned in Table 9.6.

Table 9.5   Initial Drill Down Log for Aggregate ADE Data

Our Theory	How Will We Test Our Theory?	Actual Results	Next Steps
1. The rate of ADEs will be statistically stable when we view it at the aggregate (corporate) level.	1. Corporate aggregate Shewhart chart (U chart) would help us learn whether or not our system is stable (only common cause) or whether we have a signal of special cause impacting our system performance. Plot all eight hospitals' data aggregated per month.		

Drill Down Log for: ADE Rate

Indicator: ADE per 1,000 doses per month [# ADE / (# doses administered/1,000)]

FIGURE 9.6   Shewhart Chart at the Aggregate Level

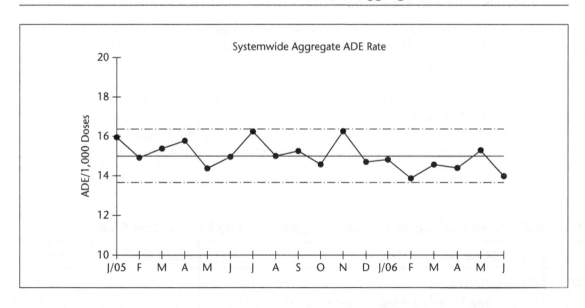

Table 9.6   Completed Drill Down Log for Aggregate ADE Data

Our Theory	How Will We Test Our Theory?	Actual Results	Next Steps
1. Our rate of ADEs is statistically stable when we view it at the aggregate (corporate) level.	1. Corporate aggregate Shewhart chart (U chart) would help us learn whether or not our system is stable (only common cause) or whether we have a signal of special cause impacting our system performance. Plot all eight hospitals' data aggregated per month.	1. Aggregate U chart shows that our system is stable at this aggregate level (no special causes).	1. Look at ADE rates for each of our eight hospitals to see if special cause exists that was hidden by the aggregation of the data.

Drill Down Log for: ADE Rate

Indicator: ADE per 1,000 doses per month [# ADE / (# doses administered/1,000)]

Drill Down Pathway Step Three

- Begin by disaggregating the data by organizational unit and placing all organizational units on a single Shewhart chart.
- Drill down by organizational unit.

Comparing all units on a single Shewhart chart is a valuable step often overlooked by those using data for improvement. The team could disaggregate the data readily as each hospital submitted their data monthly to the corporate office. A useful design principle for Shewhart charts is to limit the number of data points plotted on the chart in order to improve "legibility." If the team displayed the data monthly for each of the eight hospitals they would have 144 data points (18 months × 8 hospitals = 144). Shewhart charts are easier to view and interpret when around 20 to 80 data points are displayed. Grouping the data by quarter rather than by month (8 hospitals × 6 quarters = 48) enabled the team to adhere to the "legibility" design principle. Their drill down log is shown in Table 9.7.

The data were arranged on a spreadsheet as shown in Table 9.8.

The resulting Shewhart chart (Figure 9.7) reveals that a number of their hospitals are special cause to the system when viewed as a system.

The team's next drill down log (Table 9.9) summarizes what they learned.

Drill Down Pathway Step Three, Continued

- Begin by disaggregating the data by organizational unit and placing all organizational units on a single Shewhart chart. If one or more units exhibit special cause when viewed as a system, investigate to learn about the special cause(s).

The team had completed this step and did discover that some units were special cause to the rest of the system. The Drill Down Pathway then aids in searching for reasons for the special cause signals. We may see special cause between units in the same organization because they define ADEs differently, sample differently, have other differences in

Table 9.7   Initial Drill Down Log for Disaggregation by Unit on One Chart

Our Theory	How Will We Test Our Theory?	Actual Results	Next Steps
2. The aggregation of the data at the system level may smooth out important variation from which we could learn.	Drill down step: a. Drill down by disaggregating the data. Stratify the data by our eight hospitals. • Place all hospitals on a single Shewhart chart to determine whether any hospital is special cause when viewed as part of our larger system. • Group data by quarter. • Sequence the data on the Shewhart chart by Hospital A, quarters 1–6, then Hospital B, quarters 1–6, and so on.		

Drill Down Log for: ADE Rate

Indicator: ADE per 1,000 doses month (# ADE / # doses administered/1,000)

Table 9.8 ADE Data Disaggregated for Eight Hospitals and Subgrouped by Quarter

Hospital/ Quarter	ADEs	Doses Dispensed/1,000	Hospital/ Quarter	ADEs	Doses Dispensed/1,000
Hospital A Qtr 1	101	24.254	Hospital E Qtr 1	826	44.072
2	97	23.219	2	798	43.714
3	88	25.196	3	855	44.883
4	88	24.877	4	859	49.021
5	72	25.484	5	871	44.225
6	100	21.602	6	678	49.743
Hospital B Qtr 1	176	11.786	Hospital F Qtr 1	271	17.56
2	152	11.55	2	269	18.869
3	192	11.989	3	264	18.958
4	183	11.729	4	286	17.476
5	177	11.685	5	260	19.003
6	191	10.868	6	265	16.996
Hospital C Qtr 1	431	26.641	Hospital G Qtr 1	627	40.035
2	405	24.228	2	624	39.457
3	409	24.232	3	629	39.956
4	457	27.665	4	635	41.441
5	370	27.405	5	666	47.249
6	338	24.881	6	607	39.184
Hospital D Qtr 1	573	35.423	Hospital H Qtr 1	476	25.528
2	588	43.458	2	478	22.505
3	585	39.748	3	503	22.989
4	604	40.771	4	460	22.729
5	556	40.498	5	520	26.685
6	598	39.35	6	483	21.724

FIGURE 9.7   Shewhart Chart Displaying All Eight Hospitals on the Same Chart

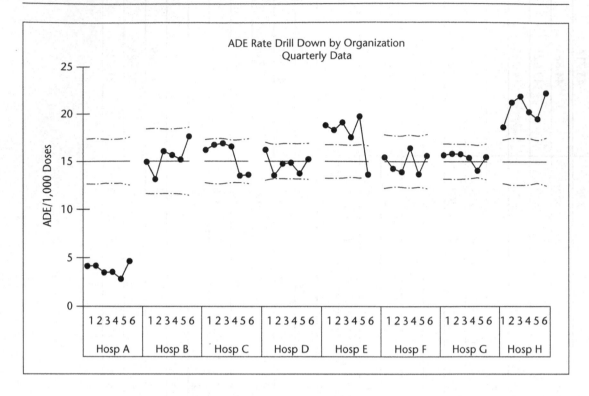

Table 9.9   Completed Drill Down Log for Disaggregation by Unit on One Chart

Our Theory	How Will We Test Our Theory?	Actual Results	Next Steps
2. The aggregation of the data at the system level may smooth out important variation from which we could learn.	Drill down step: b. Drill down by disaggregating the data. Stratify the data by our eight hospitals. • Place all hospitals on a single Shewhart chart to determine whether any hospital is special cause when viewed as part of our larger system. • Group data by quarter. • Sequence the data on the Shewhart chart by Hospital A, quarters 1–6, then Hospital B, quarters 1–6, and so on.	2. Some hospitals are special cause to our system: • Hospital A: special cause low • Hospital C: not stable (2 out of 3 rule) • Hospital E: not stable (high), but most recent quarter much lower. • Hospital H: special cause high	2. Investigate and learn from organizational units that are special cause to the rest of the system.

Drill Down Log for: ADE Rate

Indicator: ADE per 1,000 doses per month (# ADE / # doses administered/1,000)

the way they report their data, or because they practice differently from one another. Stratification between units, or within a unit, using other tools such as a Pareto chart or frequency plot aid in comparing and contrasting data to better understand special cause. For example, this organization may choose to use a Pareto chart to compare types of medications involved in the ADEs between the special cause and non–special cause units in their organization.

One fundamental approach at this point that the Drill Down Pathway suggests to enhance learning about special cause in the system is to view each special cause unit on its own Shewhart chart. This allows us to determine whether:

a. The unit is special cause to the system but internally stable. If so, this is a system or process design issue for that organization.
b. The unit is special cause to the system and unstable internally. The organizational unit may have had special cause occur. The Shewhart chart enables one to pinpoint when the special cause occurred so that more useful questions can be asked. The goal is to understand the special cause and use what is learned for improvement. If the special cause is good, we may decide to test, adapt, and implement it in the other units. If the special cause is bad, the organization may decide to assist the unit in preventing reoccurrence and spread that prevention system to the other units in our system. The ADE Team's Drill Down Log for this step is shown in Table 9.10 and Table 9.11.

The Shewhart charts they made are presented in Figure 9.8. The team utilized small multiples to display the data (the concept of small multiples is discussed in Chapter Three). The team recorded the results of their investigation of the special cause in their drill down log.

The ADE team may have enough to work on at this point with what they have learned from their drill down. Once an improvement strategy is clear there is no need to complete the entire Drill Down Pathway; its purpose is to act as a guide in searching for changes that might yield improvement for the system by making use of aggregated data in a structured way. This team decided to continue further in its use of the Drill Down Pathway.

Drill Down Pathway Step Three Continued

- Begin by disaggregating the data by organizational unit and placing all organizational units on a single Shewhart chart. Units that are not special cause when viewed as a system should then be viewed by placing each unit on its own separate Shewhart chart.

Table 9.10   Initial Drill Down Log Studying Special Cause Units

Our Theory	How Will We Test Our Theory?	Actual Results	Next Steps
Special cause may have been evident on the Shewhart chart displaying all units on one chart because: a. The unit is stable but its performance is special cause when viewed in the context of the rest of the system's performance b. Special cause has occurred inside that organizational unit	Drill down step: Create a separate Shewhart chart for each of the special cause hospitals (A, C, E, H) • Group data by month • Sequence the data in time order (Hospital A, months 1–18.) • Display as small multiples		

Drill Down Log for: ADE Rate

Indicator: ADE per 1,000 doses per month (# ADE / # doses administered/1,000)

Table 9.11   Completed Drill Down Log Studying Special Cause Units

Our Theory	How Will We Test Our Theory?	Actual Results	Next Steps
Special cause may have been evident on the Shewhart chart displaying all units on one chart because: a. The unit is stable but its performance is special cause when viewed in the context of the rest of the system's performance b. Special cause has occurred inside that organizational unit	Drill down step: Create a separate Shewhart chart for each of the special cause hospitals (A, C, E, H) • Group data by month • Sequence the data in time order (Hospital A, months 1–18.) Display as small multiples	• Hospital A stable internally at low rate—why? • Hospital C not exhibiting special cause internally, but close—any insights? • Hospital E special cause last six months • Hospital H stable internally at high rate—why?	Investigate and learn from special cause. **Summary:** Hospital A. Data self reported only. Not using computerized trigger system to discover ADE. Need to help them adapt it. Hospital C. Of note: Heparin protocol used throughout the rest of the system started by Hospital C in Nov. Will watch to see if obtain clearer evidence of improvement. Hospital E. Began using standardized IV start system in Jan. Need to plan to spread this protocol to other hospitals. Hospital H. Entered our system only 10 months ago. They still used original pharmaceutical vendor so packaging identity problems worked out by other facilities still an issue here. Also still use original pharmacy formulary. Have not adopted system formulary designed to reduce medication errors. Need to help them adopt system formulary and solve vendor packaging issue.

Drill Down Log for: ADE Rate

Indicator: ADE per 1,000 doses month (# ADE / # doses administered/1,000)

FIGURE 9.8   Separate Shewhart Chart for Each Unit Special Cause to the System

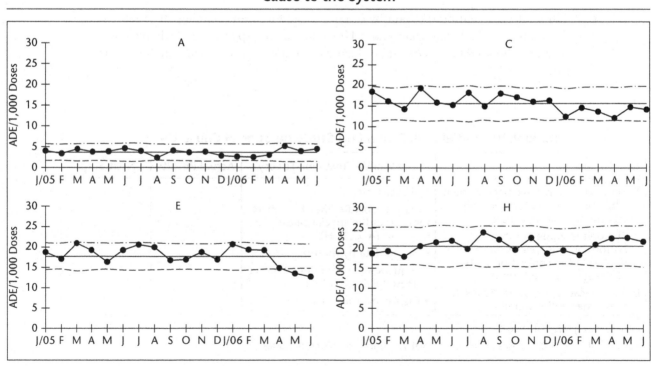

The ADE team planned their next step as recorded on their drill down log (Table 9.12). The Shewhart charts for these four hospitals are displayed in Figure 9.9. The team recorded their findings on the learning log shown in Table 9.13.

Drill Down Pathway Step Four

● Make Shewhart charts by rationally subgrouping or stratifying by other process variable
● At the aggregate level or organizational unit level, group data by treatment method, care provider, day of the week, severity status, or some other logical grouping different from the way the data were disaggregated

As noted earlier, rational subgrouping involves posing a question about what is causing variation in the data and then subgrouping the data to help answer that question. Data are grouped for Shewhart chart analysis in a way that is likely to give the greatest chance

Table 9.12   Initial Drill Down Log with Each Unit on Separate Chart

Our Theory	How Will We Test Our Theory?	Actual Result	Next Steps
Hospitals that were not special cause to the system using the U chart displaying all organizations on one chart may still have special cause occurring at that hospital when viewed on a separate U chart constructed using only that organizational unit's data to calculate mean and limits.	Drill down step: • Create a separate U chart for each of the common cause hospitals (B, D, F, G) • Group data by month • Sequence data in time order (Hospital B, months 1–18) • Display as small multiples		

Drill Down Log for: ADE Rate

Indicator: ADE per 1,000 doses per month (# ADE / # doses administered/1,000)

FIGURE 9.9   Separate Shewhart Chart for Each Unit Common Cause to the System

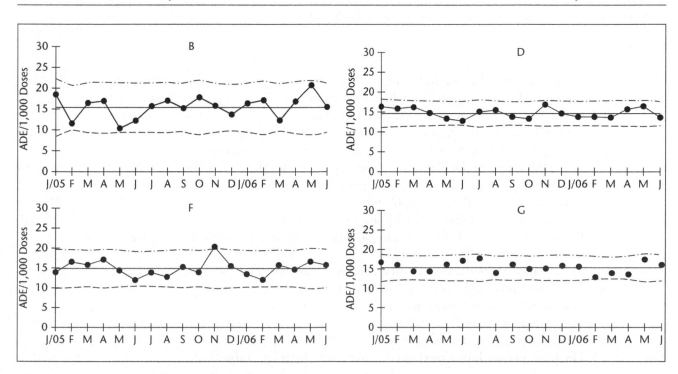

Table 9.13 Completed Drill Down Log with Each Unit on Separate Chart

Our Theory	How Will We Test Our Theory?	Actual Results	Next Steps
Hospitals that were not special cause to the system using the U chart displaying all organizations on one chart may still have special cause occurring at that hospital when viewed on a separate U chart constructed using only that organizational unit's data to calculate mean and limits.	Drill down step: • Create a separate U chart for each of the common cause hospitals (B, D, F, G) • Group data by month • Sequence data in time order (Hospital B, months 1–18) • Display as small multiples	• Hospitals B, D, G stable internally • Hospital F special cause Nov.	Investigate and learn from special cause **Summary** Hospital F. Problem with new PCA pumps in Nov. Problem resolved. *Need to see if lessons learned could be used elsewhere in our system.*

Drill Down Log for: ADE Rate

Indicator: ADE per 1,000 doses per month (# ADE / # doses administered/1,000)

Table 9.14 Initial Drill Down Log Rationally Subgrouping Aggregate Data by Day of Week

Our Theory	How Will We Test Our Theory?	Actual Results	Next Steps
ADEs may occur much more frequently on certain days of the week.	Combine remaining common cause hospitals' data (B; last six months of C; D; F with Nov. removed; G; and H) to create a U chart that will rationally subgroup the number of ADEs by day of the week at the aggregate system level. • Group data in six month subgroups • Sequence data in time order (Monday (6 mo. 1–3, Tuesday 6 mo. 1–3, and so on)		

Drill Down Log for: ADE Rate

Indicator: ADE per 1,000 doses per month (# ADE / # doses administered/1,000)

for the data in each subgroup to be alike and greatest chance for data in other subgroups to be different. In the example involving mortality earlier in this chapter, the theory that ICU-related deaths were at quite a different rate from non-ICU-related deaths resulted in grouping ICU deaths in subgroups separate from non-ICU deaths. This was done each quarter and the resulting Shewhart chart studied in light of their theory.

The ADE team decided that they had some theories they would like to explore. Fortunately, they had additional information by which to rationally subgroup their data. Their Drill Down log is shown in Table 9.14.

The Shewhart chart they created is shown in Figure 9.10.

The team recorded what they learned and planned to do next on their drill down log (Table 9.15).

The team developed a plan to rationally subgroup the data to test their next theory about shifts and recorded it on their drill down log (Table 9.16).

The Shewhart chart they created is shown in Figure 9.11.

The team was excited by what they saw on the Shewhart chart and recorded what they learned and planned to do next on their drill down log (Table 9.17).

The team planned their next steps on their drill down log (Table 9.18).

FIGURE 9.10 Aggregate U Chart Rationally Subgrouping Common Cause Data by Day of the Week in Six-Month Subgroups

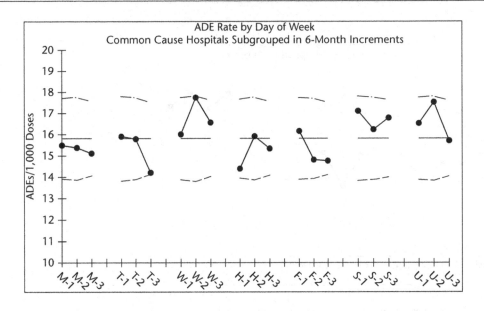

Table 9.15 Completed Drill Down Log Rationally Subgrouping Aggregate Data by Day of Week

Our Theory	How Will We Test Our Theory?	Actual Results	Next Steps
ADEs may occur much more frequently on certain days of the week.	Combine remaining common cause hospitals' data (B; last six months of C; D; F with Nov. removed; G; and H) to create a Shewhart chart that will rationally subgroup the number of ADEs by day of the week at the aggregate system level. • Group data in six month subgroups • Sequence data in time order (Monday 6 mo. 1–3, Tuesday 6 mo. 1–3, and so on)	No day of the week shows up as special cause.	Articulate another theory that our existing data will allow us to test.

Drill Down Log for: ADE Rate

Indicator: ADE per 1,000 doses per month (# ADE / # doses administered/1,000)

Table 9.16 Initial Drill Down Log Rationally Subgrouping Aggregate Data by Shift

Our Theory	How Will We Test Our Theory?	Actual Results	Next Steps
ADEs may occur much more frequently on certain shifts.	Combine remaining common cause hospitals' data (B; last six months of C; D; F with Nov. removed; G; and H) to create a Shewhart chart at the aggregate system level that will rationally subgroup the number of ADE by day, evening or night shift. • Group data quarterly • Sequence data in time order (Days Qtr. 1–6, Evenings Qtr. 1–6, then Nights Qtr. 1–6)		

Drill Down Log for: ADE Rate

Indicator: ADE per 1,000 doses per month (# ADE / # doses administered/1,000)

FIGURE 9.11 Aggregate Shewhart Chart Rationally Subgrouping Common Cause Data by Shift

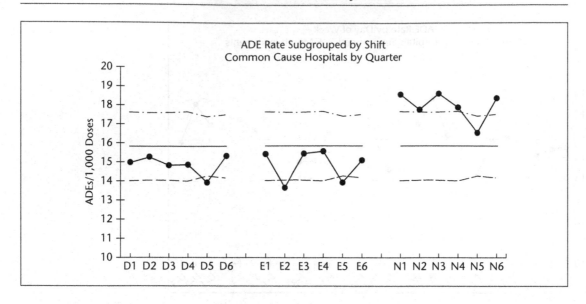

Table 9.17 Completed Drill Down Log Rationally Subgrouping Aggregate Data by Shift

Our Theory	How Will We Test Our Theory?	Actual Results	Next Steps
ADEs may occur much more frequently on certain shifts.	Combine remaining common cause hospitals' data (B; last six months of C; D; F with Nov. removed; G; and H) to create a U chart at the aggregate system level that will rationally subgroup the # of ADE by day, evening, or night shift. • Group data quarterly • Sequence data in time order (Days Qtr. 1–6, Evenings Qtr. 1–6, then Nights Qtr. 1–6)	Night shift is special cause within our system. Note: Day and evening shift appear to be special cause with a low ADE rate. This is because night shift is elevating the mean. If night shift data are excluded, day and evening shifts are stable.	• Investigate and learn from special cause.

Drill Down Log for: ADE Rate

Indicator: ADE per 1,000 doses per month (# ADE / # doses administered/1,000)

Table 9.18 Initial Drill Down Log by Unit Rationally Subgrouping Shift

Our Theory	How Will We Test Our Theory?	Actual Results	Next Steps
The higher rate of ADEs on night shift may be a special cause associated with just one or two of our hospitals.	Create separate U chart for each of our remaining common cause hospitals. Rationally subgroup the data by shift and: • Group data monthly • Sequence data in time order (Days Mo. 1–18, Evenings Mo. 1–18, then Nights Mo. 1–18) • Display as small multiples		

Drill Down Log for: ADE Rate

Indicator: ADE per 1,000 doses per month (# ADE / # doses administered/1,000)

The Shewhart charts they created are in Figure 9.12.

The team was intrigued by the Shewhart charts. After much thinking, discussion, and learning, they summarized their work on the learning log (Table 9.19).

The ADE team learned a great deal about their system by drilling down into their aggregated data using statistical process control methods. They could stop the use of

FIGURE 9.12   U Charts Placing Each Hospital on Separate Graph to Study Special Cause in Night Shift ADE Rate

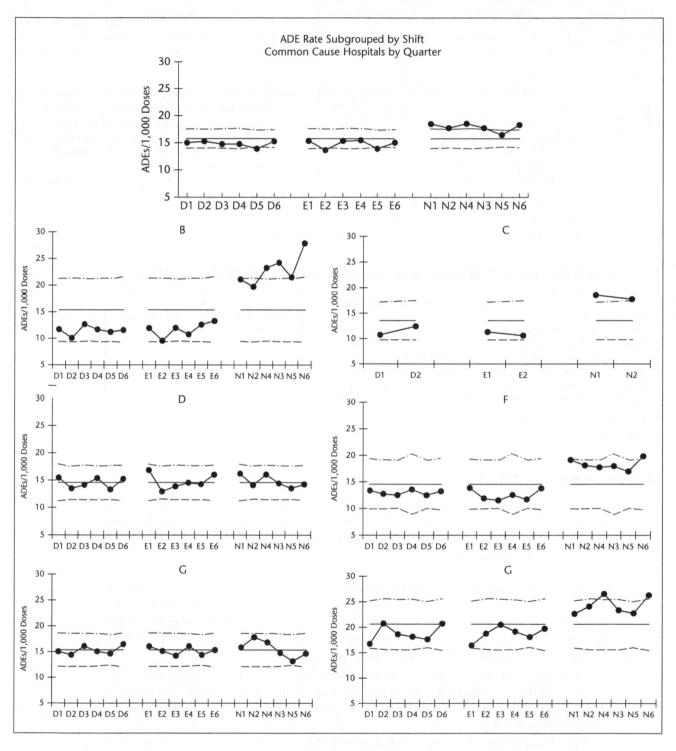

the Drill Down Pathway at any point where they believed they had enough ideas for improvement. After rationally subgrouping by day of the week and by shift the team determined that it had no other ways to rationally subgroup their data. Rather than stop, however, they returned to the Drill Down Pathway and reviewed the next step in the pathway.

Table 9.19   Completed Drill Down Log by Unit Rationally Subgrouping by Shift

Our Theory	How Will We Test Our Theory?	Actual Results	Next Steps
The higher rate of ADEs on night shift may be a special cause associated with just one or two of our hospitals.	Create separate Shewhart charts for each of our remaining common cause hospitals. Rationally subgroup the data by shift and: • Group data monthly • Sequence data in time order (Days Mo. 1–18, Evenings Mo. 1–18, then Nights Mo. 1–18) • Display as small multiples	Hospitals B, C, F, and H show night shift as special cause. Hospitals D and G do not show night shift as special cause.	Investigate and learn from special cause. What is different about hospitals showing special cause from those that do not? **Summary:** • The four hospitals with the night shift as special cause are all small, the ones without are large hospitals. • Practice difference: small hospitals did not have 24-hour pharmacy whereas large hospitals did. Evidence is clear that lack of 24-hour pharmacy results in more errors. • We need to test impact of adding 24-hour pharmacy capability.

Drill Down Log for: ADE Rate

Indicator: ADE per 1,000 doses per month (# ADE / # doses administered/1,000)

Table 9.20   Initial Drill Down Log Studying Medications Related to ADEs

Our Theory	How Will We Test Our Theory?	Actual Results	Next Steps
Studying the remaining common cause hospitals to learn more about the types of ADEs we are having would be helpful to our entire system.	Combine data from hospitals that are common cause (D and G) and create Pareto chart categorizing most common ADEs by medication name.		

Drill Down Log for: ADE Rate

Indicator: ADE per 1,000 doses per month (# ADE / # doses administered/1,000)

Drill Down Pathway Step Five

- Study the common cause system for ideas for improvement and test changes
- Use approaches such as Pareto charts, frequency plots, scatter plots, or planned experiments to learn about the common cause system. Plan and test changes using the Model for Improvement.

This is often where teams start in their use of data in their improvement projects. The ADE team decided that they had some data readily available. The team had data related to type of drug involved in each ADE and "related causal factors" they would like to explore. They planned their next step using the Drill down log as shown in Table 9.20.

Figure 9.13 shows the Pareto chart the team created.

The ADE team recorded their results and planned their next steps as shown in Table 9.21.

The ADE team also had data related to causal factors associated with each known ADE. They had a theory about a certain causal factor. Table 9.22 shows their plan for learning from this data.

The Pareto chart they created is in Figure 9.14.

The ADE team was intrigued to learn that communication and labeling issues were such prevalent factors in their ADEs. They recorded their results and planned their next steps (Table 9.23).

The ADE team returned to the Drill Down Pathway to obtain guidance for their next step.

FIGURE 9.13   Pareto Chart of ADE Occurrence by Medication Name

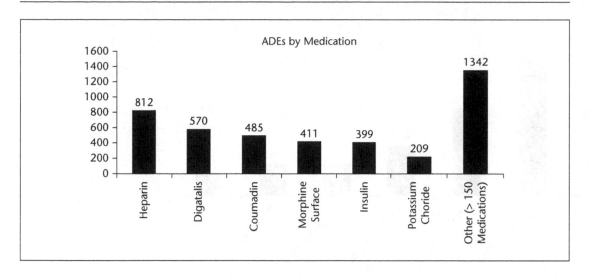

Table 9.21   Completed Drill Down Log Studying Medications Related to ADEs

Our Theory	How Will We Test Our Theory?	Actual Results	Next Steps

Studying the remaining common cause hospitals to learn more about the types of ADEs we are having would be helpful to our entire system.	Combine data from hospitals that are common cause (D and G) and create Pareto chart categorizing most common ADEs by Medication.	The data revealed a helpful Pareto effect. Of the 165 drugs tracked, five were associated with 63.9% of the ADEs:
		
		• Heparin
		• Digoxin
		• Coumadin
		• Morphine sulfate
		• Insulin
			Use change concepts in the literature or best practice already proven to work and adapt to our eight hospitals using Model for Improvement; such as:
			A. Heparin:
			  • Test changes:
			    1. Use low molecular weight Heparin
			    2. Use weight-based protocol (limit to one or two protocols)
			    3. Use pre-mixed Heparin solutions with standard concentrations
			B. Coumadin
			  • Use Coumadin dosing service
			  • Use dosing software

Drill Down Log for: ADE Rate

Indicator: ADE per 1,000 doses per month (# ADE / # doses administered/1,000)

Table 9.22   Initial Drill Down Log Studying Common Factors Related to ADEs

Our Theory	How Will We Test Our Theory?	Actual Results	Next Steps
Studying the remaining common cause hospitals to learn more about the types of ADEs we are having would be helpful to our entire system.	Combine data from hospitals that are common cause (D and G) and create Pareto chart categorizing most common factors associated with ADEs.		

Drill Down Log for: ADE Rate

Indicator: ADE per 1,000 doses per month (# ADE / # doses administered/1,000)

FIGURE 9.14   Pareto Chart of ADE Occurrence by Associated Factors

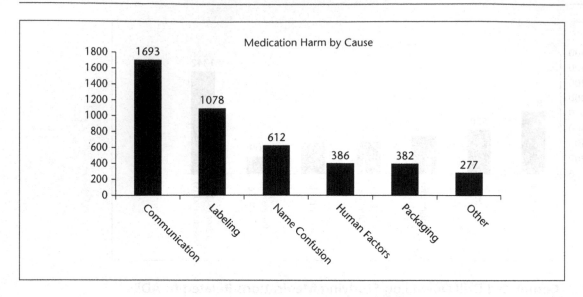

Table 9.23   Completed Drill Down Log Studying Common Factors Related to ADEs

Our Theory	How Will We Test Our Theory?	Actual Results	Next Steps
Studying the remaining common cause hospitals to learn more about the types of ADEs we are having would be helpful to our entire system.	Combine data from hospitals that are common cause (D and G) and create Pareto chart categorizing most common factors associated with ADEs.	The Pareto chart revealed two major causal factors associated with their ADEs. Communication and Labeling resulted in 62.5% of the ADEs.	A. Create a sub-team to study communication problems and adapt proven changes such as: standardizing abbreviations, using leading zeros but not trailing zeros. B. Create a sub-team to study labeling problems and adapt proven changes such as: separate look-a-likes and sound-a-likes by label, by time, and by distance.

Drill Down Log for: ADE Rate

Indicator: ADE per 1,000 doses per month (# ADE / # doses administered/1,000)

Drill Down Pathway Step Six

- Implement changes proven successful during testing
- Track aggregate data and display on Shewhart chart to determine impact of changes implemented.

The ADE team tested and implemented a number of changes. They continued to collect and display aggregate data on their Shewhart chart. Their data is presented in Figure 9.15. This chart indicates that the changes implemented have resulted in a real improvement. The safety leaders on the team confirmed this was a clinically desirable change in the ADE rate.

FIGURE 9.15   Shewhart Chart Used to Determine Impact of Changes Implemented

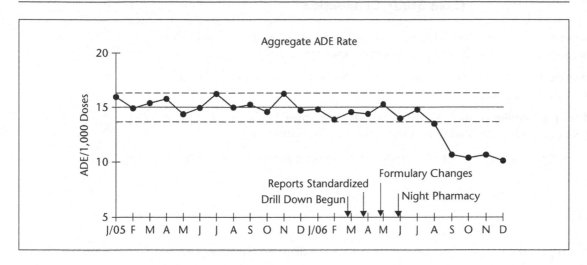

SUMMARY

Like the ADE team, those in health care are often asked to do something about a problem revealed by highly aggregated data. We currently see great variation in how this challenge is approached. Most typically the approach selected does not include much use of Statistical Process Control (SPC). The Drill Down Pathway offers guidance for using SPC tools, and particularly an understanding of special and common cause, for learning and developing changes that may lead to system improvement.

Using the Drill Down Pathway will not lead to the same journey each time. Sometimes the entire pathway will be used, other times a portion of it. The purpose of drilling down is to develop changes that might lead to improvement, not to complete the pathway. How far down the pathway we travel may, at times, depend on the organization structure and the data available. Sometimes a step in the pathway will not be used because it doesn't make sense to do so. Case study D, involving the percentage of C-sections, provides an example. In this case study we will note that the team did not drill down by multiple organization units because it was studying a single hospital.

When drilling down into aggregate data, it is important to use the principles for good Shewhart chart design and use (presented in Chapters Five and Six). Case study E, related to accidental punctures and lacerations, is one in which special cause occurred in the data. After understanding the special cause and taking appropriate action, the team was careful to remove the special cause data from the mean and calculation of the limits so that the special cause already acted on would not continue to influence their limits. When studying the common cause system it is important to use all of the data available without knowingly contaminating the study with the special cause data we have already found. In the ADE example in this chapter the team was careful to use only the data from hospitals that exhibited nothing by common cause variation (Hospitals D and G) in studying the types of medications and types of causal factors associated with ADEs. The team did not want to contaminate data by including the other hospitals' data when it had already established that data contained special causes and therefore were not expressing only the variation in the common cause system.

Case Study Connection

For further learning related to the Drill Down Pathway and the use of disaggregation, sequencing, and rational subgrouping with Shewhart charts the reader can turn to:

Case Study D illustrates the use of the Drill Down Pathway with classification data (percentage of C-sections).

Case Study E highlights the use of Shewhart charts in drilling down into aggregate data (count data on U charts related to accidental puncture/laceration rate).

KEY TERMS

Aggregate data

Disaggregation

Drill Down Pathway

Rational subgrouping

Sequencing

Stratification

APPLICATIONS OF SHEWHART CHARTS IN HEALTH CARE

## CHAPTER 10

LEARNING FROM INDIVIDUAL PATIENT DATA

Health care is about caring for patients by helping them maintain their health and diagnosing and curing health problems when they occur. When patients interact with the health system at a clinic visit or hospital stay, many measurements are obtained to learn about each individual patient's health. The methods to learn from variation described in this book can be used to aid clinicians in gaining insight and making decisions from these data.

This chapter presents examples of applying the methods presented in earlier chapters (focusing on run charts and Shewhart charts) to data from individual patients. The objective is to inspire clinicians to use these methods to better learn from the variation of measures they manage for patients in their practice. Physicians could also coach patients to track and analyze their own data to get them more involved in their health care.

In his classic paper on variation in health care, Don Berwick addresses the need for clinicians to understand the variation in these measures:[1]

"Where do clinicians measure and respond clinically based on that measurement?
- Measure prothrombin times and change anticoagulants.
- Measure oxygen tensions and change respirator settings.
- Measure fever and change antibiotics.
- Measure blood pressure and change antihypertensive.
- Measure leukocytes and change chemotherapies.
- Measure pain and change analgesia.
- Measure electrolytes and change IV fluids.
- Measure and change, measure and change."

The methods in this book are directly applicable to helping clinicians make these decisions. While most of the examples in the book have looked at measures of the health care system (length of stay, readmissions, compliance with guidelines, wait times, and so on) and measures for groups of patients (average registry values, patient satisfaction, and so on), this chapter focuses on the use of Shewhart's theory and methods in the care of individual patients.

A few examples of analyzing individual patient measures have previously been presented in earlier chapters of this book:

- Chapter Three, Figures 3.36 and 3.37 (run charts for weight of CHF patient)
- Chapter Seven, Figure 7.13 (Shewhart charts of twice a year HbA1c values for a patient with diabetes)

---

[1]Berwick, D. M., "Controlling Variation in Health Care: A Consultation with Walter Shewhart," *Medical Care*, December, 1991, *29*(12), 1212–1225.

Although the methodology has been known for more than thirty years, the use of Shewhart charts for a patient's data is still not commonplace in health care. Deming described the use of control charts in health care in a Japanese hospital in 1980 to monitor the progress of a patient who had to learn to walk again after an operation.[2] An $\bar{X}$ and R chart was used to analyze data collected on step time using recorded electronic pulses for 10 steps. When the $\bar{X}$ chart indicated stability, the patient was ready for discharge. This approach optimized the utilization of the physical therapists.

The health care literature has a number of examples of using Shewhart's methods with individual patient data. In 2007, Tenant and others published a systematic review of control chart applications of monitoring patients.[3] Three of the studies they found compared the use of control charts to more standard statistical methods. Although comparisons were not very rigorous, these studies showed that Shewhart charts were easy to use and effective. Four of the other studies reviewed had used Shewhart charts to monitor individual patient clinical variables and showed positive results for both patient and provider. Their article concluded that "Control charts appear to have a promising but largely under-researched role in monitoring clinical variables in individual patients. Furthermore, rigorous evaluation of control charts is required."

The measures used in the papers they selected for analysis included:

- Asthma: symptom-free days, expiratory flow rate
- Hypertension: blood pressure
- Diabetes: blood glucose levels
- Post-transplant kidney function: serum creatinine levels

The use of control charts for asthma patients is one of the most common applications cited in the literature. Daily monitoring of peak expiratory flow rate is important for effective management of asthma. Patients who are asked to monitor their asthma each day need some guidelines on when they should modify their treatment plans. Both traditional and time between control charts can be used to monitor asthma attacks.[4]

Bucuvalas and others describe the use of Shewhart's method in the care of liver transplant patients.[5] They concluded that the utilization of Statistical Process Control (SPC) increased the proportion of CNI (calcineurin inhibitor) blood levels in target range from 50% to 77% in their population of transplant patients. The authors suggested that the control chart method may be applicable to the care of other chronic health care problems.

EXAMPLES OF SHEWHART CHARTS FOR INDIVIDUAL PATIENTS

The following nine examples illustrate the use of run charts and Shewhart charts for specific patients. They are all *adapted* from real cases.

---

[2]Deming, W. E., *Out of the Crisis*, Cambridge, MA: MIT Center for Advanced Engineering Study, 1982, 252–253.

[3]Tennant, R., Mohammed, M., Coleman, J., and Martin, U., "Monitoring Patients Using Control Charts: A Systematic Review," *International Journal of Quality in Health Care*, 2007, *19*(4), 187–194.

[4]Alemi, F., and Neuhauser, D., "Time-Between Control Charts for Monitoring Asthma Attacks," *Joint Commission Journal for Quality and Safety, 2004, 30*(2), 95–102.

[5]Bucuvalas, J. et al., "A Novel Approach to Managing Variation: Outpatient Therapeutic Monitoring of Calcineurin Inhibitor Blood Levels in Liver Transplant Recipients," *Journal of Pediatrics*, 2005, *146*, 744–750.

Example 1: Temperature Readings for a Hospitalized Patient

The first example comes from Berwick's 1991 paper on variation where he describes a 16-year-old patient admitted to the hospital with possible osteomyelitis (inflammation of the bone due to infection).[6] Before admission, antibiotic therapy was started for the patient but his temperature continued to spike after a week and he was hospitalized to further understand his condition. The diagnostic strategy included careful observation, adjustments of antibiotics, imaging tests, a bone biopsy, and a bone marrow biopsy. During the 14 days in the hospital, the patient had his temperature recorded in his chart 100 times. Berwick shows the temperature readings in a table but notes that the measurements appeared on 22 separate pages of nursing notes. Could the methods presented in this book be used to learn from these temperature readings?

Figure 10.1 shows a run chart for the 100 temperatures. The run chart is annotated with the changes made in use of antibiotics and other tests done. Applying the run chart rules, there are numerous signals of nonrandom patterns, including a run of 6 points below the median at the end of the series (patient's temperature returned to normal). The pattern on the run chart shows daily temperature cycles per day of 5 to 6 degrees.

The run chart in Figure 10.1 could be turned into an I chart (Figure 10.2). This Shewhart chart shows special causes on individual readings at the beginning of the series, documenting the high temperatures that led to admission of the patient.

When enough data are available, $\overline{X}$ and S chart are preferred to the I chart for learning from continuous data. Rational subgroups for these data are the temperatures taken on the same day. But with this subgrouping strategy, the normal daily temperature cycle will be included in the S chart. Figure 10.3 shows the $\overline{X}$ and S charts for these data. Although the trends are clearer in this $\overline{X}$ chart, there are no special cause signals in either of these charts. Because the variation from daily fluctuations in body temperature are included in

FIGURE 10.1   Run Chart of Temperatures for Patient with Fever

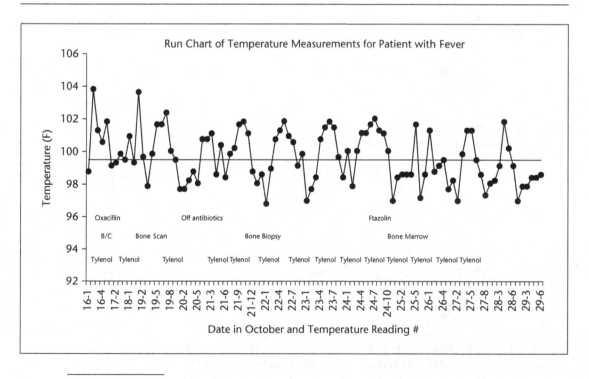

[6]Berwick, "Controlling Variation in Health Care: A Consultation with Walter Shewhart."

FIGURE 10.2   I Chart for Temperature Readings for Patient with Fever

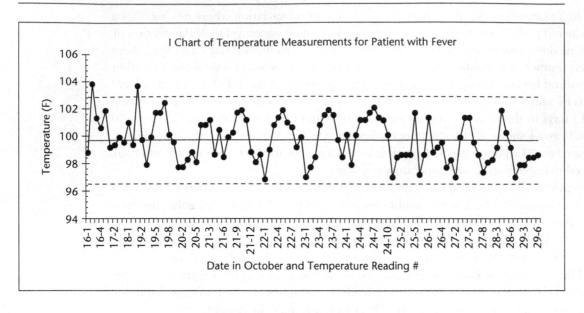

**FIGURE 10.3   X̄ and S Charts for Temperature Readings
for Patient with Fever**

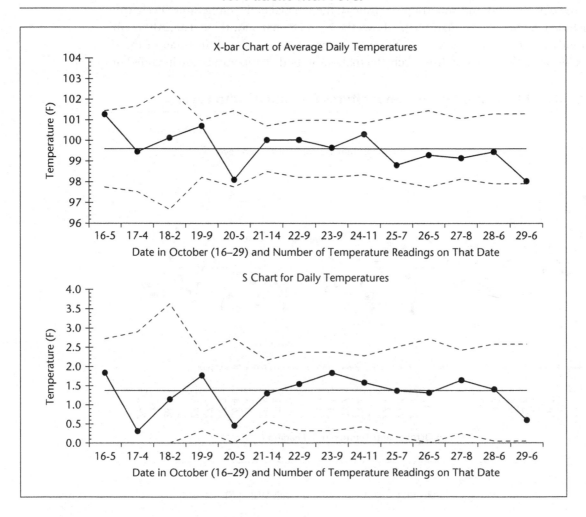

the standard deviation calculation (S chart), the wide swings of 5 to 6 degrees on many days could be making the standard deviation large and thus inflating the limits on the $\bar{X}$ chart. If there was a record of the time that each individual temperature was taken, a more sophisticated subgrouping strategy based on time of day could be explored.

This example illustrates how run charts and Shewhart charts could be easily applied to measures routinely made when patients are hospitalized. These charts can make the data accessible to anyone who wants to learn about the patient's history and conditions.

Example 2: Bone Density for a Patient Diagnosed with Osteoporosis

A BMD test uses a special machine to measure bone density or bone mass. This test indicates the amount of bone mineral in a certain area of bone. Based on a bone density test done in January 1993, a female patient was diagnosed with osteoporosis. The patient had been taking estrogen to prevent bone loss. Test results were reported at two locations—the hip neck and the spine. An increase in BMD is an indicator of improved bone strength. A repeat of the test was done in February 1993. After each test the clinician classified the results as increased, decreased, or maintained.

The results of the repeat test on the second month were interpreted by the clinician as significant improvement over the previous month. It was suggested that the patient repeat the scan tests a year later. The test done the next year was interpreted as a significant increase. After the next test, Calcetonin was prescribed, but was stopped because of side effects. Subsequently tests were continued about every 12 months with most results classified as an increase or decrease. Fosamax was recommended after a decrease in the BMD, but the patient did not want to be on an osteoclast-type drug. The patient decided to reduce the frequency of scans to every other year in 1998, then went on a treatment (Forteo) for two years from 2005 to 2007.

Figure 10.4 shows two versions of run charts for the BMD (bone mineral density) measurement for the spine (lumbar spine, L1–4) from January 1993 to March 2009. In Chapter Three, the use of a time-based scale was generally recommended when measurements are made at unequal intervals. The first chart at Figure 10.4 illustrates this approach, making it evident on the x-axis that unequal amounts of time have elapsed between scans. The second chart uses equal intervals so does not make evident this unequal time interval between scans.

As discussed, specific treatments were recommended in 1993 and again in 1995, either not started or quickly discontinued both because of patient preference. There is a significant trend of five or more increasing points starting in May 1998.

At the time of each of the tests, most were classified as an "increase" or "decrease" in BMD. How should the variation from test to test be described—common cause or special cause? Figure 10.5 shows I charts for both measurement locations constructed using the first 10 test results from 1993 to 2005, with the limits extended to future tests. Only 10 subgroups were used here so that limits could be set based on the data prior to beginning treatment in 2005.

The I charts show that both of the BMD measures indicate a stable system prior to 2005. So the changes from year to year are due to common cause variation. After the Forteo treatment began in 2005, an improvement (special cause based on rules 1, 3, and 4) is seen on the BMD for the spine location, but the BMD for the hip location remains stable.

One advantage of the Shewhart chart is that differences from patient to patient are automatically accounted for when calculating the center line and limits. Rather than use specifications (selected for an "average" patient) to define an "improvement" or "decrease"

FIGURE 10.4   Run Charts for Bone Density Test—Different Spacing on X-Axis

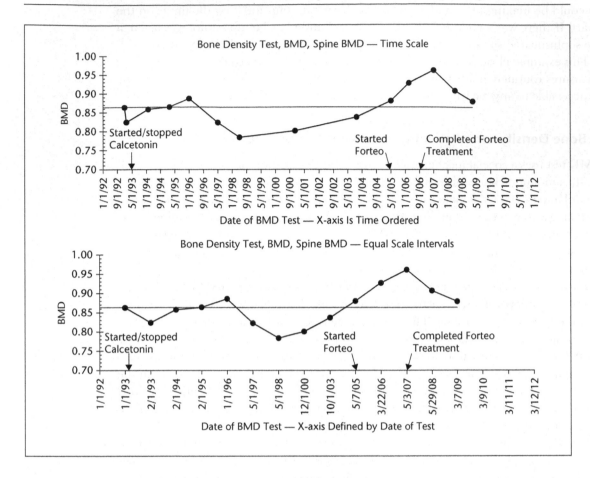

for all patients, the limits can be used to provide specific guidelines for each patient based on individual patterns of variation.

Example 3: PSA Screening for Prostate Cancer

A controversial issue for males in the United States over fifty is the PSA test used for early identification of prostate cancer. The PSA (prostate-specific antigen) test began to be used routinely in the late 1980s. There is mixed evidence on its effectiveness and recent studies suggest it leads to unnecessary treatment. Because prostate cancer grows so slowly, it often causes no problem for many of the men who have it. Many end up dying of something else without ever knowing that they had prostate cancer. Because of that, there's been an intense debate over whether routine PSA testing is warranted.

A recent study concluded that for every man whose life was saved by PSA testing, at least twenty underwent unnecessary treatment that may have left them incontinent, impotent, or suffering from other side effects.[7]

A PSA test greater than 4 ng/mL is considered abnormal. Other studies have shown that the absolute value of a test is not the key, but rather the trend over time. Even when the total PSA value isn't higher than 4, a high PSA velocity (an increase greater than 0.75 ng/mL in

---

[7]Welch, H. G., and Albertsen, P. C., "Prostate Cancer Diagnosis and Treatment after the Introduction of Prostate-Specific Antigen Screening: 1986–2005," *Journal of the National Cancer Institute*, doi:10.1093/jnci/dj, 278.

FIGURE 10.5 I Charts for Patient BMD at Two Locations

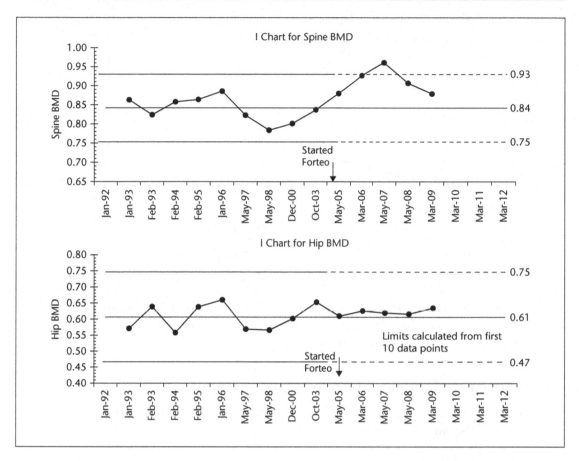

FIGURE 10.6 Run Chart for PSA Test Results for Colleague

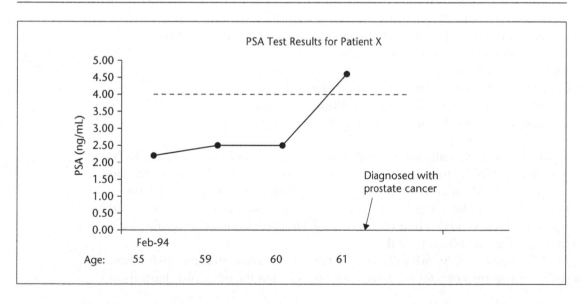

one year) suggests that cancer may be present and a biopsy should be considered. This suggests that the run chart would be a useful way for men to display their PSA test results. Figure 10.6 shows a run chart of PSA tests for a colleague of the authors. After the PSA test result exceeded 4 ng/mL in 2000 (when he was 61 years old), he was diagnosed with prostate cancer and underwent successful surgery for treatment.

FIGURE 10.7   PSA Test Results for One of the Authors

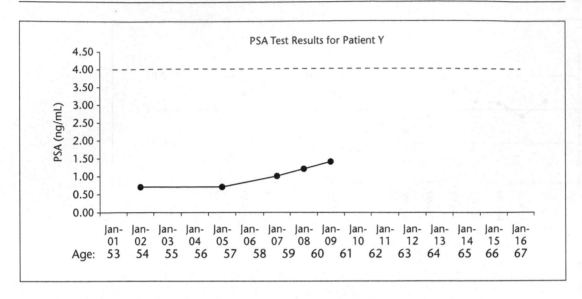

Figure 10.7 shows a run chart for PSA test results for one of the authors. He will continue to update this graph each year when PSA tests are done as part of an annual physical exam and discuss the patterns on the chart with his physician.

Example 4: Shewhart Charts for Continuous Monitoring of Patients

One of the biggest potential opportunities for use of Shewhart charts in hospitals is for analysis and presentation of the data obtained from patient monitors. Monitors have been used in intensive care units for many years and recently they have begun to be used in general medical and surgical units.[8] Patient measures monitored using these instruments include:

- Functioning of the heart (ECG/heart rate)
- Pulse oximetry: peripheral circulation and arterial blood oxygenation (SpO2)
- Non-invasive arterial blood pressure
- Skin and cavity temperature
- Breathing by impedance (breathing rate/respirogramm)
- Strength of myocardial hypoxia (ischemia) (ST-segment analysis)
- Capnography/breathing (breathing rate, capnogramm, EtCO2, FiCO2)

For heart patients, typically monitored parameters are end-diastolic volume (EDV, end-systolic volume (ESV), stroke volume (SV), ejection fraction (Ef), heart rate (HR), and cardiac output (CO). Many of these measures are continuously reported by the instruments and readings can be averaged for a minute, five minutes, 30 minutes, hour, and so on. Figure 10.8 shows a run chart of measures of blood pressure and heart rate for a patient averaged for a half-hour period.

Figure 10.9 shows three Shewhart I charts for the same measures in Figure 10.8. There are special causes on the chart for diastolic blood pressure, but the other two charts show

---

[8]Gao, H., and others, "Systematic Review and Evaluation of Physiologic Track and Trigger Warning Systems for Identifying At-Risk Patients on the Ward," *Intensive Care Medicine*, 2007, *33*, 667–679; Sandau, K., and Smith, M., "Continuous ST-Segment Monitoring: Protocol for Practice," *Critical Care Nurse*, August, 2009, *29*(4), 39–50.

FIGURE 10.8   Run Chart of Patient Monitoring Data (Half Hour Summaries)

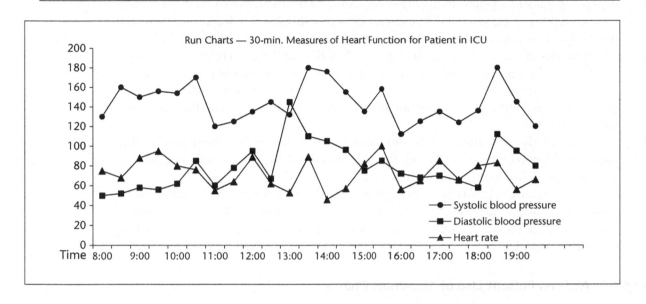

FIGURE 10.9   I Charts for Patient Heart Function Variables Monitored in the ICU

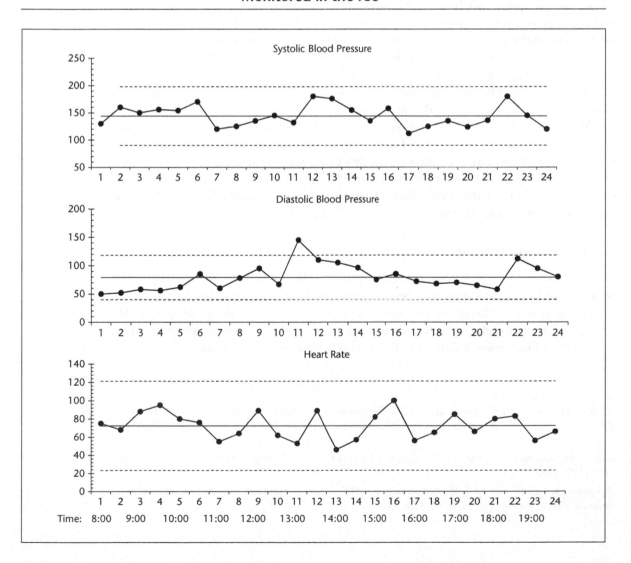

only common cause variation. Targets and critical clinical limits for these measures depend on patient age and many other conditions. Thus, a Shewhart chart with limits calculated from recent patient data can provide a very useful way to learn from the variation and to detect changes long before they reach critical values. If additional sensitivity is needed to detect small changes in the measure, $\bar{X}$ and S or CUSUM charts could be used.

One of the issues with monitors in hospitals is the number of false alarms. It would be useful to do some research on the use of Shewhart charts as a method to reduce these alarms, which can be a nuisance for nurses and reduce sensitivity to alarms that are important to respond to.[9]

Some of the measures from continuous monitors would be expected to exhibit patterns of autocorrelation.[10] The methods described in Chapter Seven for dealing with autocorrelation would be useful in these cases.

An intriguing advantage of Shewhart charts is that they reflect each person's system variation. They enable us to detect a special cause relative to the patient's own system, rather than react solely to targets or triggers that may be generalized for patient populations.

Example 5: Asthma Patient Use of Shewhart Charts

As discussed at the beginning of this chapter, an asthma patient's use of Shewhart charts is one of the most common applications reported in the medical literature. Figure 10.10 shows an example of an $\bar{X}$ and S Shewhart chart for daily readings with a peak flow meter. Subgroups were formed using three readings each day. The limits calculated using the first 20 subgroups showed a stable process, so they were extended for future monitoring. A reduction in the average value was noted during the next week. When sharing the graph with her physician, the patient noted that she traveled for business frequently. During the time frame when her average values fell she was on a business trip and had forgotten to move her inhalants from the medicine cabinet to her suitcase, a frequent problem.

When she returned home and resumed using her inhaled medication, her values returned to normal (see Figure 10.11). After discussing ways to prevent this from occurring again on business trips, the provider suggested keeping inhalant samples in her travel kit to avoid the need to transfer medications each time she traveled. The Shewhart chart clarified issues in the patient's life that interfered with optimal care and fostered patient involvement and self-management.

Example 6: Monitoring Weight

Obesity is a major health problem for many people today. In addition, many others could benefit from losing a few pounds. The measurement of weight is probably the most common measurement of health that is made. Many people weigh themselves daily or weekly to monitor their weight, but they try to track the measure in their heads rather than recording it. This makes it difficult to learn from the variation in the data.

---

[9]Clifton, D. et al., "Patient-Specific Biomedical Condition Monitoring in Post-operative Cancer Patients," *The Sixth International Conference on Condition Monitoring and Machinery Failure Prevention Technologies*, 2009, 424–443.

Imhoff, M., and Kuhls, S., "Alarm Algorithms in Critical Care Monitoring" *Anesthesia & Analgesia*, 2006, *102*, 1525–1537.

[10]Gordon, K., and Smith, A.S.M., "Modeling and Monitoring Biomedical Time Series," *Journal of the American Statistical Association*, 1990, *85*, 328–337.

FIGURE 10.10 X̄ and S Chart for Patient with Asthma Peak Flow Meter Readings

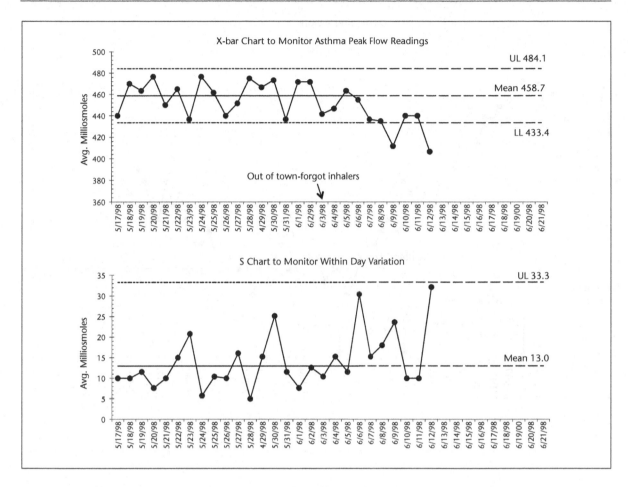

FIGURE 10.11 Continued Use of Peak Flow Meter Shewhart Charts

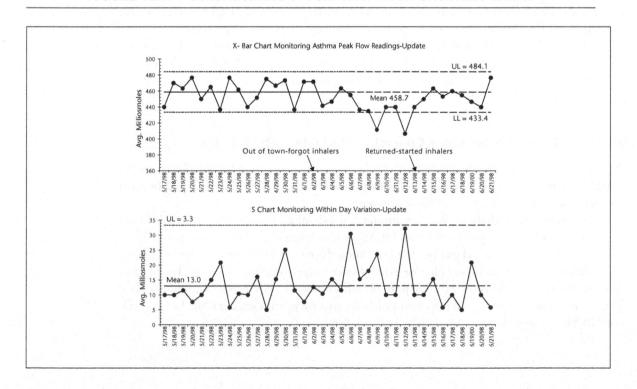

FIGURE 10.12   Run Chart and I Chart for an Individual's Weighings

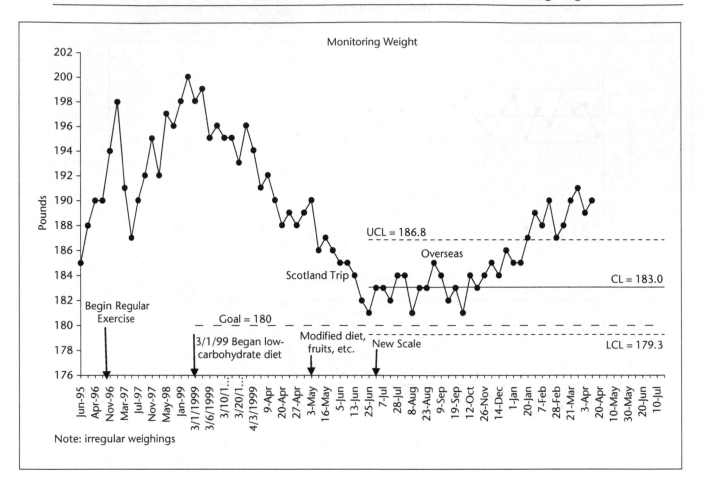

Figure 10.12 shows an example of a run chart that an individual used to monitor his weight. Note that the weights are made very irregularly, with a much higher frequency in 1999. But the individual chose to use a horizontal scale with regular intervals. Annotations of key actions (exercise and diets) are used to document approaches to control or lose weight. I chart limits were calculated in 1999 after a stable period of a desirable lower average weight.

Example 7: Monitoring Blood Sugar Control for Patients with Diabetes

Many patients with chronic diseases (diabetes, asthma, congestive heart failure, and so forth) have regular tests done to monitor their condition. Shewhart charts could be used to communicate and learn from these measures.

For patients with diabetes who are insulin dependent, an HbA1c test is a simple blood test usually done on a quarterly basis. HbA1c is also known as HgbA1c or glycosylated hemoglobin. Where a blood glucose test is an immediate measure of blood glucose control, the HbA1c test assesses blood glucose control over longer time periods. The HbA1c test is typically performed quarterly for patients with diabetes. The results can detect poor control and can be used as an important diabetes treatment-monitoring tool. Target levels for HbA1c are age dependent, usually in the 6–8 range.

FIGURE 10.13   I Chart for Monitoring HbA1c for Patient with Diabetes

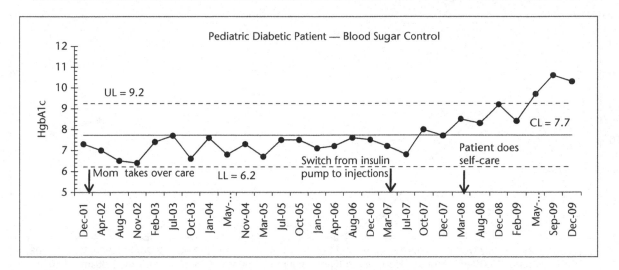

Figure 10.13 shows an I chart for a young patient with diabetes over an eight-year period (note: the limits are calculated using all of the data). The chart is annotated with key treatment events. When the child became a teenager in 2008, she took over the management of her disease from her mother. The result was an increase in the HbA1c level over the next year as indicated by the special causes on the I chart.

Example 8: Monitoring Patient Measures in the Hospital

An eight-year-old child had experienced multiple urinary tract surgeries to correct a congenital condition. He had recently experienced some narrowing of his urine stream and was scheduled to see his surgeon in a couple of weeks. After he complained to his mother in the afternoon that "no urine was coming out today," his surgeon asked that the family allow no food nor fluids and bring him directly to the nearest children's hospital. After a seven-hour drive he was treated in the emergency department with multiple attempts to catheterize him. The catheterization effort was not deemed successful. Ultrasound revealed a bit of a puzzle: only 36 cc of urine remained in the bladder at 11:30 PM yet it was clear that significant urinary tract blockage existed. The child was hospitalized for further investigation and to determine an appropriate course of action.

While in the hospital some urine flow began. Ultrasounds were performed periodically to measure the volume of urine retained after his bladder was "emptied completely" by the patient. When the data were recorded in the patient's charts, the mother began plotting the data on a run chart created on a whiteboard in the child's room. The surgical team noted the graph and discussed possible theories. Figure 10.14 shows a computer version of the run chart.

After a while the graph of the data made a clear pattern indicative of stricture that allowed only small amounts of urine to pass at a time. It took repeated attempts to urinate throughout the morning to "work down the backlog" of urine. By the end of the day the bladder was not showing residual urine present. The decision was made to perform surgery and a suprapubic catheter was placed to allow a period of urinary tract rest prior to additional reconstructive surgery.

Examples like this patient-specific measure are common for inpatients. Making the data visible on an in-room whiteboard would be beneficial to all the caretakers and aid communications with the patient.

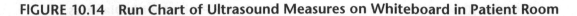

FIGURE 10.14 Run Chart of Ultrasound Measures on Whiteboard in Patient Room

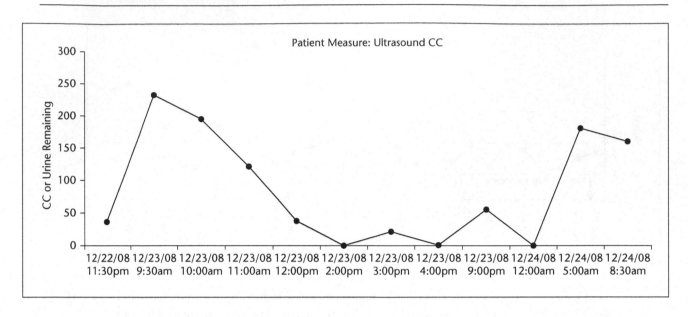

Example 9: Using Shewhart Charts in Pain Management

In 2001, the Joint Commission published standards for health care providers that included:

- Recognize the right of patients to receive appropriate assessment and management of pain.
- Establish the existence of pain and assess its nature and intensity in all patients.
- Record the results of the assessment in a way that facilitates regular reassessment and follow-up.

Regular assessment of pain and tracking the pain measures for each patient using Shewhart control charts is one way to accomplish these standards. There are a variety of tools used to measure pain from the patient's perspective. Many of these use a 0 (no pain) to 10 (extreme pain) interval scale.

The visual analog scale (VAS) is another common tool used to measure pain.[11] With the VAS, a patient is asked to indicate his or her perceived pain intensity along a 100 mm horizontal line, and this rating is then measured from the left edge (VAS score). The measure can then be treated as a continuous measure (ratio scale). Figure 10.15 shows an I chart for a patient who was regularly assessed for pain using the VAS scale during a nine-day hospitalization.

---

[11]Myles, P., and others, "The Pain Visual Analog Scale: Is It Linear or Nonlinear?" *Anesthesia & Analgesia*, 1999, *89*, 1517–1520.

FIGURE 10.15 I Chart for Patient Pain Assessments During Hospital Stay

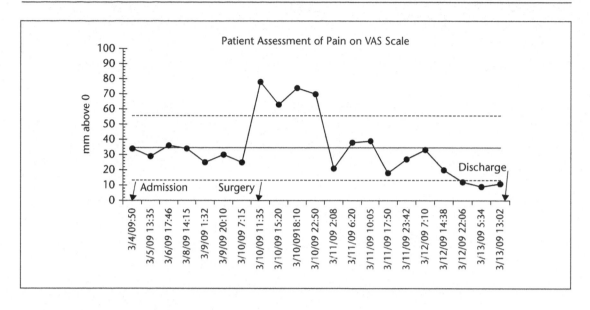

SUMMARY

This chapter illustrated nine examples of patient-specific run charts and Shewhart charts. As concluded in the research articles referenced at the beginning of the chapter, there are many opportunities to apply Shewhart's theory of variation and the simple concept of run charts to monitor and learn from clinical measures for individual patients.

Why are clinicians not making more frequent use of these methods, especially for patients with chronic diseases? We hope that this chapter will raise enough curiosity to explore an application. The expansion of electronic medical records will make more longitudinal data readily available for analysis. Health care providers should also encourage patients with chronic diseases to monitor their health and related measures using run charts or Shewhart charts.

FIGURE 10.15 Chart for Patient Pain Assessments During Hospital Stay

SUMMARY

## CHAPTER 11

LEARNING FROM PATIENT FEEDBACK TO IMPROVE CARE

This chapter focuses on using data that is obtained by direct feedback from patients (and other stakeholders) for learning and improvement. Although we use a variety of data sources in our improvement work, information from patients based on their experiences with the health care system is often pivotal. The reader of this chapter will be able to address issues such as selection of a summary statistic for patient satisfaction data and selection of the appropriate Shewhart Chart for display and analysis for that data. In addition, the reader will gain an appreciation for the use of both quantitative and qualitative patient feedback, and insight into using patient feedback data at the global project level, at the process measure level, and to "feed" learning in PDSA cycles. In addition, we will also describe the use of Shewhart charts for patient survey data and other key stakeholder feedback data to fuel the organizational planning process.

We have already illustrated the use of patient feedback data in other parts of this book. In Chapter Two, Figure 2.4, we illustrate the use of a run chart to summarize patient satisfaction and contrast summarizing by percentile and by average satisfaction. In Figure 2.27, we illustrate the use of patient satisfaction as a balancing measure for a team improvement project. In Chapter Three, Figures 3.43 and 3.44, we introduce the use of the CUSUM statistic on a run chart using patient satisfaction data. In Chapter Four, Figure 4.2 uses patient satisfaction scores on a scatter plot and Figure 4.6 illustrates the use of the Shewhart chart to track patient satisfaction after improvements were made in order to determine whether gains are being held. In Chapter Seven, Figures 7.15 and 7.16 illustrate the use of the CUSUM method with Shewhart charts and includes an example of displaying the V-mask and the use of two limits with a CUSUM chart. An exponentially weighted moving average (EWMA) Shewhart chart for patient feedback data is also introduced in Chapter Seven and shown at Figure 7.18.

Creating a good patient satisfaction feedback instrument can be difficult and expensive. We don't intend to address creating these instruments here. For further information regarding development of good survey designs see the book by Hayes[1] which also includes the use of Shewhart charts with survey data. A vast amount of work has been accomplished in this arena related to both development of instruments and creating a

---

[1] Hayes, B. E., *Measuring Customer Satisfaction: Development and Use of Questionnaires*, Milwaukee, WI: ASQC Quality Press, 1992.

culture receptive to their use.[2] This chapter is devoted to better display and understanding of patient feedback data. The following quotation from a British medical journal article captures our perspective:

> [P]ut aside preconceptions about the value of patient surveys: there now are valid and reliable instruments that ask patients objective questions about aspects of care that both clinicians and patients think represent quality . . . newer surveys and reports can provide results that are interpretable and suggest specific areas for quality improvement efforts. . . . Now that we have the right tools we should all work together to hear patients' voices clearly and meet their needs better.[3]

PATIENT SURVEYS

Most organizations make use of a commercial product or a methodology they developed internally for regularly obtaining patients' feedback related to patient experience of care or to their satisfaction. These survey instruments typically yield both quantitative data and qualitative data. The quantitative data are typically in the form of a feedback rating, such as an average of 3.7 on a scale of 1 (low) to 5 (high). Qualitative data might also be available in the form of written comments or lists of problems.

One relatively new survey used by many is CMS's Hospital Consumer Assessment of Healthcare Providers and Systems (HCAHPS).[4] It is the first national, standardized, publicly reported survey of patients' perception of their hospital care. The HCAHPS survey asks discharged patients 27 questions about their recent hospital stay. An excerpt from the HCAHPS is shown in Figure 11.1.

These survey data are summarized monthly as the percent of patients responding who rated the hospital in the "top box" indicating the highest satisfaction rating (for most questions this would be a 4 on the 1–4 scale). These data are currently publicly displayed comparing states or specific hospitals to one another by presenting an annual average of the percentage of patients who rated the hospital(s) in the top box.[5]

Figure 11.2 shows an example of questions yielding both quantitative and qualitative data from some NRC-Picker survey instruments.[6] Both of these data types are potentially

[2]Seid, M. et al., "Parents' Perceptions of Primary Care: Measuring Parents' Experiences of Pediatric Primary Care Quality," *Pediatrics*, 2001, *108*(2).

Ruta, D. et al., "SF 36 Health Survey Questionnaire: I. Reliability in Two Patient Based Studies," *Quality in Health Care*, 1994, *3*, 180–185.

Davies, E., and Cleary, P., "Hearing the Patient's Voice? Factors Affecting the Use of Patient Survey Data in Quality Improvement," *Quality and Safety in Health Care*, 2005, *14*, 428–432.

Colla, B. et al., "Measuring Patient Safety Climate: A Review of Surveys," *Quality and Safety in Health Care*, 2005, *14*, 364–366.

[3]Cleary, P. D., Professor, Department of Health Care Policy, Boston: Harvard Medical School, Boston.

[4]CMS HCAHPS: Patients' Perspectives of Care Survey, http://www.cms.gov/HospitalQualityInits/30_HospitalHCAHPS.asp.

[5]Ibid.

[6]NRC Picker, http://www.NRCPicker.com.

FIGURE 11.1   Excerpts from HCAHPS Survey

1. During this hospital stay, how often did nurses treat you with courtesy and respect?

       1   Never   2   Sometimes   3   Usually   4   Always

7. During this hospital stay, how often did doctors explain things in a way you could understand?

       1   Never   2   Sometimes   3   Usually   4   Always

13. During this hospital stay, how often was your pain well controlled?

       1   Never   2   Sometimes   3   Usually   4   Always

14. During this hospital stay, how often did the hospital staff do everything they could to help you with your pain?

       1   Never   2   Sometimes   3   Usually   4   Always

22. Would you recommend this hospital to your friends and family?

       1   Definitely no 2   Probably no 3   Probably yes 4   Definitely yes

useful for focusing improvement work. Some organizations routinely share only the quantitative data and ignore or even discard the qualitative feedback. Combining qualitative and quantitative data is a stronger approach to learning from patients or clients.

These formal patient written surveys can be expensive and time consuming and sometimes the response rate is low. Farrokh et al. have proposed a less formal two-question survey, called the "Minute Survey," to assess patient's satisfaction:[7]

- The patient's rating of overall satisfaction with the care (5 option Likert scale)
- The patient's explanation of what worked well and what needed improvement

The survey can be completed and returned at the end of a clinic or hospital visit or could be mailed back after returning home. The two questions could also be asked by phone. This approach potentially reduces cost of conducting satisfaction surveys and reduces delays in feedback and reporting.

Data from formal patient experience or satisfaction surveys is the most common source of patient feedback information. In addition, there are numerous other potential sources of patient feedback data, such as complaint systems, in-person and phone personal interviews, and group interviews. Most health care organizations also get feedback from employees, contract and referring physicians, partners, and suppliers. Data such as feedback on patient pain levels, employee issues surfaced during exit interviews, and provider issues raised via focus groups are examples of feedback obtained by other than patient experience/satisfaction surveys. All these feedback sources may prove very useful in improvement projects as data for measures of progress or balancing measures. They also can be used for generating focus areas for aims and ideas for improvement. The points made in this chapter related to methods for summarizing and displaying patient satisfaction data obtained via a variety of methods also apply to using feedback from patients and these other stakeholder groups.

An important consideration in designing systems for patient feedback is to obtain and analyze the data over time rather than aggregating the data for special quarterly or

---

[7]Alemi, F., Badr, N., Kulesz, S., Walsh, C., and Neuhauser, D., "Rethinking Satisfaction Surveys: Minute Survey." *Quality Management in Health Care*, 2008, *17*(4), 280–291.

FIGURE 11.2 Excerpts NRC-Picker Survey and CG HCAHPS Survey

Emergency Department (Adult) Survey NRC Picker

27. How often were the different doctors and nurses consistent with each other in providing you information and care?

    Never   Sometimes   Usually   Always

34. How often did you have enough input or say in your care?

    Never   Sometimes   Usually   Always

GOING HOME FROM THIS EMERGENCY DEPARTMENT

35. Did someone on the staff explain what to do if problems or symptoms continued, got worse, or came back?

    No   Yes, somewhat   Yes, mostly   Yes, definitely

36. Did someone on the staff talk with you about whether you would have the help you needed when you left the emergency department?

    No   Yes, somewhat   Yes, mostly   Yes, definitely

37. Did you know who to call if you needed help or had more questions after you left the emergency department?

    No   Yes, somewhat   Yes, mostly   Yes, definitely

40. Is there anything else you would like to say about the care you received during this visit?

(Please print your answer on the lines provided below.)

HCAHPS® Clinician & Group Survey

Version: Adult Primary Care Visit Questionnaire

Please answer only for your own health care. Do not include care you got when you stayed overnight in a hospital. Do not include the times you went for dental care visits.

22. During your most recent visit, did this doctor seem to know the important information about your medical history?

    1 Yes, definitely   2 Yes, somewhat   3 No

23. During your most recent visit, did this doctor show respect for what you had to say?

    1 Yes, definitely   2 Yes, somewhat   3 No

24. During your most recent visit, did this doctor spend enough time with you?

    1 Yes, definitely   2 Yes, somewhat   3 No

27. Please tell us how this doctor's office could have improved the care you received during your visit. Please print _____

---

annual events. Currently many forms of feedback, such as that from employees or other stakeholders, are obtained only once a year. Obtaining data annually makes patient satisfaction a special event rather than an ongoing measure. In order to better learn from these data we suggest obtaining data more frequently. If the desire is to survey individuals only once per year, one approach to achieving this is to divide the population being surveyed into monthly increments. Rather than survey all at one point in the year, survey 1/12 of the population each month. This supports learning about the impact of changes being made to better serve this population as well as the impact of other parts of the system on these individuals.

SUMMARIZING PATIENT FEEDBACK DATA

Patient feedback data from surveys is summarized to make it useful for those utilizing the data. Many different approaches for summarizing patient satisfaction data are used. Should an organization analyze and summarize quantitative patient satisfaction by charting the average satisfaction score? Perhaps they'd learn more by tracking the median satisfaction score? What about summarizing the data by tracking the percentage of patients who report that they are satisfied or very satisfied, or even dissatisfied? Some organizations use percentile rankings of patient satisfaction scores. Is this useful for improvement? Another popular summary statistic is called the Net Promoter Score.[8] Some track the receipt of qualitative data such as the number of patient complaints. Each of these statistics has advantages and disadvantages. Each of these statistics requires careful selection of the appropriate Shewhart chart if we are to learn accurately from this patient satisfaction data. Table 11.1 summarizes some of the assumptions and issues around various statistics used to summarize patient feedback data.

Table 11.1   Summary Statistics, Issues, and Tools Used with Patient Satisfaction Data

Summary Statistic	Assumptions	Advantages	Issues	Shewhart Chart
Average Patient Satisfaction Score	Have scale data (e.g., using scale 1–5 Likert scale and record score for each response)	Easily understood by users Detect improvement sooner than % satisfied	Controversial with researchers when using average of Likert scale data	$\bar{X}$ and S charts
Median Patient Satisfaction Score	Have small odd-sized samples (e.g., 3, 5, 7, 9) of scaled data (e.g., using scale such as 1–10)	May be more acceptable to researchers than average	Less sensitive to changes than average Median not useful for discrete data (e.g.,1–5 ratings)	Median and range chart I chart
Percentage Satisfied	Have scaled data that we have chosen to treat as classification data **or** have classification data (two choices— satisfied or dissatisfied)	Focuses on positive measure Percentage data well understood Focus on positive (those satisfied)	Must determine which categories constitute satisfied More difficult to detect improvement	P chart
Percentage Dissatisfied	Have scaled data that we have chosen to treat as classification data **or** have classification data (two choices- either satisfied or dissatisfied)	Focus on dissatisfaction may create sense of urgency Percent data are well understood Leverage to improve rapidly by dealing with the extreme sources of dissatisfaction	More difficult to detect improvement when this percentage in this category is small	P chart

(continued)

---

[8]Reichheld, F., "The One Number You Need to Grow," *Harvard Business Review*, December 2003.

Table 11.1   Continued

Summary Statistic	Assumptions	Advantages	Issues	Shewhart Chart
Percentile Ranking of Satisfaction	Have comparative peer group Data treated as classification	Measures direct comparison to other organizations	Can be misleading and not useful to improvement teams working to track impact of changes	I chart
Net Promoter Score	Data treated as multiple classifications (e.g., 1–5 or 1–10 Likert scale)	Summarizes all satisfaction data into one statistic Factors both good and bad responses into the statistic	New statistic that many are not familiar with	I chart
Number of Complaints or Negative Replies	Have count of volume of qualitative data received Can capture how many complaints or negative replies made on each survey	Captures the magnitude of dissatisfaction (rather than 1 patient being dissatisfied we know that they expressed dissatisfaction 4 times) Can be stratified to study sources of dissatisfaction	Must determine what comprises dissatisfaction or a negative reply Number of responders must be relatively the same for each time period summarized	C chart
Complaint or Negative Reply Rate	Can count how many complaints or negative replies made on each survey	Captures the magnitude of dissatisfaction Can be stratified to study sources of dissatisfaction Can be used with widely varying number of responders for each period summarized	Must determine what comprises dissatisfaction or a negative reply	U chart
Type of Negative (or Positive) Comments	Have qualitative data in form of comments Have clear/useful way to categorize each comment	Can identify things that may lead to ideas for improvement team to test or areas for leadership to focus	Focuses improvement effort on specific areas with highest potential gain	Pareto chart

Figure 11.3 illustrates patient satisfaction data from one organization working hard to improve patient satisfaction. These graphs summarize replies to the HCAHPS question "Would you recommend this hospital to your friends and family?" In this illustration they have summarized the patient satisfaction data using a variety of statistics. Summarizing their *average patient satisfaction* involved using the survey's 1–4 scale, obtaining each patient's response to this question, and selecting an $\bar{X}$ and S chart to display the average score for the question. (For the first chart at Figure 11.3 we have chosen to display the $\bar{X}$ chart only rather than both the $\bar{X}$ and S charts.)

The $\bar{X}$ chart shows a special cause is occurring in September 2009 (a point above the upper limit). This special cause was also ultimately part of a shift of 8 consecutive points above the mean. This organization chose not to summarize their data as the *median patient satisfaction* because the median was not useful for detecting improvement. As most of the

**FIGURE 11.3   Shewhart Charts for One Question from Patient
Satisfaction Survey**

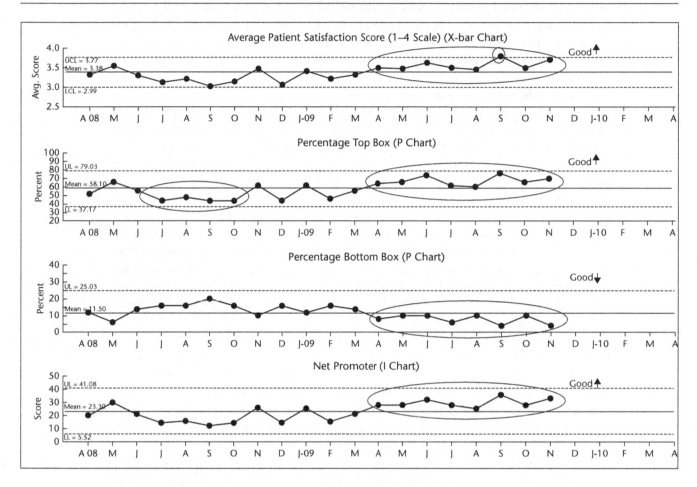

patient responses were 4 each month, the median each month was 4. Working to reduce bad satisfaction (a score of 1) or to improve ratings from 3 to 4 would not change the median a bit. Ironically, those with a strong research background may express discomfort with using the average for Likert score data and suggest the use of the median.[9] If our purpose, however, is to detect improvement, we need to be able to see the variation in the data. The average satisfaction score outperforms the median satisfaction score when using data from a survey response scale.

The appropriate Shewhart chart for analyzing the *percentage of patients selecting* the highest satisfaction rating (often called "top box") is the P chart. Sometimes working to move from so-so to extreme satisfaction can be a very motivating and creative approach to improving satisfaction. The P chart of "Top Box" in Figure 11.3 also reveals special cause. From July to October 2008 the P chart shows special cause (2 out of 3 consecutive points 2 sigma or beyond) indicative of undesirable special cause. This is then followed by special cause indicative of improvement by November 2009 (8 consecutive points above the center line). The overall message in this P chart is of two different systems, an old poorly performing system and a new system performing at a better level. The $\bar{X}$ chart, graphing

---

[9]Carifio, J., and Perla, R., "Ten Common Misunderstandings, Misconceptions, Persistent Myths and Urban Legends about Likert Scales and Likert Response Formats and their Antidotes." *Journal of Social Sciences*, 2007, *3*(3), 106–116.

the average, revealed the improvement two months earlier due to its greater sensitivity. Summarizing the responses as the *percentage of patients selecting* the lowest satisfaction rating on the scale (or "bottom box"), also requires the use of a P chart. Sometimes working to decrease sources of extreme dissatisfaction can be a rewarding approach. The P chart for percentage "Bottom Box" also reveals improvement but again not until November 2009 (8 consecutive points below the mean).

The last chart in Figure 11.3 summarizes the satisfaction data using the *Net Promoter Score* (NPS). The NPS is based on the concept that an organization's customers can be divided into three categories: Promoters, Passives, and Detractors.[10] The NPS suggests asking customers a single question: "How likely is it that you would you recommend our company to a friend or colleague?" The NPS is calculated by asking customers to answer this question using a 0–10 point scale. It then classifies them as promoters, passives, or detractors. *Promoters* are categorized based on a score of 9 or 10. They are viewed as loyal enthusiasts who will keep using the organization and referring others to it. *Passives*, with a score of 7 or 8 are satisfied but not enthusiastic customer; they are viewed as being a population that may switch readily to a competitor. *Detractors*, with a score of 0 to 6 are viewed as unhappy customers who can damage your organization's reputation and slow the organization's growth through negative word-of-mouth. To obtain an NPS one takes the percentage of customers who are Promoters and subtracts the percentage of customers who are Detractors. An NPS of 75–80% is considered reflective of world-class loyalty on the part of the organization's customers.

For the chart seen in Figure 11.3 we adapted the NPS methodology a bit. To obtain the NPS for this chart, the number of patients replying that they definitely *would not* recommend the hospital (a score of 1 on the 1–4 scale) is subtracted from the number of patients replying that they definitely *would* recommend the hospital (a score of 4 on the 1–4 scale). For example, in the first month (April 08) 26 patients replied that they definitely would recommend the hospital while six replied that they definitely would not recommend the hospital. Using an approach similar to the Net Promoter methodology would yield a Net Promoter score of 20 for April. These data would best be analyzed on an I chart. The I chart also reveals improvement (8 consecutive points above the mean) but again not until November of 2009. For these data, the chart for the Net Promoter statistic is very similar to the percentage Top Box P chart.

In summary, a variety of charts are available for use with these patient feedback data. The $\overline{X}$ chart for the average of the patients' ratings was most helpful for those in this organization working to detect improvement from their patient satisfaction efforts. Table 11.2 shows an excerpt of the data for these graphs.

Summarizing the responses for a single question on a survey has the risk of missing the whole message about the patient's experience. For example, HCAHPS publicly reports results for 10 survey questions. Each patient completing a survey could be dissatisfied with multiple areas reflected on this survey. Patient A may have replied negatively (selecting a 1 or 2 on the 1–4 scale) for 8 of the 10 questions while Patient B may have rated only 1 of the 10 questions a 1 or a 2.

Another option for analysis is for the organization to track the number of negative replies (for example, a question rated 1 or 2) that they receive per month. In this example the organization obtained 50 completed surveys a month. They used a C chart to display the total number of negatively answered questions from these surveys each month. The C chart was appropriate because they had count data and they had a consistent area of

[10]Reichheld, "The One Number You Need to Grow."

Table 11.2   Shewhart Charts for One Question from Patient Satisfaction Survey

Month	Patient Score 1	P2	P3	P4	P5	P 6 . . .	P50	Average	Median	% Satisfied (# Top Box)	% Dissatisfied (# Bottom Box)	Net Promoter (Number of 4s minus number of 1s)
A 08	4	1	4	4	4	4	4	3.22	4	26	6	20
M	4	4	3	4	4	4	1	3.42	4	32	3	29
J	4	2	4	4	3	4	3	3.18	4	28	7	21
J	3	1	4	4	2	4	4	3.02	3	23	9	14
A	4	3	3	4	3	4	4	3.18	4	26	7	19
S	2	4	1	4	3	4	2	3.00	3	24	9	15
O	4	4	4	3	4	4	4	3.06	3	22	8	14
N	3	4	4	4	4	4	4	3.38	4	32	5	27
D	4	2	4	4	4	4	3	2.96	3	22	8	14
J-09	4	4	3	4	3	4	4	3.30	4	31	6	25
F	4	2	4	4	4	4	4	3.12	3	23	8	15
M	3	4	4	4	4	4	1	3.22	4	29	7	22
A	4	4	2	4	4	4	4	3.40	4	32	4	28
M	3	4	4	4	3	4	4	3.38	4	34	5	29
J	4	4	3	4	4	4	4	3.52	4	37	5	32
J	4	4	1	4	4	4	3	3.40	4	31	3	28
A	2	4	4	4	4	4	4	3.36	4	31	5	26
S	4	4	4	4	4	4	4	3.68	4	38	2	36
O	4	2	4	4	4	4	4	3.40	4	33	5	28
N	4	4	3	4	4	4	4	3.60	4	35	2	33
D												
J-10												

FIGURE 11.4   Patient Satisfaction Data Summarized with Multiple Negative Replies

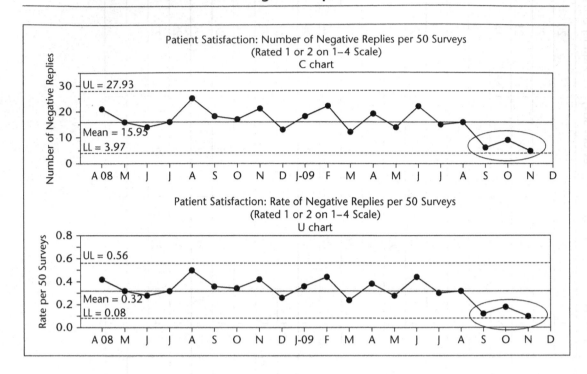

opportunity (50 surveys a month). Figure 11.4 shows that the number of negative answers per 50 surveys had been around 15. By November 2009 it had improved (two out of three consecutive points in the outer third of the limits) to a level closer to 5.

The organization also summarized these data as the rate of negative replies per 50 surveys using a U chart. Although right now they obtained 50 completed surveys per month, in the future they planned to use an approach that would result in unequal numbers of surveys returned each month. Unlike the C chart, the U does not require an equal area of opportunity (from Chapter Five). Summarizing the data on the U chart reveals the same signal of improvement and sets the organization up with a measure that is robust in regard to the area of opportunity (number of returned surveys).

Another popular method of summarizing patient feedback data is to graph **percentile rankings**. Percentile rankings go beyond just the organization's performance by comparing the organization's performance to that of other organizations in a given peer group and determining the percentile that its performance has reached (the percentage of organizations that your organizations ranks above). For example, 70% of an organization's patients rate themselves as "very satisfied" with the organization, yet that organization may only be at the 30th percentile when compared to other organizations.

Though useful for understanding how the organization compares to others, percentile rankings are less helpful, and even potentially misleading, when using patient satisfaction data for improvement (see discussion in Chapter Two, Figure 2.4 on the use of percentile data). Percentiles are influenced not only by the performance of one organization, but by all organizations in the comparison group. An organization's percentile ranking could remain unchanged, even though its performance has improved. This could occur because other organizations' performances have also improved or because there has been a change in the peer group (such as new organizations added or previous organizations dropped

FIGURE 11.5   Patient Satisfaction Percentile Ranking

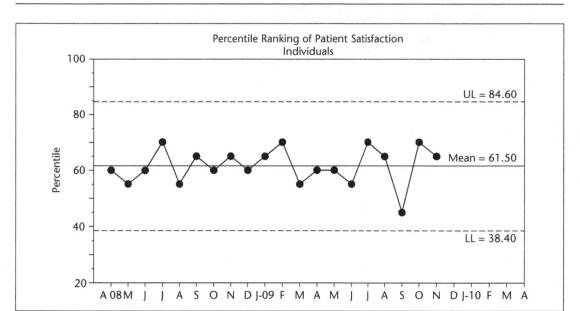

out). Figure 11.5 illustrates a stable percentile ranking for the organization when compared to its peer group of 40 other hospitals. Note that when the organization's own data were summarized in a variety of ways in Figure 11.3 they clearly revealed improvement.

The important concept here is that percentile rankings are influenced by several factors: the performance of the reporting organization, the performance of the other organizations in the comparison group, and the number of organizations in the comparison group. Improvements in an organization's percentile ranking can occur then because it improved, others in the comparison group worsened, or the peer group size changed. Thus, although percentile rankings may be useful for judging performance compared to others, they are not useful for guiding improvement efforts. Leadership may well need two or more views of the patient feedback data: a graph of performance over time as percentile rankings when they want to see how they compare to others *and* one or more appropriate Shewhart charts of their actual patient satisfaction levels when they want to learn and improve their organization's performance.

Improvement teams should not use percentile ranking data to determine whether the changes they are testing are resulting in improvement, as doing so can be misleading. It is possible for a team to see an increase in their organization's percentile ranking of patient satisfaction and to think their changes worked. However, the increase in the percentile ranking of patient satisfaction could have nothing to do with the changes they tested but rather with poorer performance by another organization(s) in the comparison group. This makes it difficult for improvement teams to learn accurately about the impact of changes they are testing. An improvement team needs an appropriate chart(s) of the *actual* patient satisfaction data rather than percentile rankings. The team will be testing changes and needs to see the actual data to determine if these changes are leading to improvement.

Qualitative patient feedback data in the form of *negative or positive comments*, such as complaints or compliments, can also be summarized to aid improvement efforts. A number of tools for organizing qualitative feedback are listed in Table 1.4. One such tool is the Pareto chart, another is the affinity diagram. Figure 11.6 shows data from an organization that received written comments from patients, used affinity analysis to develop categories

FIGURE 11.6   Pareto Chart of Types of Patient Complaints

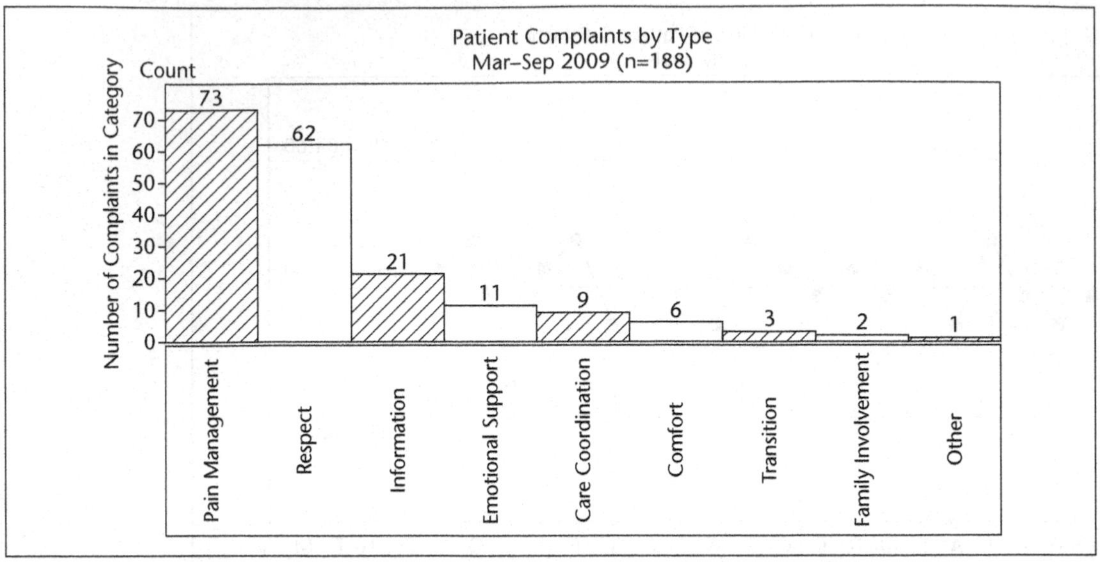

Patient Complaints by Type
Mar–Sep 2009 (n=188)

of the comments, and then organized all the comments by "type" using the categories. The Pareto chart in Figure 11.6 summarizes the patient complaints received over the most recent seven months for each type.

The Pareto chart identifies two areas in which to focus work to improve patient experience: pain management and lack of respect. The improvement team can then read all the verbatim patient comments in these two categories to develop ideas for improvement. Summarizing data by viewing the average satisfaction score or by tracking the percentage of satisfaction is important but does not tell the organization *what* patients are happy or unhappy about. Obtaining and summarizing qualitative data is important in working to improve satisfaction.

PRESENTATION OF PATIENT SATISFACTION DATA

The concept of **small multiples**, as discussed in Chapter Three, may be very useful when displaying patient satisfaction data. Small multiples of run or Shewhart charts consist of a set of run or Shewhart charts. Each chart is of the same measure but for a different location, segment of the organization, or provider. All of these charts are presented on the same "page" and with the same scale for rapid visual comparison. Another version of small multiples would be graphs of data from multiple questions in the same survey. For example, the 10 questions on the HCAHPS survey that are publicly reported could be presented as small multiple run charts.

The small multiple in Figure 11.7 reveals that the overall satisfaction with the ABC Outpatient Health Care System is stable. However, satisfaction with the Imaging Department shows recent special cause to the bad. Investigating the special cause in Imaging would be advisable. OB-GYN clinic is stable and performing near the system average. Orthopedics clinic is also stable, but at a substantially lower level of satisfaction than the rest of the system. How could Orthopedics redesign their stable system to result in improved patient satisfaction? Pediatrics and Primary Care clinics have both shown special

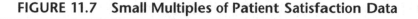

FIGURE 11.7   Small Multiples of Patient Satisfaction Data

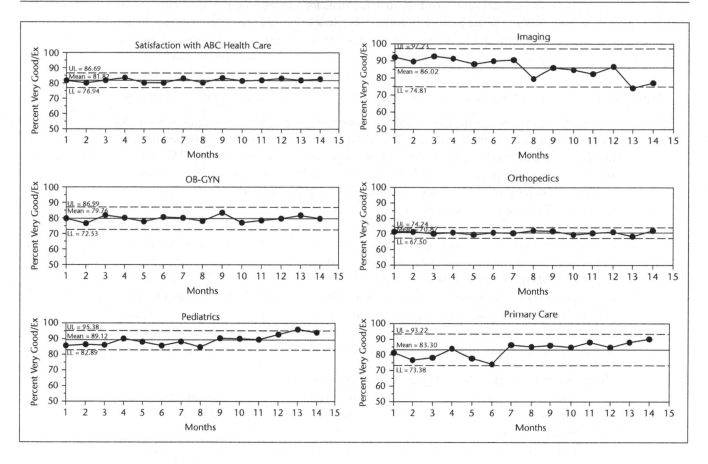

cause indicative of improvement. What are they doing that may be useful elsewhere in the system? The use of small multiples with this patient satisfaction data makes it possible to determine how parts of the system compare to the rest of the system. They also make it possible to distinguish special from common cause variation so that leadership may take the appropriate action for the type of variation observed.

USING PATIENT FEEDBACK FOR IMPROVEMENT

Improvement teams can make great use of patient feedback data. The Model for Improvement described in Chapter One includes three key questions and the Plan-Do-Study-Act cycle. Each of these components can make use of patient feedback:

1. What are we trying to accomplish?

    Patient feedback can be useful in identifying aspects of care that are important and currently have low levels of patient dissatisfaction. This information can be useful in determining which project selection, prioritization and in shaping the scope of a project (see later discussion of using patient feedback in planning).

2. How will we know a change is an improvement?

    Patient feedback data can be turned into measures to provide outcome and process measures for improvement projects.

3. What change can we make that will result in improvement?

   Patient feedback may contain specific ideas for improvement (e.g., please put an additional chair in the providers' offices). Feedback may also provide common themes around which the team can generate specific ideas to take to testing (for example, "My family wasn't provided with adequate information on my care after discharge").

The Plan-Do-Study-Act Cycles (PDSA) Cycle for Testing and Implementing Changes

Some PDSA cycles benefit from—or are completely dependent on—patient feedback as the team runs specific tests of an idea. Both quantitative and qualitative patient feedback data can be used in Plan-Do-Study-Act cycles as a team tests changes. What do the patients say when that idea is tested? Do they like it, dislike it, or bring up issues or barriers to its use? Do patients have suggestions for modifying the idea prior to the next test? All of this feedback can be helpful in improvement projects.

One organization obtained real-time patient feedback when testing a change by posting a question in a visible spot with a bowl of poker chips and containers marked "highly satisfied," "somewhat satisfied," "neither satisfied nor dissatisfied," "somewhat dissatisfied," or "very dissatisfied." Patients indicated their feedback by placing a poker chip in the container corresponding to their opinion. Using this method they were able to obtain patient feedback on a daily basis regarding the change tested. Another organization uses patient rounding to ask a question specifically related to a change being tested to collect data daily and summarize it rapidly. We offer here three examples of using patient feedback in improvement projects.

Improvement Team Working on Clinic Satisfaction

A team in a specialty clinic working to improve patient satisfaction used a 1–7 Likert scale to track responses to "Would you recommend this clinic?" as their project's key outcome measure. As illustrated in the previous section, patient feedback data are not always quantitative. Summarizing qualitative patient feedback data such as patient comments or complaints can provide much-needed direction for channeling improvement efforts. It can also stimulate specific ideas to take to testing with Plan-Do-Study-Act cycles.

The team had access to both patient comments from a year's worth of surveys and patient complaint data from the complaint system. However, without some means of summarizing these data, they were of limited utility. The team chose to summarize the data by using a Pareto chart. They used existing operational definitions to categorize the negative survey comments and patient complaints (Chapter Two provides additional guidance related to operational definitions). The Pareto chart in Figure 11.8 revealed several major categories of patient dissatisfaction with the clinic.

The clinic already knew about dissatisfaction related to the length of time patients had to wait for an appointment and were currently working on this issue. Clinic leadership had the resources for another improvement effort, and they chartered a team to start working to reduce the dissatisfaction related to several other areas made evident by the Pareto chart. They targeted lack of provider respect, lack of information provided during visit, and confusion over who to call with questions after a visit.

Each month, the team tracked the percentage satisfied (the percent replying 6 or 7) for the overall question "Would you recommend this clinic?" and for three other related to survey questions:

- Were you treated with respect by the provider?
- Did you receive enough information from the provider?
- Do you know who to call with questions?

FIGURE 11.8   Pareto Chart of Clinic Patient Feedback

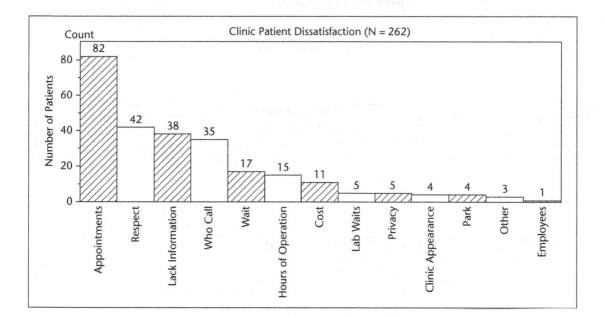

The team had historical data from 2007 and was able to create a baseline P chart for each question with data from 12 months. This baseline analysis showed that each measure was stable, so the team extended the baseline limits into the future to detect the impact of their changes (note: Chapter Four provides more detail related to this technique with Shewhart charts). The team next tested three changes to improve the satisfaction ratings. The first two ideas came from literature review of best practices. The third idea was taken directly from a patient comment: "Why don't you give me your card so I have your number in case of questions? Other people in business use business cards for this purpose." The three changes were:

1. The physician asked the patient if he had any more questions prior to ending the appointment
2. The physician walked the patient out from the exam room
3. The physician provided her card with a phone number to call if questions arose

The team annotated their tests of these changes and detected improvement after six months in the graphs at Figure 11.9.

The team also used scatter plots (Figure 11.10) to relate the monthly patient's satisfaction score on the question reflecting their change (for example, "Were you treated with respect?") to the monthly percentage for overall clinic satisfaction (note: Chapter Four discusses use of scatter plots in more depth). They determined that being treated with respect and being provided with enough information were areas more closely related to overall satisfaction with the clinic than was the third area: knowing who to call in case of questions. The team decided to continue providing cards with information on who to call in case of questions as it was inexpensive and fit well into the flow of the visit. In addition the team viewed this change as another means of communicating their respect for the patient.

The team was encouraged that their three process measures had shown evidence of improvement, but what about the outcome measure *Willingness to Recommend the Clinic to Others*? The team realized that this outcome measure was influenced by many factors in addition to their three areas of focus. Although they had clear evidence of improvement in

**FIGURE 11.9   Clinic Patient Feedback Shewhart Charts for
Three Areas of Focus**

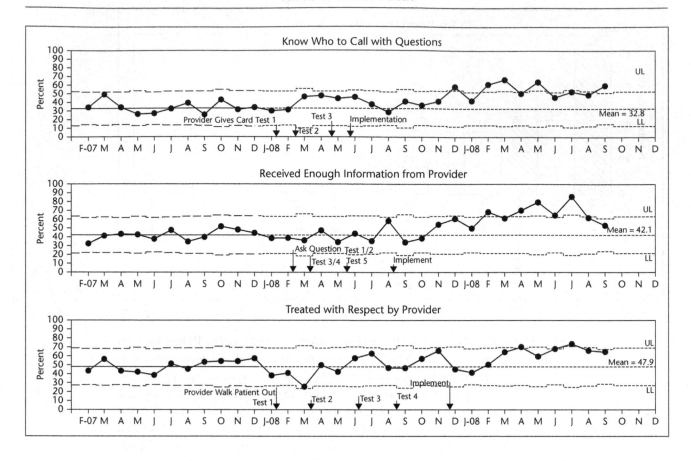

FIGURE 11.10   Scatter Plots for Three Areas of Focus

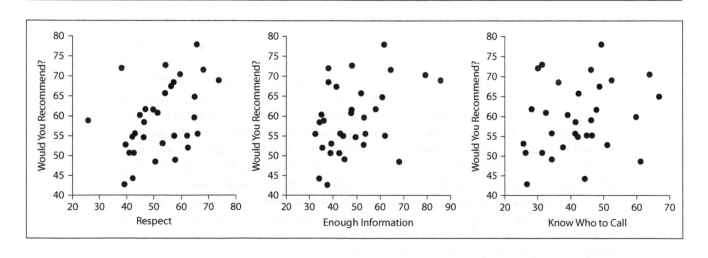

FIGURE 11.11   Shewhart Chart of Willingness to Recommend the Clinic

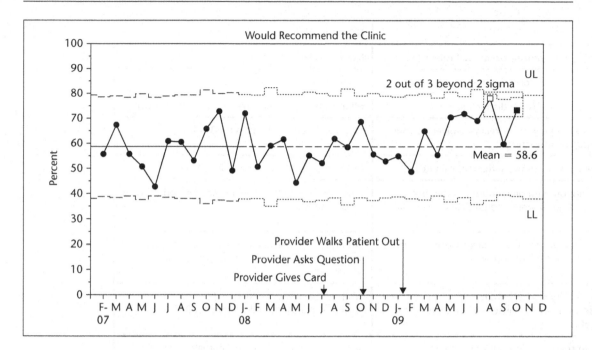

some of their process measures as early as January 2009, they did not yet have a signal of improvement in overall satisfaction. They thought it reasonable that a signal of improvement may well be delayed due to the many variables influencing this measure. By October of 2009 special cause (a shift and 2 out of 3) was detected, indicating improvement in this measure as shown in Figure 11.11.

Improvement Team Working on Pain

Feedback from patients may deal with issues other than satisfaction. Patient self reported perception of their pain level is an example. Many organizations use a pain rating scale such as that shown in Figure 11.12.[11] This measurement of pain is often recorded as a "5th vital sign" and is tracked over time for inpatients. Similar scales are used for outpatient chronic care involving pain. Patient feedback such as this may use a scale (as do most patient surveys) and be summarized quantitatively.

Pain assessment data can be summarized in a number of ways. For example, each patient with elective hip replacement surgery is asked to assess his pain multiple times during the hospital stay. These scores could be averaged to obtain the average pain rating reported by that patient during their stay. These data are best displayed using an $\bar{X}$ and S chart. The $\bar{X}$ chart in Figure 11.13 shows the average pain assessment for each patient.

Viewing the $\bar{X}$ chart, we can see that the pain control for elective hip surgery patients is stable. The S chart displays the variation within the patient's pain ratings making up that average. It reveals that the average pain scores do not include any unusually high or low ratings. The variation within each subgroup is also stable. (Chapter Five provides more detail related to the $\bar{X}$ and S chart.) If the organization wanted to work to improve pain levels the $\bar{X}$ and S chart could be very useful. This $\bar{X}$ and S chart has an upper and a

---

[11]Mankoski, A., *Mankoski Pain Scale*, http://www.wemsi.org/painscale.html.

FIGURE 11.12 Mankoski Pain Scale

0	Pain Free	No medication needed.
1	Very minor annoyance—occasional minor twinges.	No medication needed.
2	Minor annoyance—occasional strong twinges.	No medication needed.
3	Annoying enough to be distracting.	Mild painkillers are effective (Aspirin, Ibuprofen)
4	Can be ignored if you are really involved in your work, but still distracting.	Mild painkillers relieve pain for 3–4 hours.
5	Can't be ignored for more than 30 minutes.	Mild painkillers reduce pain for 3–4 hours.
6	Can't be ignored for any length of time, but you can still go to work and participate in social activities.	Stronger painkillers (Codeine, Vicodin) reduce pain for 3–4 hours.
7	Makes it difficult to concentrate, interferes with sleep. You can still function with effort.	Stronger painkillers are only partially effective. Strongest painkillers relieve pain (Oxycontin, Morphine).
8	Physical activity severely limited. You can read and converse with effort. Nausea and dizziness set in as factors of pain.	Stronger painkillers are minimally effective. Strongest painkillers reduce pain for 3–4 hours.
9	Unable to speak. Crying out or moaning uncontrollably—near delirium.	Strongest painkillers are only partially effective.
10	Unconscious. Pain makes you pass out.	Strongest painkillers are only partially effective.

Source: Andrea Mankoski. All rights reserved. Used by permission.

FIGURE 11.13   X̄ and S Chart of Average Self-Reported Patient Pain Assessment

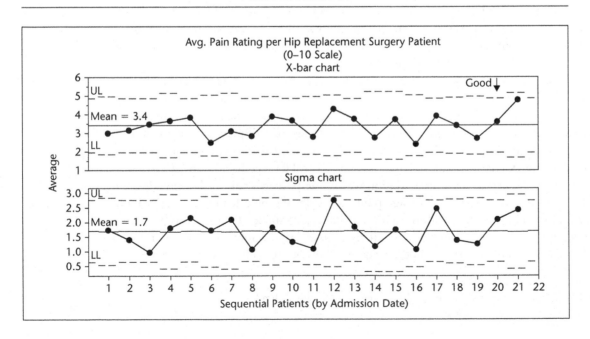

FIGURE 11.14   P Chart Summarizing Patient Feedback Regarding Pain

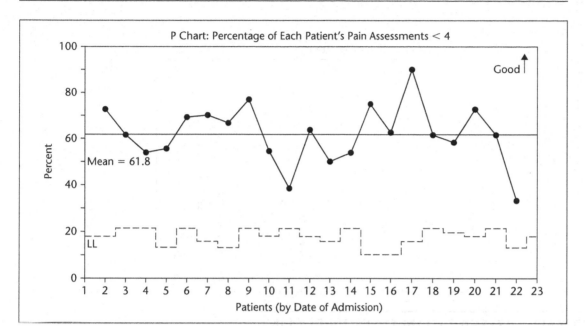

lower limit; patients whose average pain level improved could be readily detected as they dropped below the lower limit.

Although not generally recommended, it is also possible to summarize patient feedback related to pain level as the percentage of patient pain assessments that are considered "acceptable" (such as 0–3 on the pain scale) and display this using a P chart. To summarize these data, the organization would count the number of "acceptable" pain assessments scores each patient reported and divide this by the total number of pain assessments that patient completed. The percentages would be analyzed using a P chart, as shown in Figure 11.14. The pain assessment appears stable analyzing the data using a P chart.

This analysis of the pain ratings changed the data from continuous to classification data in order to obtain the percentage "acceptable." In addition, the sample size is small with patients having 6–13 pain assessments during their stay. As discussed in Chapter Two, it is almost always better to use the continuous scale for data when it is available. Note that the P chart created from these data does not have an upper limit. As a result it will not be as useful to those assessing the impact of changes they are testing. It typically takes longer to detect improvement with the P chart (attribute data) than with the $\overline{X}$ and S chart (variables data).

Feedback from Employees

An organization was concerned about employee turnover. Methods of summarizing qualitative or quantitative feedback data addressed in this chapter also apply to feedback from patient families, employees, providers, suppliers, the community, or other stakeholders. This type of data can be very useful for improvement. This organization had data from exit interviews conducted by their human resources department. The exit interviews asked departing employees why they were leaving. These data were readily summarized into the Pareto chart in Figure 11.15. By summarizing and sharing the data in the Pareto chart format, the organization realized that they had an opportunity to influence employee retention by developing better career pathways (to address growth issues) within their organization.

FIGURE 11.15   Employee Feedback upon Exit Interview

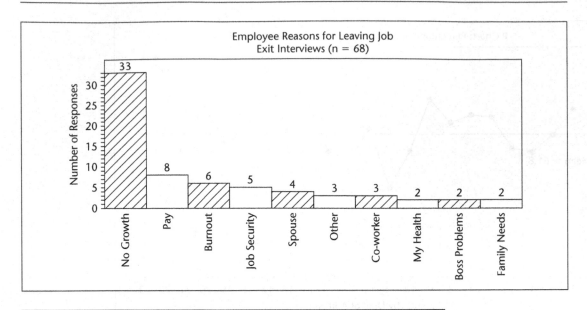

USING PATIENT SATISFACTION DATA IN PLANNING FOR IMPROVEMENT

For patient-oriented organizations, information obtained from patients should carry a lot of weight when decisions are made as to which parts of the system to improve. Both qualitative and quantitative data are valuable in helping organizations maintain focus on their mission when planning for improvement. These data also aid in identifying specific areas for improvement. Useful information from patient studies such as patient market research, patient satisfaction measures, patient complaints, and suggestion data should all be included as inputs when planning for improvement. The information in these data need to be summarized effectively to be useful to those in the planning process. The middle of a planning session is no time for leaders to be asked to sort through stacks of surveys or other forms. Key qualitative data are often displayed using Pareto charts such as those in Figures 11.6 and 11.8.

In addition to using patient comments and complaints in planning, patient satisfaction survey data may offer important information about elements of care that correlate closely to overall patient satisfaction. For example, an organization using the HCAHPS (see Figure 11.1) may have found that questions 1 ("How often did nurses treat you with courtesy and respect?") and 7 ("How often did doctors explain things in a way you could understand?") correlated closely to question 22 regarding their overall measure of patient satisfaction ("Would you recommend this hospital to your friends and family?"). Bringing this correlation information into planning would be a good idea. Figure 11.10 illustrates the use of scatter plots to display correlation among data used for clinic improvement planning.

A potentially useful way to bring patient feedback into a planning session involves obtaining information from patients about both the importance of a particular aspect of care and their satisfaction with that same aspect of care. A patient could appreciate some aspect of their experience (such as parking), but may not feel that it is important to their overall care experience. We illustrate this by obtaining both their satisfaction score with an element of care (illustrated here by the patient's rating on a 1–4 scale for each of the HCAHPS survey questions) and, in addition, the importance they place on the aspect of care represented by that HCAHPS question. In this example, importance was expressed

FIGURE 11.16 Importance and Satisfaction Matrix

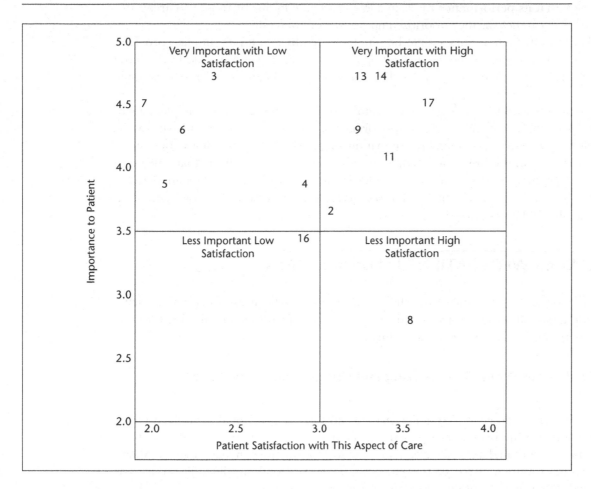

using a 5-point scale (1 unimportant, 2 slightly important, 3 somewhat important, 4 very important, and 5 extremely important).

Figure 11.16 illustrates placing annual summaries of these data on a scatter plot by placing the HCAHPS survey question number in the quadrant corresponding to the average importance and satisfaction rating that the patients gave it. This plot could be used to develop or prioritize potential improvement projects during the planning process. For example, the HCAHPS questions placed in the upper left-hand quadrant indicate that patients believe these are highly important but rated their satisfaction low in these areas. Questions 3 and 7—"During this hospital stay, how often did nurses *explain things* in a way you could understand?" and "During this hospital stay, how often did doctors *explain things* in a way you could understand?"—both measured areas of high importance and low satisfaction to patients. This quadrant is a ripe area for consideration in prioritizing improvement projects. The lower left quadrant of the scatter plot includes areas of low importance and low satisfaction. These may not be areas in which the organization invests much. The upper right quadrant indicates areas of high importance and high satisfaction. This may be valuable marketing information for the organization.

Planning for improvement can make use of percentile ranking satisfaction data such as that shown at Figure 11.5. It can be powerful to combine patient feedback related to aspects of care with an understanding of how the organization compares to others in those aspects of care. Patients may be dissatisfied with two aspects of care.; if the organization discovers that its performance ranks in a low percentile in one of those two areas, this information can help as they prioritize improvement resources.

Patient satisfaction data should be supplemented by employee, supplier, provider, financial, governance, and other data appropriately summarized and graphically displayed as part of a robust planning process. The Pareto chart in Figure 11.15 is one example of summarizing some employee information. Including data from each of these sources leads to a better understanding of the system throughout planning. For example, patient feedback may indicate that lack of respect from providers is a moderate source of dissatisfaction. Employee surveys may reveal that nursing staff is providing information about lack of respect in the workplace. Employee exit interviews may indicate that a negative work environment is a key reason for employee turnover. Respect may be a moderately important issue for patients but could be selected as a major focus for improvement when viewing all the data pointing in that direction.

SPECIAL ISSUES WITH PATIENT FEEDBACK DATA

This section addresses some of the challenges of which to be aware when summarizing and using patient satisfaction survey data and some considerations on selecting the scale for patient satisfaction or experience ratings.

Are There Challenges When Summarizing and Using Patient Satisfaction Survey Data?

Some challenges do exist in tracking patient satisfaction as a global measure used for improvement. One issue is that patient satisfaction data are often reported by date of response rather than date of service. If we want to know whether changes tested in March were an improvement, we need the data grouped by the month in which the service was received rather than month in which the survey was returned.

Another issue is that patient satisfaction data may be organization-wide although the improvement effort is being piloted on just one unit or with one patient population. Teams need to be able to disaggregate the patient satisfaction data specific to their test population so that the impact of their change(s) is not obscured. Chapter Nine addresses disaggregation of measures.

A third challenge is that patient satisfaction data from formal surveys often lag several months behind real time. This makes it difficult for teams to tell if their changes are yielding improvements in a timely fashion. How does a team determine whether the four changes tested in March resulted in improvement and should be tested more widely, or even implemented, when they have to wait three months to see the patient satisfaction data?

To address this issue, improvement teams often create a satisfaction measure that they can obtain in real time in order to determine the impact of changes tested. They may do this by using the same survey tool on a small sample of patients from the unit or population in which they are testing changes and then processing them by hand in real time. Another approach is to use a simpler survey or method that they can obtain weekly or monthly that is logically related to their formal patient survey results (see earlier discussion in this chapter of the "Minute Survey").

One outpatient clinic created a short patient survey for their department and asked patients to complete it as they were checking out. As they piloted changes each month,

FIGURE 11.17   Using an Interim of Surrogate Measure to Avoid Lag Time

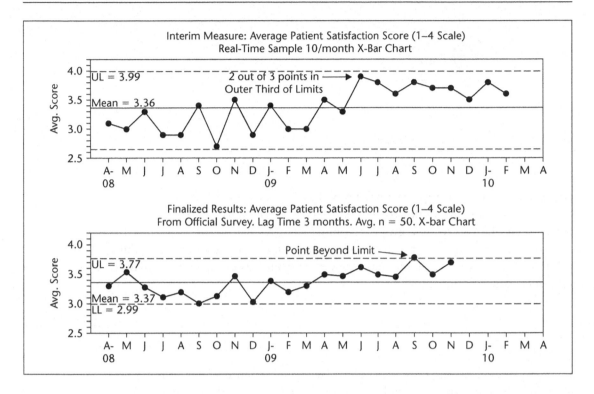

they would obtain a sample of 10 surveys from that department and plot the results on an $\overline{X}$ and S chart. Figure 11.17 shows their $\overline{X}$ chart for this measure. When the organization-wide patient survey data arrived three months later, with a typical sample size of 50 or more from their department, they would chart this on another $\overline{X}$ and S chart (see bottom chart in Figure 11.17). Using this method they could tell in real time if the changes they were testing worked or not. Figure 11.17 illustrates that they found that results of both methods were similar enough to be useful.

Does Survey Scale Matter?

The selection of a response scale may make it difficult to see improvement when using patient feedback data. A general principle to remember is that the more options on the scale, the more important it is to display the data as continuous rather than classification data. Figure 11.18 contains several examples of Likert scales and illustrates this concept. Note that the top one or two scores of each scale are usually treated as "good." In summarizing the percentage of responses that are "good" we can see that the more rating options on the scale, the more data are excluded when treating the data as classification rather than continuous data. Treating the data as continuous will result in all the data being used to create the summary statistic and result in a more sensitive measure better suited to detecting improvement.

Some scales are problematic by their design. It is not our intent to discuss this in depth but to point out that using a flawed scale can make it difficult for an improvement team to detect the impact of their changes. For example, a home health care organization designed a survey that had only three options: very dissatisfied, dissatisfied, and satisfied. With a three-option scale such as this, and a process that is generally meeting the patients' needs, nearly all responses will cluster around the top box. Using this scale, the average

FIGURE 11.18   Data Not Used When Treating Continuous Data as Classification

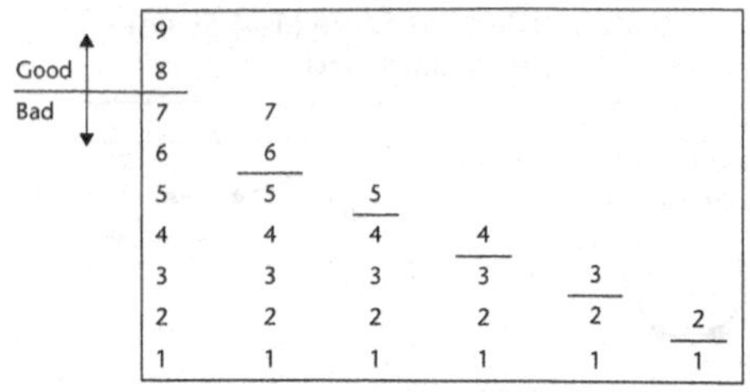

or percentage of satisfaction reported will be high, so it may look like improvement isn't necessary. If an improvement project is started, it will be hard for a team to see the impact of their changes using a graph stemming from the flawed survey design. In general, as the number of increments in a scale increases, the usefulness increases. This trend tends to level off around 7 increments. Above 11 increments there is little gain and additional unnecessary complexity.[12]

SUMMARY

This chapter focuses on learning from patient feedback data for improvement. It is important to summarize quantitative data with the appropriate statistic and view that statistic on the correct Shewhart chart. Scatter diagrams may be used to learn of relationships between various components of patient feedback. Qualitative data is a vital source of learning, and it may be summarized by using the Pareto Chart. This chapter illustrated using patient feedback data at the global project level, at the process measure level, and to "feed" PDSA cycles. Bringing quantitative and qualitative patient and staff feedback effectively into organizational planning sessions is of extreme importance.

Case Study Connection

Case Study A illustrates the use of run charts with an improvement project. It also provides an example of the use of multiple project measures graphically displayed on a single page. Some of these measures deal with patient and staff satisfaction.

KEY TERMS

Net Promoter Score

Percentile rankings

Small multiples

[12]Page-Bucci, H., "The Value of Likert Scales in Measuring Attitudes of Online Learners," http://www.hkadesigns.co.uk/websites/msc/reme/Likert.htm, 2003.

## CHAPTER 12

USING SHEWHART CHARTS IN HEALTH CARE LEADERSHIP

The usefulness of Shewhart charts extends beyond the project level and into the realm of senior leadership. This chapter discusses how leaders can use a set of measures for learning about and improving their organization as a system. In some organizations, system-level data are primarily used to set targets linked to senior leadership accountability and financial compensation. This chapter illustrates a different use for key system-level data.

In order to improve the system, it is vital that senior leaders and board members view key measures of the organization's status in ways that further their ability to ask pivotal questions, draw valid conclusions, and make insightful decisions. Often senior leadership is presented data for system-level measures in a tabular summary or other relatively flat ways that are of limited utility for learning. How should leaders view data in a way that fosters system learning and improvement?

Chapter Two addressed the use of a set of multiple measures for improvement projects. In this chapter we extend that concept to the system level and focus on using a set of measures useful to leadership in understanding, planning, and predicting the impact of changes made to improve the system.[1] Displaying vital organizational measures using run charts or Shewhart charts is far more useful for learning by senior leaders. In addition, understanding the performance of a system requires the use of multiple measures; no single measure is adequate to inform leadership of the system performance. Creating and displaying a set of multiple measures with each measure on the appropriate Shewhart chart is a strategic move that enhances leadership's ability to manage, lead, and improve the entire system for which they are responsible.

A HEALTH CARE ORGANIZATION'S VECTOR OF MEASURES

Many frameworks are available for developing a set of measures for an organization. These include the Balanced Scorecard,[2] Clinical Values Compass,[3] and Quality as a Business Strategy.[4] Each may be used to help those in health care to develop a useful set of measures for the various systems of interest. Our focus here is not to provide in-depth

---

[1]Provost, L., and Leddick, S., "How to Take Multiple Measures to Get a Complete Picture of Organizational Performance," *National Productivity Review*, 1993, Autumn, 477–490.

[2]Kaplan, R., and Norton, D., *Balanced Scorecard: Translating Strategy into Action*, Cambridge, MA: MBS Press, 1996.

[3]Nelson, E., Batalden, P., and Ryer, J., *Clinical Improvement Action Guide*, Chicago: The Joint Commission, 1998.

[4]Associates in Process Improvement, *Quality as a Business Strategy*. Austin, TX: API, 1999.

guidance on how to develop this measurement set, but rather to focus on using the measures to a better advantage.

Hospitals, payers, primary networks, and other health care systems are made up of many departments, functions, and services so that any single measure is not adequate to understand the detailed complexity of the system; thus, multiple measures are required. In addition, these functions and organizations are interconnected through a series of processes that create dynamic complexity as the various processes change over time. For learning about systems, measures must be displayed in a way to understand this dynamic complexity. For example, a small change in scheduling surgeries this month may have a significant impact on emergency room use next month.

The set of measures for learning from a system has been called different names including a family of measures, balanced scorecard, report card, dashboard, instrument panel, and vector of measures. The term we will use in this chapter is a **vector of measures** (VOM) or just a vector. The concept of a vector provides a good analogy when we consider the purpose of this family of measures. A vector is an engineering concept that describes both magnitude and direction. The individual components of the vector may not be tremendously useful by themselves, but when the components are combined, useful information is obtained. Like the various dials in a cockpit, some measures describe the past (for example, tachometer to measure hours of engine time used); some describe the present (for example, speedometer, altimeter); some are there to indicate problems (for example; fluid pressure gauges); and some describe the future (for example, fuel gauge).

The vector of measures brings together information from all parts and perspectives of the organization and thus provides a tool for leaders to focus planning and decisions on the whole system. The effect of changes to parts of the organization can be assessed for their impact on the whole. The vector for an organization should serve as an indicator of the present performance of the system and as a predictor of how the system will act in the future. It is the responsibility of the leaders of the organization to plan and manage improvement efforts and operate the system to improve the entire vector of measures. Managers in departments and divisions of the organization can often create vectors for their parts of the organization that roll up to the system level measures.

DEVELOPING A VECTOR OF MEASURES

A vector of measures, then, is a set of key organizational measures that are balanced across the dimensions and stakeholders of the organization. Although as individual measures they are inadequate to describe the system, together they are very useful to senior leaders to learn about, manage, and improve their system. A vector can be developed at a variety of levels. The Clinical Values Compass is often used to develop a vector of measures at the micro-system level.[5]

One key principle in developing a VOM is that the measures selected should reflect a balanced view of the purpose (or mission) of the organization. There should be a direct relationship between the key ideas in the organization's purpose statement and the measures in the vector.

A second key principle in developing a VOM is that it needs to bring together information from all parts and perspectives of the organization. Doing so provides a tool for the leaders to focus planning and decisions on the whole system. The effect of changes to

---

[5]Nelson, G., Mohr, J., Batalden, P., and Plume, S., "Improving Health Care, Part 1: The Clinical Value Compass," *The Joint Commission Journal on Quality Improvement*, 1996, *22*(4).

Table 12.1   A Summary of Some of the Categories Used to Develop a Vector of Measures

Framework	Balanced Scorecard	Clinical Values Compass	IOM Dimensions of Quality[6]	Quality as a Business Strategy	HEDIS[7]	Hospital (Example)
Major Focus	Organization	Patient Population	Organization	Organization	Health Plan	Hospital
Categories	Customers	Functional	Safety	Customers	Effectiveness of Care	Employee
	Learning and Growth	Satisfaction	Effectiveness	Employees	Access to Care	Clinical Excellence
	Financial	Costs	Patient Centeredness	Owners or Stockholders	Satisfaction	Safety
	Internal Business Processes	Clinical	Timeliness	Operations (including suppliers)	Use of Services	Operational
			Efficiency	Outside Environment (including the community)	Health Plan Descriptive Information	Patient Perspective (Service)
					Cost of Care	Community
					Health Plan Stability	Finance
					Informed Health Choices	

parts of the organization can be assessed for their impact on the whole. This means that the measures selected should also relate to the organization from a variety of stakeholder perspectives. The perspectives selected may depend on the framework used and the organizational level for which they are being developed. Table 12.1 provides a summary of some of the categories others have used in framing their vector of measures.

A third key principle in developing a VOM is to select a relatively small number of measures that are pivotal to understanding and improving the system. Table 12.2 contains examples of some of the measures being used in health care organizations from a variety of perspectives and in a variety of health care settings. This list includes some **composite measures**. Composite measures combine more than one measure into a single measure. The use of composite measures is a useful strategy for limiting the size of the vector while including a great deal of information.

DISPLAYING AND LEARNING FROM A VECTOR OF MEASURES

Effective leadership of an organization requires making predictions on the future performance of the organization. The directional aspect of the organization's vector of measures provides the focus for learning and making predictions. Using a VOM enables

---

[6]Institute of Medicine, Committee on Quality of Health Care in America, *Crossing the Quality Chasm: A New Health System for the 21st Century*, Washington, D.C.: National Academies Press, 2001.

[7]National Committee for Quality Assurance, 2010 Measures, *HEDIS 2010 Summary Table of Measures, Product Lines and Changes*, http://www.ncqa.org/Portals/0/HEDISQM/HEDIS2010/2010_Measures.pdf.

Table 12.2 Potential Measures of a System from Different Perspectives

Employee	Clinical Excellence
Voluntary Employee Turnover Employee Satisfaction Employee Injury Rate Nursing Time at the Bedside Sick Time Overtime Days to Fill Vacancies	Composite Index: Core Measures Timely Childhood Immunization Rates Unplanned Readmissions Percentage of Population with Breast Cancer Screening Composite Index of Cancer Screening Performance Index: Diabetes Control (Timely Care and HbA1c) Percentage of Patients Receiving Ideal Care Tobacco Use Rates Ages 15 and Over Newly Reported HIV Infections Mental Health 30-Day Follow-Up Rate
Safety	**Operational**
Adverse Events Percentage of Patients Developing a Pressure Ulcer Hand Hygiene Compliance Days Between Ventilator-Acquired Pneumonia Codes Outside the ICU Falls Bloodstream Infections Surgical Site Infections Total Infections Hospital Standardized Mortality Ratio (HSMR)	New Patients Number of Surgical Procedures Physician Recruitment Adjusted Admissions-Percentage of Budget Average Length of Stay Caseload Average Occupancy Physician Satisfaction Success Rating of Key Improvement Projects
Patient Perspective (Service)	**Community**
Days Wait for Third Next Available Appointment "Would You Recommend?" Score Overall Patient Satisfaction Score Satisfaction with Emergency Services	Community Service Budget Spent on Community Programs Media Coverage
Finance	
Operating Margin Man-Hours per Adjusted Patient Day Cost per Adjusted Patient Day Days in Accounts Receivable Days of Cash on Hand Investment Earnings	

leadership to track their predictions and effectively study the impact of their changes on the organization. Creating a vector of measures is a substantial investment for the organization. The return on that investment is earned when the vector is properly displayed and used for learning. How a vector is displayed affects our ability to make predictions and learn about the impact of deliberate changes as well as a host of other key interactions in the system.

Most system measures used in health care organizations today are not effectively displayed for learning. It's common to see a VOM displayed as a list of measures with the goal and the most current value noted. Some organizations add to this tabular display by including a comparison to the value from one year earlier or possibly a rating of progress toward the goal associated with the measure. Figure 12.1 illustrates one very typical method of displaying a VOM. It includes a scale to rate the performance of each measure by color coding the measure as green (met goal), yellow (75% of the way to goal) or red (not meeting goal). (The colors are represented in shades of gray.)

FIGURE 12.1 Tabular Vector of Measures Using Green, Yellow, and Red Indicators

Legend for Status of Goals (Based on Annual Goal)
- ☐ Goal Met (Green)
- ▨ Goal 75% Met (Yellow)
- ▓ Goal Not Met (Red)

FY 2009 HOSPITAL SYSTEM-LEVEL MEASURES

	Good	Goals		FY 2007	FY 2008	FY 2009 Q1	FY 2009 Q2	FY 2009 Q3
		FY 09 Goal	Long-Term Goal					
Patient Perspective								
1. Overall Satisfaction Rating: Percentage Who Would Recommend (Includes inpatient, outpatient, ED, and Home Health)	↑	60%	80%	37.98%	48.98%	57.19%	56.25%	51.69%
2. Wait for 3rd Next Available Appointment: Percentage of Areas with appointment available in less than or equal to 7 business days (n = 43)	↑	65%	100%	53.5%	51.2%	54.3%	61.20%	65.1%
Patient Safety								
3. Safety Events per 10,000 Adjusted Patient Days	↓	0.28	0.20	0.35	0.31	0.31	0.30	0.28
4. Percentage Mortality	↓	3.50	3.00	4.00	4.00	3.48	3.50	3.42
5. Total Infections per 1,000 Patient Days	↓	2	0	3.37	4.33	4.39	2.56	1.95

(continued)

FIGURE 12.1 Continued

Clinical								
6. Percentage Unplanned Readmissions	↓	3.5%	1.5%	6.1%	4.8%	4.6%	4.1%	3.5%
7. Percentage of Eligible Patients Receiving Perfect Care—Evidence = Based Care (Inpatient and ED)	↑	95%	100%	46%	74.1%	88.0%	91.7%	88.7%
Employee Perspective								
8. Percentage Voluntary Employee Turnover	↓	5.80%	5.20%	5.20%	6.38%	6.10%	6.33%	6.30%
9. Employees Satisfaction: Average Rating Using 1–5 Scale (5 Best Possible)	↑	4.00	4.25	3.90	3.80	3.96	3.95	3.95
Operational Performance								
10. Percentage of Occupancy	↑	88.0%	90.0%	81.3%	84.0%	91.3%	85.6%	87.2%
11. Average Length of Stay	↓	4.30	3.80	5.20	4.90	4.60	4.70	4.30
12. Physician Satisfaction: Average Rating Using 1–5 Scale (5 Best Possible)	↑	4.00	4.25	3.80	3.84	3.96	3.80	3.87
Community Perspective								
13. Percentage of Budget Allocated to Non-Recompensed Care	↗	7.00%	7.00%	5.91%	7.00%	6.90%	6.93%	7.00%
14. Percentage of Budget Spent on Community Health Promotion Programs	↗	0.30%	0.30%	0.32%	0.29%	0.28%	0.31%	0.29%
Financial Perspective								
15. Operating Margin-Percentage	↑	1.2%	1.5%	-0.5%	0.7%	0.9%	0.4%	0.7%
16. Monthly Revenue (Million)—change so shows red—but special cause good related to occupancy	↑	20.0	20.6	17.6	16.9	17.5	18.3	19.2

FIGURE 12.2   Shewhart Chart of Safety Error Rate

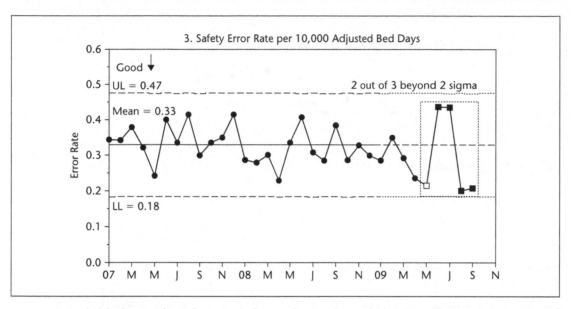

A tabular version of a vector that evaluates the variation in each measure compared to a goal can lead to erroneous conclusions and missed opportunities for learning. For example, an organization looking at Figure 12.1 would likely conclude that measure 3, Safety Events per 1,000 Patient Days, is in good shape and moving in the right direction. It used to be red but has moved to green this most recent quarter. This measure might not merit attention as it is improving nicely. But is it? Figure 12.2 displays the data for this measure more appropriately using a Shewhart chart. On this graph, special cause (2 out of 3 consecutive points close to or beyond a limit) is clearly evident. Data from June and July are special cause in an undesirable direction. August and September data indicate special cause in a desirable direction. The measure reflective of safety is unstable with multiple signals of special cause. By viewing the data in a flat tabular view, leadership would easily have made Mistake Two, treating an outcome as if it came from common causes of variation, when actually it came from a special cause (Chapter Four discusses Mistakes One and Two in detail). The costs associated with making Mistake Two include failing to learn from the special cause. What happened in June and July of 2009? How could this special cause increase in safety errors be prevented in the future? What happened in August and September? Data displayed in tabular form cannot reveal the information needed to understand or predict the performance of the organization.

Similarly, Measure 7, The Percentage of Patients Receiving Perfect Care, looks to be performing poorly. It has been red or yellow all year despite the efforts of an improvement team chartered two years ago to focus on this measure. Should the leadership team take another direction in working to improve in this area? Perhaps they need to invest a great deal more resources? Do they need a change in the manager who is the sponsor to help the team meet the target? When viewing this measure more appropriately on a Shewhart chart, Figure 12.3 reveals a very different picture. Although they have not yet met the goal of 95%, the Shewhart chart reveals clear evidence of improvement in the processes represented by this measure. The measures revealed a positive shift beginning in January 2008 that was sustained long enough to warrant the calculation of new limits for the improved measure. In addition, they currently have another shift indicative of further improvement in this measure beginning as of October 2008. They are waiting for a few more months and then will calculate a new set of limits for the current improved performance of the processes as reflected by this measure. Again, the tabular data with

FIGURE 12.3 Percentage Perfect Care Displayed on a Shewhart Chart

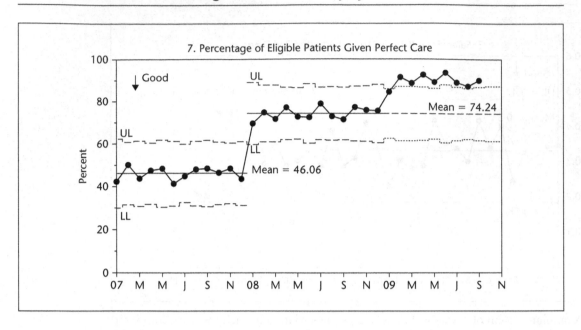

FIGURE 12.4 Shewhart Chart of Percentage of Areas Meeting Appointment Goal

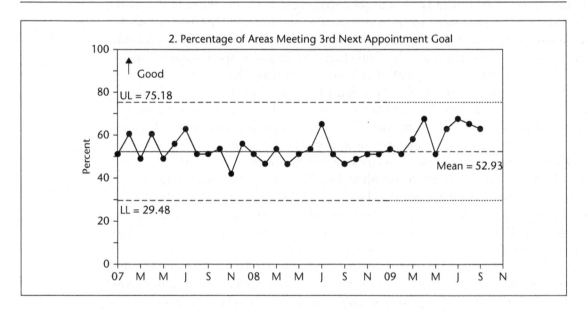

the coding of green, yellow, or red was simply not robust enough to provide insight into this measure. Leadership is better able to assess and make appropriate decisions when viewing the data on a Shewhart chart.

Measure 2, The Percent of Areas Meeting Goal for 3rd Next Available Appointment, has moved from red to yellow to green in the most recent quarter. Most would conclude that something very special is going on in the organization resulting in improvement in this measure. Leadership may well decide that we need to invest in studying and replicating what we have been doing to improve these processes related to access to appointments the last few months. Again, by looking at the data displayed monthly on a Shewhart chart (Figure 12.4) we learn something very different. The more recent data are higher and therefore closer to the target, but there is not a statistical signal that anything special is going on. This measure is stable; there is no improvement here yet. If leadership took action to investigate the most recent data as if it were somehow special, it would be making Mistake One—reacting to an outcome as if it came from a special cause when actually it came from common causes of variation—and incurring losses. Losses here include the resources spent erroneously investigating something special that is really not special. In addition, there are opportunity costs inherent in failing to push for the changes needed to the underlying processes. Again, looking at a table of numbers, even with an attempt to rate progress of the data toward a goal, simply doesn't provide leadership with the information needed for accurate assessment and action.

The tabular view of a vector of measures at Figure 12.1 displays data quarterly. Some organizations display tabular data monthly rather than quarterly and code that monthly data as red, yellow, or green (colors are represented in shades of gray). They then react to each month's data. Without an understanding of the common cause variation in the measure, this can lead to chaos. Figure 12.5, Measure 5, Total Infections per 1,000 Patient Days, has been adapted by overlaying a red, yellow, or green circle on each month's data to

FIGURE 12.5 Infection Rate Data Color-Coded Monthly

Month	Infection Rate per 100 Patient Days	Month	Infection Rate per 100 Patient Days	Month	Infection Rate per 100 Patient Days
J 07	1.43	J 08	3.97	J 09	3.20
F	3.46	F	2.48	F	4.48
M	1.04	M	2.43	M	5.38
A	2.32	A	4.67	A	2.00
M	4.39	M	5.88	M	4.50
J	6.83	J	6.66	J	1.60
J	5.41	J	2.20	J	2.30
A	2.12	A	4.17	A	1.10
S	4.71	S	6.83	S	2.60
O	3.30	O	2.34		
N	3.50	N	6.69		
D	3.13	D	4.39		

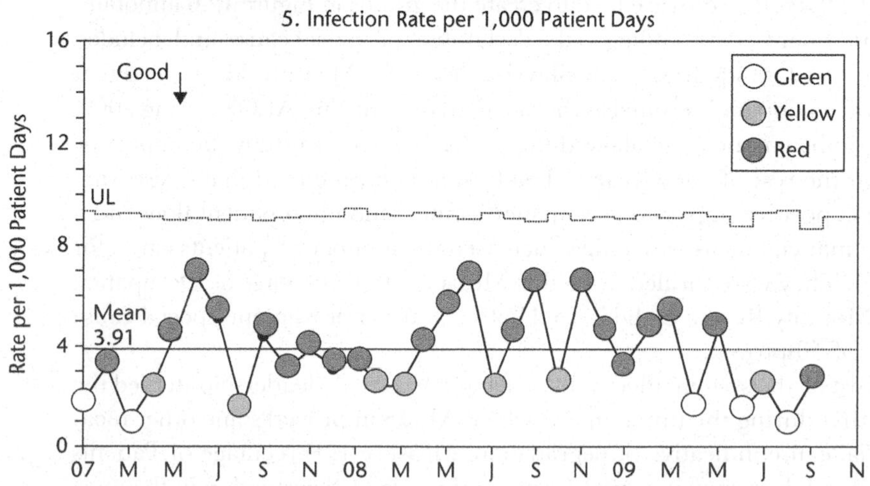

5. Infection Rate per 1,000 Patient Days

illustrate this potential chaos. This measure is statistically stable. All of the months are common cause. There is no evidence of improvement or of degradation in the infection rate.

However, if an organization used only the tabular view and classified each month as red, yellow, or green they would rate April 2009 as a great month (it was green). Perhaps they would reward the manager or invest in attempting to find out why April was so good and introduce some practices from this process into other processes in their system. May, however, would be seen as a terrible (red) month. Leadership may ask "What happened?!" Perhaps they would decide that it's time to investigate May and take some action. June was green. It appears to leadership as much improved; problem solved! But wait, July showed the infection rate slipping again (yellow). Perhaps the organization should renew work on these processes? August was green. It looks like leaderships' decision to renew work on key processes worked out well. September is red. "How can this be happening?!" By this time people could be confused, a bit worn out and perhaps even angry with conflicting messages. When appropriately displaying these on a Shewhart chart we can see that this measure is stable. It exhibits only inherent, common cause variation. Reacting to common cause variation as if it is special (Mistake One) incurs cost, which could be in both financial and emotional capital.

"So How Do We Best Display a Vector of Measures?"

Clearly displaying each measure on the appropriate time series graph allows leadership to correctly interpret, learn from, and react to variation for each measure. But, given the dynamic nature and complexity of systems, it's entirely possible for an improvement evident in one part of the system to result in a negative consequence in another aspect of system performance (note: balancing measures were introduced in Chapter Two as a method for improvement teams to address this issue). This could happen in the current time period or may show up in a later time period (dynamic complexity). This is very difficult to detect by looking at each graph separately.

Best practice, then, in displaying a vector of measures is for each measure to be displayed on the appropriate time series graph, typically a Shewhart chart, *and* presented all on the same page. Displaying them all on one page fosters learning about each individual measure as well as about vital interactions and the dynamic complexity of our health care system. Figure 12.6 illustrates an example of this best practice.

This organization's strategic plan called for a reduction in Measure number 11, Average Length of Stay (ALOS), from its 2008 average of 4.9 to a lower average of 4.3 by the end of 2009. (Note: the software used to create the graphs in Figure 12.6 annotates special cause in dark squares, data leading to the declaration of special cause, and included in the special cause, in white squares.) The Shewhart chart for Measure 11 revealed that special cause (improvement) had resulted as they focused on reducing ALOS during 2009. Seeing all of the graphs on one page allowed the leadership team to study the impact of reducing ALOS on the rest of their system. Leadership had predicted that decreasing ALOS would have a positive impact on occupancy as they smoothed patient flow and a positive impact on financial measures as they increased the number of patients cared for by the organization. They were thrilled to see that Measure 10, Percentage of Occupancy, and Measure 16, Monthly Revenue, did indeed both exhibit improvement (special cause to the good) as ALOS improved.

How was the rest of the system affected by reducing ALOS? As leadership studied the vector they noted that during the timeframe in which ALOS improved some other measures showed special cause indicative of degradation. Measure 1, Percentage of Patients Willing to Recommend, had shown a special cause indicative of degradation in the most recent quarter. Feedback from patients indicated that staff were slow to respond to their

FIGURE 12.6   Appropriate Display of Vector of Measures

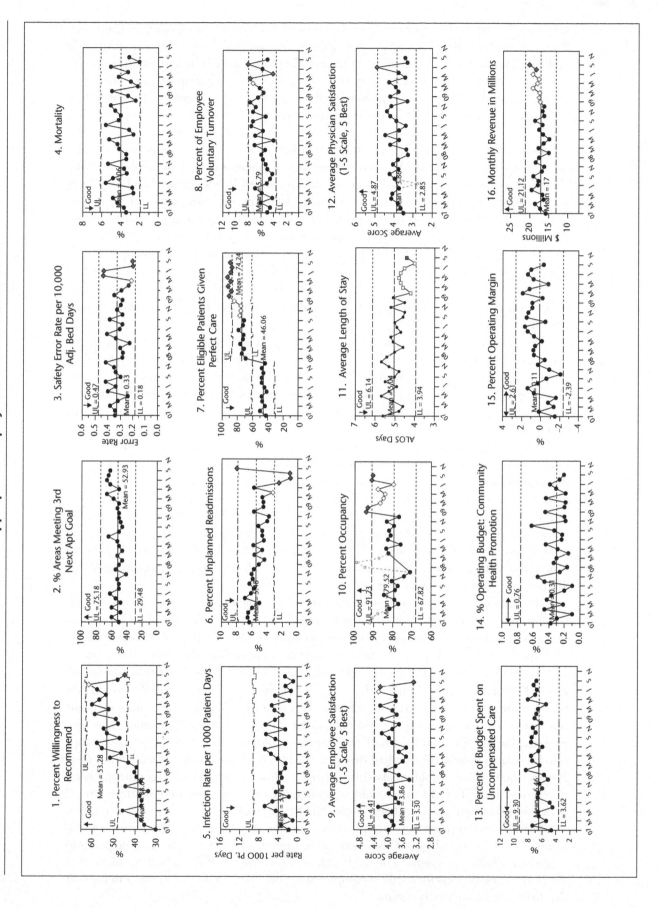

needs and insensitive or rude at times. Leadership also noted that Measure 9, Employee Satisfaction, had shown a similar special cause (worsening) during this time frame. In addition Measure 8, Percentage of Voluntary Employee Turnover, had multiple special cause signals indicative of rising employee turnover. In following up on these employee issues, leadership obtained employee feedback from multiple sources. This feedback indicated that shorter ALOS and increased occupancy created an enormous paperwork challenge related to admitting, assessing, and discharging patients. In follow-up interviews, employees stated that they felt like they hardly had time to care for the patients as they were so busy taking care of the required paperwork inherent in each admission and discharge. In addition, Measure 6, Percentage of Unplanned Readmissions, had been doing fine, but was now showing special causes in the undesirable direction. Leadership realized that losing employees, creating dissatisfied patients, and increasing unplanned readmissions might well be unintended consequences of reducing ALOS. Although decreased ALOS was good news, the leadership team felt that these unintended consequences to their system, if not addressed, would more than offset any advantage gained. Leadership determined that efforts to reduce the burden of admitting and discharge paperwork and to better prepare and support patients being discharged were necessary if they were to optimize the system as a whole.

The leaders came to realize a vital point through this experience. Learning about these key system interactions would be nearly impossible for them if they were using tabular data such as that in Figure 12.1. It would also be nearly impossible if they had viewed each graph separately. Seeing the data on appropriate graphs *and* all together on one page was essential for the level of learning and decision making required of them as leaders.

It is obviously impossible for an organization's vector of measures to contain all of the information needed by leadership. Follow-up data and analysis are often needed, including disaggregation (see Chapter Nine) and looking at additional measures. It is common for leadership to need to drill down into another level of the organization in order to appropriately learn from their vector of measures. For example, Measure 3, Safety Error Rate, exhibited special cause to the bad in June and July of 2009. Analyzing the data on the appropriate Shewhart chart allowed leadership to detect this. Leadership still didn't know much about the problem though. Where were these safety problems happening? What kind of safety problems were they?

By drilling down into the organization they were able to learn more. After review of small multiple graphs for each unit (small multiples as described in Chapter Three), they discovered that the special cause in safety errors was related to one part of the organization, the surgical unit. In following the trail of information leadership they learned that medication errors specific to intravenous (IV) medications were the issue (Pareto analysis of types of errors). New IV pumps had been placed on this unit in June. It was discovered that pump settings subtly differed from those of the previous style of pumps. Employees had not received any training on the new equipment. The unit manager fully understood the problem by July. She obtained staff training for employees working with the new pumps and by August their error rate had dropped. The leadership team was alarmed that their system would allow a problem like this to happen. How had new medical equipment been purchased that differed from the old equipment in a way that resulted in safety errors? Why had equipment users not been involved in the purchase? Why had appropriate training not been provided prior to pump placement on the surgical unit? Were more of these same pumps slated to be used elsewhere in the organization? If so, was training going to be provided with placement? The safety manager on the leadership team determined that the purchasing process for medical equipment needed to be improved in order to prevent this from happening in the future.

Using data from different levels of the organization in pursuing an understanding of the organization's vector of measures is common. No set of measures, no matter how well designed and appropriately displayed, will convey all of the information necessary for appropriate leadership understanding and action.

ADMINISTRATIVE ISSUES WITH VECTOR OF MEASURES

Leadership's job is to optimize their system to accomplish their mission. To do this they regularly plan strategic changes aimed at improving the system. As with change strategy, prediction is important. The use of the vector of measures provides a method for leadership to predict the impact of these strategic changes on their system, study the effect of their changes as reflected in their VOM, and compare the actual impact to their predictions. A vector of measures should become a key leadership tool for learning and for managing into the future. Good graphical display helps the vector become future oriented. As such, it is good practice to always include room on the graphs for future data. Figure 12.7 illustrates this practice. By leaving room and labels for future data, the organization makes it easier to focus their analysis and discussions on the performance of the measures in the future. Regardless of current performance, where do we expect to see the measure next month or next quarter?

A vector of measures requires a number of administrative decisions. How often do we add data to the graphs? When do we update the limits on the graphs? When do we remove older data from the graphs, and so on?

Ideally each graph in a vector should be updated monthly. Viewing the data monthly, rather than quarterly, allows leadership to detect patterns of special cause more readily. In some cases data will only be available quarterly, semi-annually, or even annually. While this is less desirable than monthly data, we still suggest making use of these data by plotting them on the appropriate graph. There is nothing to lose by doing so. Such graphs still afford us an opportunity to learn about our system.

FIGURE 12.7   Graph with Appropriate Space for Future Data

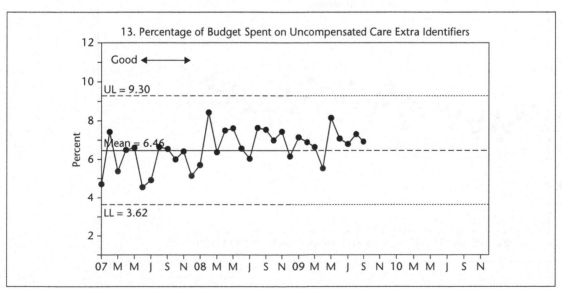

In general, we can follow guidance for creating and updating limits as detailed in Chapter Four.

1. When beginning a graph for our vector, if fewer than 12 data points are available the graph is usually best displayed as a run chart.
2. When the graph has 12 data points, a mean and trial limits may be made and extended into the future. (Note: with I and T charts we suggest waiting to create limits until enough data are available to produce initial limits.)
3. When the graph has 20–30 data points the trial limits should be updated to create what are termed initial limits.
4. Update limits when special cause has indicated a new level of sustained system performance (typically, 12 data points representative of the new level of system performance before revising the limits).

Shewhart charts can effectively display around 80 data points. If we are working with monthly data, this amounts to six or seven years of data. This rich data resource supports leadership in their deep learning about the system. When the Shewhart chart becomes too crowded, as seen in the chart in Figure 12.8, it's appropriate to reduce the number of data points on the graph. In reducing the amount of data on a too busy graph we suggest always showing a minimum of 24 data points. Figure 12.9 illustrates this approach. We chose to update the limits using two years, 2008 and 2009, as the new baseline. Another option, rather than removing the old data completely from the graph, is to summarize the old data and include it on the existing graph as a single dot for the entire year. Figure 12.10 illustrates this approach.

SOME EXAMPLES OF OTHER VECTORS OF MEASURES

This chapter has focused on an example of one hospital-based vector of measures. We thought it useful to include a few examples of the types of measures included in vectors of measures from other hospitals, clinics, departments, or other entities.

FIGURE 12.8   Graph with Excessive Number of Data Points

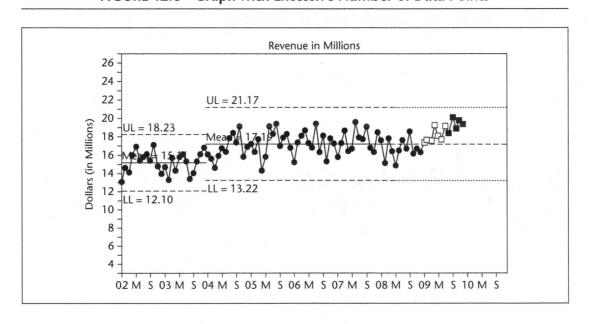

FIGURE 12.9   Graph Updated to Provide More Readable Number of Data Points

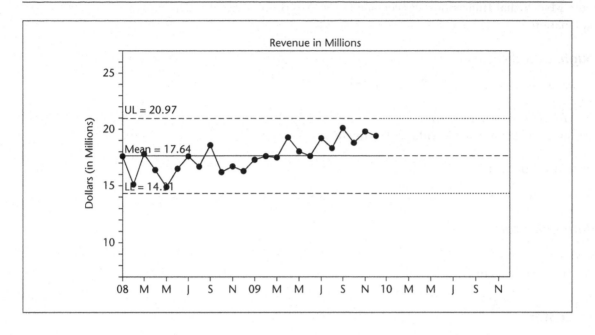

FIGURE 12.10   Graph with Historical Data Summarized

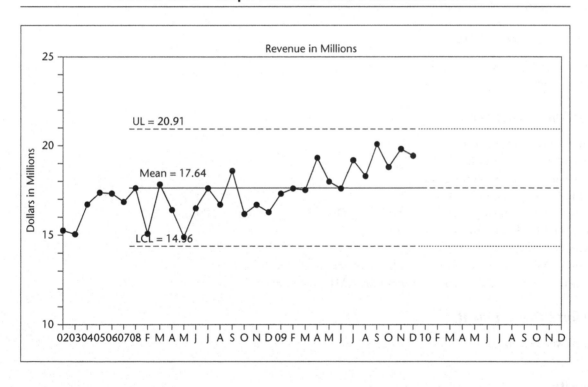

Emergency Department:

Quality Indicators:

- Pneumonia—Percentage Given Antibiotics (ATB) Within 6 Hours of Admission
- Percentage of Appropriate ATB Ordered/Administered

- Percentage of Blood Cultures Obtained Prior to ATB
- Acute Myocardial Infarction—Percentage Given Aspirin on Arrival or Documented Explanation

Throughput Indicators

- Average Length of Stay (ALOS) Discharge
- ALOS Admitted
- Time from Door to Physician
- Percentage of Patients Left Without Treatment

Patient Satisfaction

- Likelihood of Recommending (Percentage Top Box)

Staffing Indicators

- Physician Staffing Level
- Patients per Physician Hour

Primary Care Center

Customer/Owner

- Overall Rating of Care (Customer Satisfaction)

Financial and Workload

- Investment Earnings
- Net Margin

Operational Effectiveness

- Childhood Immunizations
- Breast Cancer Screening Rate
- Cervical Cancer Screening Rate
- Colon Cancer Screening Rate
- Diabetic Cholesterol in Good Control (Low Density Lipoprotein < 100)
- Diabetic On-Time HbA1c Screening
- Diabetics HbA1c in Poor Control
- Cholesterol Control for Patients with Cardiovascular Conditions
- Persistence of Beta Blocker Treatment for AMI Customers

Workforce Development

- Employee Satisfaction

Health Authority

Wellness

- Residential Care Influenza Immunization Rate
- Immunization Rate for Children at 24 Months of Age December 2008
- Screening Mammography—Rate of Participation

Health Promotion

- Tobacco Use Rates Ages 15 and Over
- Rate of Newly Reported HIV

Access

- Percent Health Services Self-Sufficiency
- Assisted Living, Supportive Living and Residential Spaces
- Percentage of Community-Based Clients Admitted to Residential Care < 30 Days
- Average Length of Stay
- Home Care Client Rate—Age 65+
- Alternate Level of Care as a Percentage of Acute Patient Days

Wait Times

- Computerized Tomography (CT) Wait Time
- Magnetic Resonance Imaging (MRI) Wait Time
- Surgical Wait Time—Total Hip Replacement
- Surgical Wait Time—Total Knee Replacement
- Surgical Wait Time—Cataracts
- Percentage of Cases Admitted from Emergency Department Within 10 Hours
- Surgical Wait Time—Hip Fracture Repair
- Percentage of Coronary Artery Bypass Graft Cases Waiting Longer Than Six Weeks

Appropriate

- Ambulatory Care Sensitive Conditions Rate
- Readmission Rate
- Mental Health 30-Day Follow-Up Rate—All Ages
- Mental Health 30-Day Follow-Up Rate (65+)
- Percentage of Cancer Deaths Occurring Outside Hospital
- Percentage of Non-Cancer Natural Deaths Occurring Outside Hospital
- Hospital Standardized Mortality Ratio
- Percentage with Diabetes HbA1c Testing
- Percentage of Patients Assessed Within Canadian Triage Acuity Scale (CTAS) Guidelines
- Percentage of In-Hospital Mortality—Acute Myocardial Infarction
- Percentage of In-Hospital Mortality—Stroke

Safety

- Hospital Infectious Organisms Rate
- In-Hospital Hip Fracture Rate
- Housekeeping Quality
- Food Safety

Satisfaction

- Food Satisfaction—Contracted Acute Care Sites
- Satisfaction—Emergency Services

Work Life

- Sick Time Rate
- Overtime Rate

- Staff Injury Rate (Time Loss Only)
- Days Paid per Injury Claim
- Long Term Disability Rate (Own Occupation Only)
- Staff Influenza Immunization Rate
- Difficult to Fill Rate

Sustainability

- Year End Surplus (or Deficit)
- Working Capital Ratio
- Facility Condition Index
- Return on Investments
- Equipment Depreciation Index
- Revenue Generation

Large Urban Hospital

Clinical Excellence

- Acute Myocardial Infarction: Appropriate Care Score
- Community-Acquired Pneumonia: Appropriate Care
- Heart Failure: Appropriate Care
- Surgical Care Improvement Project: Appropriate Care

Patient Safety

- Percentage of Patients with Pressure Ulcer
- Percentage of Appropriate Hand Hygiene

Service Pathway

- Main Campus Hospital Consumer Assessment of Healthcare Providers and Systems (HCAHPS Percentile Rank)
- Specialty Campus (Mean Score)
- Emergency Department (Press Ganey Percentile Rank)
- Physician Satisfaction (Percentile Rank) Reported Annually

Staff Pathway

- Agency Utilization—Percentage of Budget
- Staff Satisfaction
- Registered Nursing Recruitment

Finance Pathway

- Net Income—Percentage of Budget

Growth Pathway

- Adjusted Admissions MC—Percent of Budget
- Physician Recruitment

The Institute for Healthcare Improvement (IHI) developed a balanced set of system-level measures to provide health care leaders and other stakeholders with data that:

Table 12.3 Institute for Healthcare Improvement Whole System Measure

System Measure	IOM Dimension	Outpatient Care	Inpatient Care	Regional Care
1. Rate of Adverse Events	Safe	X	X	
2. Incidence of Nonfatal Occupational Injuries and Illnesses	Safe	X	X	
3. Hospital Standardized Mortality Ratio (HSMR)	Effective		X	
4. Unadjusted Raw Mortality Percentage	Effective		X	
5. Functional Health Outcomes Score	Effective	X	X	
6. Hospital Readmission Percentage	Effective	X	X	
7. Reliability of Core Measures	Effective	X	X	
8. Patient Satisfaction with Care Score	Patient Centered	X	X	
9. Patient Experience Score	Patient Centered	X		
10. Days to Third Next Available Appointment	Timely	X		
11. Inpatient Days During the Last Six Months of Life	Efficient		X	X
12. Health Care Costs per Capita	Efficient	X	X	X
Stratification of Measures	Equitable	X	X	X

- Show performance of their health care system over time;
- Allow the organization to see how it is performing relative to its plans for improvement;
- Allow comparisons to other similar organizations; and
- Serve as inputs to strategic quality improvement planning.[8]

The aim of IHI's Whole System Measures initiative was to develop, test, and use a small set of measures that focuses on quality of care and is aligned with the Institute of Medicine's (IOM's) six dimensions of quality (that is, care that is safe, effective, patient-centered, timely, efficient, and equitable). Table 12.3 shows these measures. This family of measures was constructed to complement existing measures (for example, utilization, program growth, finance, workforce satisfaction, and so forth) that organizations use to evaluate the performance of their heath care system. Not all of the measures are applicable to every health care organization.

---

[8]Martin L., Nelson, E., Lloyd, R., and Nolan, T., *Whole System Measures,* IHI Innovation Series Whitepaper, Cambridge, MA: Institute for Healthcare Improvement, 2007, (available from www.IHI.org).

SUMMARY

The usefulness of Shewhart charts extends beyond the improvement project level and into the realm of senior leadership. Creating a vector of measures and displaying them each on Shewhart charts enhances senior leadership's ability to manage, lead, and improve the entire system for which they are responsible.

- A vector of measures is a set of key organizational measures that, although inadequate as individual measures to describe the system, together are very useful to senior leaders to learn about, manage, and improve their system.
- Each measure in the vector should be displayed on the appropriate Shewhart chart or, if more appropriate, on a run chart.
- Each measure in the vector should be updated monthly in order to learn about system performance in a timely fashion. Data for some measures may only be available quarterly or even annually, but these should be the exception.
- A vector of measures appropriately displayed using Shewhart charts is an essential senior leadership tool for an organization focused on improvement. It is a more efficient and effective way for senior leadership to view key data than are tabular summaries, bar charts, or stoplight signals.
- Shewhart charts for use in the vector of measures should be placed on the same page so that leaders can more readily see system interactions and relationships. Viewing each Shewhart chart serially, rather than all on one page, is far less effective for understanding key relationships in the system.

KEY TERMS

Composite measures

Vector of measures

CASE STUDIES

## CHAPTER 13

CASE STUDIES USING SHEWHART CHARTS

This chapter consists of a variety of case studies illustrating the use of Shewhart and other charts.

- **Case Study A** illustrates the use of run charts with an improvement project. It also provides an example of multiple project measures graphically displayed on a single page.
- **Case Study B** illustrates the use of data to support improvement projects in a radiology department. This case study addresses using rare event data, capability analysis, and examples of updating charts after improvements have been made.
- **Case Study C** illustrates the use of a Shewhart chart to track the impact of a change. It also highlights using disaggregation, stratification, and rational subgrouping techniques to learn about the process.
- **Case Study D** illustrates the use of the Drill Down Pathway from Chapter Nine with classification data (percentage of C-sections).
- **Case Study E** highlights the use of Shewhart charts in drilling down into aggregate data (count data on U charts).
- **Case Study F** addresses using Shewhart charts as a central part of an improvement effort. It also illustrates updating and revising Shewhart chart limits.
- **Case Study G** illustrates the use of Shewhart charts with routine financial data. It highlights the value of posing questions and using the appropriate Shewhart chart to aid in answering that question. In addition, it provides an example of using scatter plots.

These case studies build on the examples of applications offered in the previous chapters and offer the reader additional opportunity to further explore the use of methods to learn from variation in health care. The case studies spend more time placing the application of the method into the specific improvement context in the case. They also discuss the implications of the case on leadership issues in the organization. Please note that these case studies have been adapted from the authors' experiences. Data, changes tested, team decisions, outcomes, and other case details have been altered to optimize the teaching points.

For a quick reference, Table 13.1 illustrates the specific tools and methods used in each case study.

Table 13.1   Summary of Use of Tools and Methods in the Case Studies

Tools and Methods to Learn from Variation	Case Study A	Case Study B	Case Study C	Case Study D	Case Study E	Case Study F	Case Study G
Run Chart	x						x
I Chart							x
X-bar/S chart		x					x
C Chart			x				
U Chart					x		
P Chart		x		x		x	
G Chart		x					
T Chart		x					
X-bar/R Chart							x
Pareto Chart				x			
Frequency Plot		x	x				
Scatter Plot							x
Drill Down Pathway				x	x		
Rational Subgrouping			x	x			x
Stratification			x				x

CASE STUDY A: IMPROVING ACCESS TO A SPECIALTY CARE CLINIC

Key Points for This Case Study

1. Using data for improvement
2. Using run charts for an improvement project
3. Summarizing and displaying data when only a small amount of data are available
4. Graphical display of a set of project measures on one page

Situation

The organization in this case study was part of a large single-payer health care system with regional oversight. Regional medical leadership noted a problem with the time it was taking for those referred to the urology specialty clinics to obtain an appointment. Wait time was around three months for elective referrals. This wait time concerned the urologists in the specialty clinic who recognized that delay in treatment increased patient suffering and escalated the severity of the issue by the time the patient was able to be seen. The clinic staff was stressed with juggling appointments, generating letters for future appointment schedules, and handling heartfelt pleas from patients for earlier appointments. The specialists were frustrated with schedules locked up for three months. The organization recognized that it had substantial issues related both to quality of care due to scheduling delays and significant costs in dealing with no-shows, rebookings, and communications with patients.

Regional leadership offered to support a team improvement effort using the Model for Improvement as a guide. The team had an eager urologist as team leader, but not all of the urologists were willing to support this project. The regional improvement adviser suggested a lunch and learn session with a urologist from another region who had great success with this issue and was willing to come to describe the changes their clinic made and answer questions. After the lunch and learn all physicians were supportive of this project. The team was formed and developed an aim to "reduce the time to third next available appointment" to 10 days within one year. To answer the Model question, "How do we know if a change is an improvement?" the team developed a family of measures (with goals):

Outcome

1. Average Days Until Third Next Available Appointment (Goal 10)
2. Patient Satisfaction with Access to Clinic (Goal 50% top box)
3. Staff and Provider Satisfaction (Goal 3.6 or greater)

Process

4. Demand Versus Capacity (Goal to match demand and capacity)
5. Percent of Referrals Sent to Unspecified Provider (Goal 60%)
6. Percentage of Urology Clinics No-Shows (Goal 10%)

Balancing

7. Number of Referrals Weekly (remain same)
8. Number of Referrals from Outside the Region (remain same)

The team had some historical data for some of these measures and the team leader, with help from team members, was able to collect additional baseline data. Meanwhile, the entire team was learning about and planning for changes they could test from the plentiful literature on access best practices. Their baseline data are shown in Figure 13.1, displayed on run charts with all graphs on a single page.

Questions

1. The team chose to display their data on run charts. Do you think this was an appropriate choice?
2. What do these run charts reveal about current performance?

Analysis and Interpretation

These graphs could readily have been displayed on appropriate Shewhart charts. With 12 data points the team could have created trial limits for each graph (Chapter Four provides additional guidance on Shewhart chart limits). This team chose not to use Shewhart charts for several reasons. Their improvement adviser was aware that several key team members were concerned that data display would be so complex that the team would have a hard time understanding it and communicating it to others. Run charts alleviated this concern. In addition, the practice had no software for building Shewhart charts. Finally, run charts are well suited to improvement projects. The run rules rapidly detect signals of improvement without introducing additional complexity into the team's measurement system.

The run charts do inform the team as to the current performance of their system relative to each project measure. They don't indicate any early evidence of improvement nor degradation in the measures. This gives the team a baseline from which to track improvement and answer the question "How will we know that the change(s) is an improvement?"

FIGURE 13.1 Baseline Data for Clinic Access Project

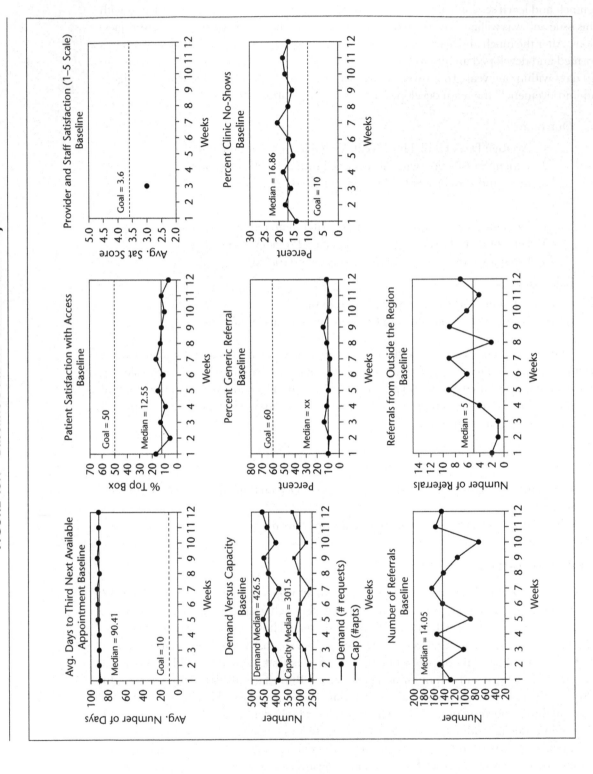

Situation

The team rapidly got busy testing changes. Their skilled improvement adviser guided them to work in multiple areas simultaneously in order to increase the rate of improvement. Changes the team started testing were annotated on their graphs with "(T)" to indicate that testing had begun or "(I)" to indicate that testing was complete and implementation begun. See Chapter One for additional information about the difference between testing and implementation. The changes included:

Related to patient satisfaction with access:
- Began six-month contract to increase appointments available
- Started testing patients choosing appointment time and day rather than being informed of appointment by letter

Related to shaping demand:
- Tested and implemented new process for "generic" referrals with one primary care clinic
- Testing referral agreement with one primary care clinic regarding referral criteria and work up for several diagnoses

Related to improving clinic capacity:
- Began six-month contract to increase appointments available
- Testing reduction in appointment categories
- Began working down backlog (weekend clinics)

Related to primary care sending generic referrals (not specifying a particular urologist):
- Testing new process for generic referrals with one primary care clinic
- Revised and implemented process in that clinic
- Testing process in three primary care clinics

Related to reducing clinic no-shows:
- Tested and implemented new no-show policy for urology clinics in region
- Started testing having patients choose appointment time and day rather than being informed of appointment by letter

Questions

3. Are any of the team's outcome or process measures indicating that the tests of change have resulted in improvement yet? (See Figure 13.2.) Will process or outcome measures be likely to show improvement first?
4. If improvement was not yet evident, would you suggest the team abandon the changes they are testing?

Analysis and Interpretation

Some of the measures include signals indicating improvement. In general, process measures will show evidence of improvement before outcome measures. Typically an outcome measure may need several process measures to show improvement before the changes are powerful enough to move an outcome measure. The team's process measure of capacity shows a signal

FIGURE 13.2 24 Week Data for Clinic Access Project

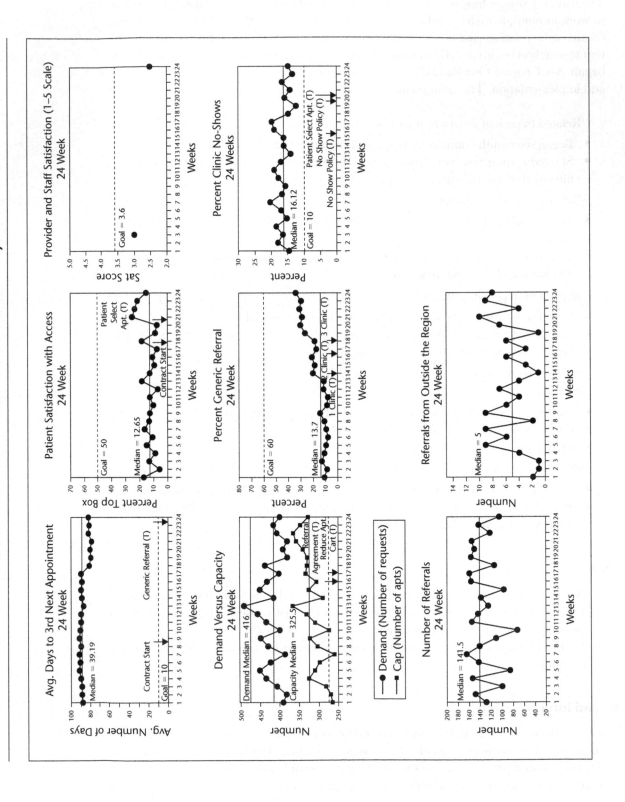

of improvement (6 or more consecutive points above the median) as they start testing a new approach to scheduling in which they reduced the number of appointment types. They also initiated a contract, started working down the backlog and started testing a referral agreement with one of the primary care clinics.

It looks like these changes are adding up to produce a signal of improvement in capacity. In addition, the Percentage of Generic Referrals exhibit a signal of improvement (6 or more consecutive points above the median) as the clinic tests a change asking one, then three, primary care clinics to request a referral nonspecifically (that is, with the first available urologist). This change permitted the clinic to reduce some of the patient's long waits. When we look at the entire set of measures we note that so far these changes don't appear to have changed the percentage of appointment no-shows or patient satisfaction. Also, overall clinic referrals and out-of-region referrals have held steady. These last two measures make it clear that they are improving despite continuing demand.

One of the outcome measures, Days to Third Next Available Appointment, shows a signal of improvement (6 or more consecutive points below the median). This early evidence of improvement is encouraging to the team, although they have a long way to go yet to reach their goal!

Is there any indication here to suggest that the team abandon the changes they are testing? It's typical for early tests of change to affect relatively small numbers of patients. Not until changes are tested on a wide scale, or even implemented, do some teams see changes in their measurement sets. This highlights the pivotal role of the PDSA cycle throughout testing. When testing a change on a small, moderate, or even a large scale, obtaining quantitative and qualitative data during the cycle is pivotal in helping the team to assess the usefulness of the change. Another factor that would lead this team to continue with the changes they are testing, even if their measurements had not indicated improvement, is the fact that this team was testing evidence-based changes that simply have a substantial body of literature and best practice that supports continued use.

Situation

The team has been busy testing, adapting, implementing, and spreading numerous changes including those:

Related to patient satisfaction with access:
- Completed six-month contract to increase appointments available
- Implemented practice where patients choose appointment time and day rather than being informed of appointment by letter

Related to Staff/Provider Satisfaction:
- Tested and implemented expansion in PA and RN roles so they can handle portion of referral work up rather than physician

Related to shaping demand:
- Implemented new process for generic referrals with three primary care clinics and spread begun to all in region
- Completed testing and implemented referral agreement with all primary care clinics regarding referral criteria and work up for several diagnosis

Related to improving clinic capacity:

- Tested and implemented expansion in PA and RN roles so that they can handle portion of referral work up rather than physician
- Completed and stopped six-month contract to increase appointments available
- Completed testing and implemented the reduction in appointment categories
- Tested and implemented a change to reduce frequency of return for routine patients
- Tested and implemented process to return stable patients to primary care

Related to primary care sending generic referrals (not specifying a particular urologist):

- Completed testing and implemented new process for generic referrals with three primary care clinics and began spread in region

Related to reducing clinic no-shows:

- Completed testing and implemented a practice where patients choose appointment time and day rather than being informed of appointment by letter
- Tested and implemented a telephone appointment reminder system

Questions

5. What has the impact been on Demand Versus Capacity (Figure 13.3)? Are the urology services in this region now capable of meeting demand?
6. How are the other process measures doing (the Percentage of Generic Referrals and Percentage of No-Shows)?
7. How are outcome measures performing (Days to Third Next Available Appointment, Percentage of Patients Rating Access "Top Box," Staff and Provider Satisfaction)? Was the small amount of staff/provider satisfaction data useful?

FIGURE 13.3   Urology Services Regional Demand Versus Capacity

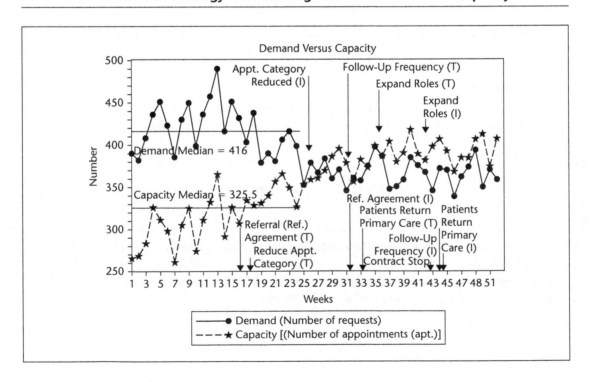

8. Is the clinic performing better because workload (new referrals and referrals from outside the region) has decreased or because of their internal process changes?

Analysis and Interpretation

The first question deals with demand versus capacity in Figure 13.2. Urology demand and capacity have both shown signals of improvement. We could use the run rules to analyze the chart, but visual interpretation alone is adequate given this magnitude of change. The urology services now have a match between capacity and demand. They have adequate appointment availability to provide for requests for appointments.

Figure 13.4 provides insights to question 6. Generic referrals jumped rapidly to the goal of 60% and this measure is now holding its own nicely. "The Percentage of Clinic No-Shows" have met the goal and been reduced from 16 to 10%. This improvement has been sustained at that level for several months. This is a tremendous aid to capacity as the unused appointment resulting from a no-show is typically wasted.

Question 7 asked how the team's outcome measures are performing. Third next available appointment has been at the goal of 10 days for the past month. Patient satisfaction with access has reached the goal of 50% for the last three weeks. The team had little data on provider/staff satisfaction. They decided that obtaining survey data four times during the year was as much as they could manage. They believed that monthly surveys would have been difficult for the team to obtain and would have annoyed the staff and providers. Even though the team had little data on staff/provider satisfaction it still appeared useful when viewed on a run chart and in context with the rest of the measurement set. Provider and staff satisfaction fell initially. This came as no surprise to the team as improving access involved working down the backlog and a large amount of other hard work. As a host of changes began yielding improvement, provider and staff satisfaction rose.

Question 8 asked if the improvement was due to a decrease in demand for services. Improved clinic access does not appear to be due to a decrease in in-region or out-of-region referrals. The two run charts graphing these measures show no signals. Volume of external workload appears to have remained about the same. Demand did decrease, but not external demand. Clinic process changes included a reduction in follow up appointment frequency for returning patients. This, and other changes, reduced repeat workload (internal demand) and freed up availability for referral demand. Improved clinic access was the result of the hard work of the team and clinic colleagues who tested and implemented many changes.

Leadership Issues

1. Management's role in targeting areas for improvement and then providing political, financial, and other resources is key.
2. Sustainability of any improvement project is always a management issue. Access improvements are particularly vulnerable to degradation. Poor planning resulting in several physicians being gone at the same time can rapidly increase the wait for an appointment. The loss of a single physician or key physician assistant or nurse without rapid replacement can do the same. It is important for management to designate an owner for the system, and vital that management continue to monitor access data, routinely see access graphs, and listen to physicians and staff.

FIGURE 13.4 One Year Data for Clinic Access Project

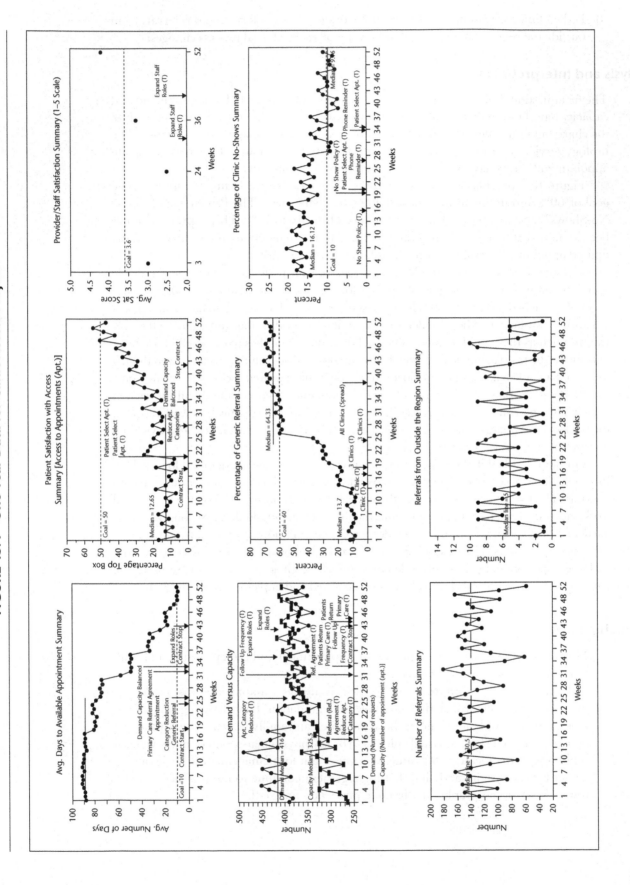

CASE STUDY B: RADIOLOGY IMPROVEMENT PROJECTS

Key Points for This Case Study

1. Using data to help scope and guide an improvement project
2. Developing appropriate charts to learn from count data
3. Using Shewhart charts to understand and report the impact of improvements to a system

Background

The quality improvement team in the radiology department was working on improvement projects in a number of areas using the Model for Improvement as a roadmap. During the last six months, one project focused on reducing the number of significant revisions (after review by a radiologist of initial diagnosis done by a resident) on all exams. Another project focused on turn-around time for reporting routine x-rays. A third project dealt with the start time for radiological intervention procedures. The Department had recently collected data to look at baseline conditions for each of these measures.

Question

1. What type of Shewhart chart would you chose to evaluate baseline data for the key measures for each of the projects?

Analysis and Interpretation

The team developed the following charts to analyze the baseline data:

a. *Significant revisions*—the team collected historical monthly data since January 2006 on the total number of radiology exams and the number that had significant revisions after review by a radiologist. Figure 13.5 shows the P chart for these data.

b. *Turn-around time*—For the past three weeks, the team collected the time from scan to reporting for all routine x-rays. The hospital had a standard of 48-hour turn-around for reporting on these films. Figure 13.6 shows the $\bar{X}$ and S chart for these data with subgroups formed from the x-rays which were done on each of the days.

FIGURE 13.5   P Chart for Significant Errors in Reading Films

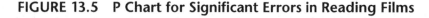

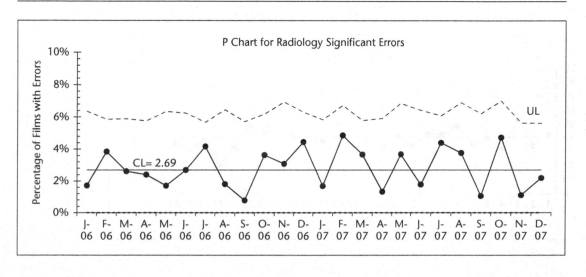

FIGURE 13.6   X̄ and S Charts for Turn-Around Times for Routine X-Rays

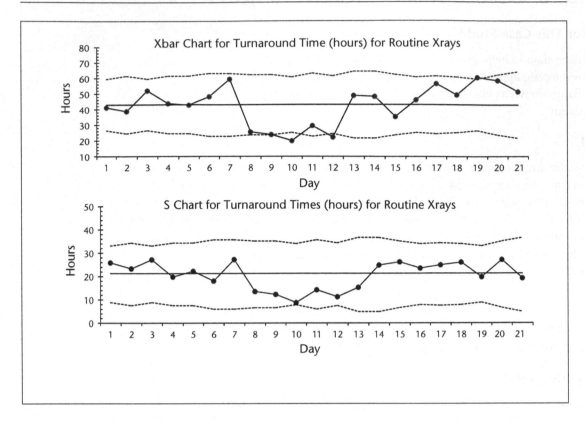

FIGURE 13.7   X̄ and S Charts for CT Scan Start Times (Actual—Scheduled)

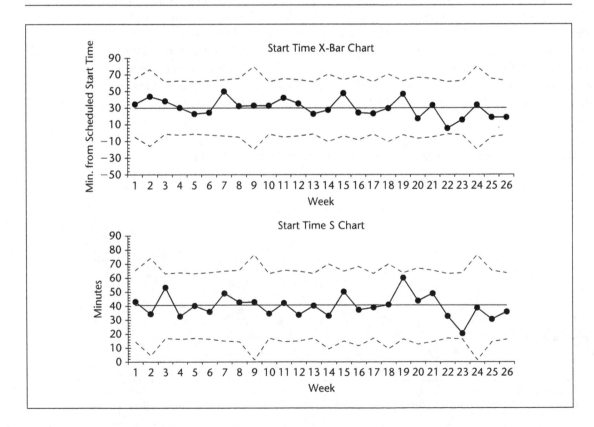

c. *Start time for CT scans*—The team collected weekly data available for the previous six months on the scheduled and actual start time for each CT scan. Figure 13.7 shows the $\bar{X}$ and S charts for these data.

Question

2. How could the Shewhart charts be used to focus the team's improvement efforts?

Analysis and Interpretation

The P chart for significant errors shows a stable process for this attribute. The chart did not have a lower control limit; thus, it would be possible to have zero errors in any given month. Thus the chart was not ideal for quickly signaling an improvement when the team began testing changes. The subgroup sizes (number of films read during the month) ranged from 133 to 274.

Question

3. How could the team develop a Shewhart chart that would quickly give a signal when improvement occurred?

Analysis and Interpretation

From Table 5.5 (Chapter Five), with a Pbar (center line) of about 3%, a subgroup size of more than 300 would be required to obtain a lower limit for a P chart. One way to do this would be to use subgroups of two months for the P chart. Another option would be to develop a "time or number of films" between errors for this measure. Figure 13.8 shows a T chart (days between significant errors) and Figure 13.9 shows a g chart (number of films between significant errors) for the same data used to construct the P chart. The upper limits on either of these charts provide a possible signal when improvements are made.

FIGURE 13.8   T Chart for Days Between Significant Reading Errors

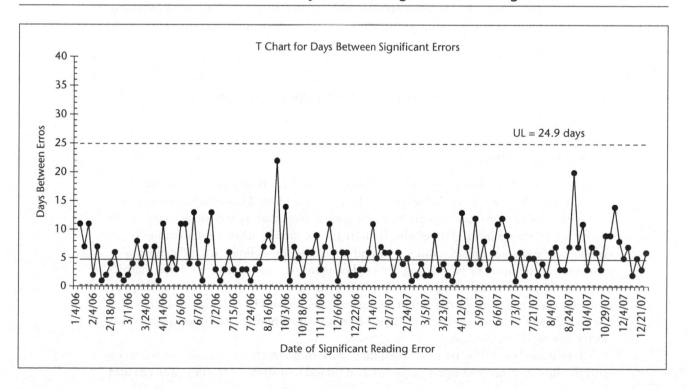

FIGURE 13.9 G Chart for Number of Films Between Significant Reading Errors

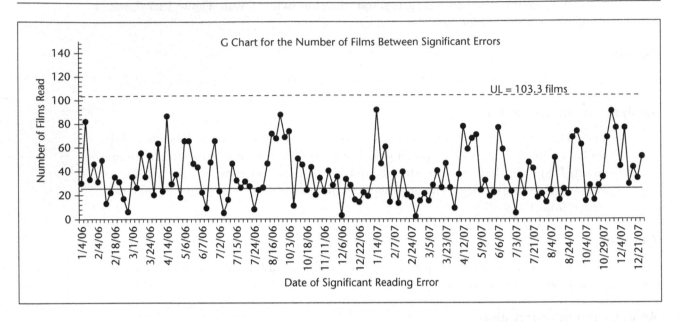

As the number of films is known, The G chart is preferred over the T chart. All three of these Shewhart charts indicate the variation in the significant reading errors is primarily due to common causes. So the team is ready to begin testing fundamental changes and use the G chart to understand the impact of the changes.

The $\bar{X}$ and S charts for turn-around times for routine x-rays show signals of special causes. The review of both the $\bar{X}$ and S charts indicate that the turn-around times were lower on days 8–12 than the other days. The improvement team should identify the special cause associated with these days to develop some ideas to reduce the turn-around times.

The $\bar{X}$ and S chart for start time of CT scans indicates a stable process. The improvement teams needs to generate some ideas for changes that could be done to reduce the number of late starts. A shift in both the average start time (which is now 30 minutes late) and a reduction in the variation in start times (average S of 40 minutes) would be useful.

Question

4. How can the Shewhart charts that the team developed be useful in understanding the impact of changes to the radiology processes?

Analysis and Interpretation

Significant reading errors: The project team working on reading errors tested and adapted the use of a checklist for use by the residents when reading films. They also began monthly case reviews with all residents to go over examples of films that were difficult to interpret. Figure 13.10 shows an update of the G chart for six months after implementing these changes. The special causes (points near and above the upper limit) are indications of a reduction in the number of reading errors. The team planned to wait until they had 15 data points for the improved process and then revise the G chart center line and upper limit. They were very encouraged that average number of films between the 10 events after the change was more than 100 days. This was a dramatic improvement from the previous center line of about 20 days.

Turn-around time: The team learned that more radiologists were available the week with the low turn-around times (days 8–12). This led to a study of staffing patterns and

FIGURE 13.10   Updated G Chart for Errors Showing Impact of Changes to the Process

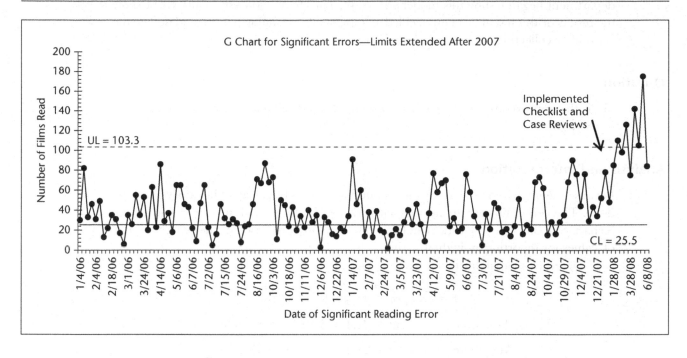

FIGURE 13.11   X̄ and S Charts for Turn-Around Times for Routine X-Rays

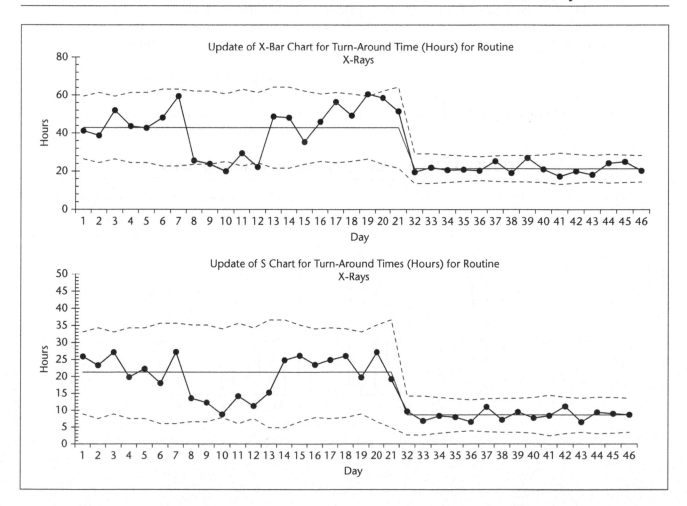

a capacity versus demand analysis. The result of this work was a new staffing model. The department began testing this model on day 32. The charts shown in Figure 13.11 show the results of this test. The team decided to implement the staffing pattern and update the chart after collecting enough data for trial limits.

Question

5. Is the improved process capable of meeting the 48-hour turn-around standard for all x-rays?

Analysis and Interpretation

Because the improved process for turn-around times is stable, a capability analysis can be done. The center line for the average chart ($\overline{X}$) is 21.5 hours and the center line for the S chart ($\overline{S}$) is 8.6. These statistics can be used to develop a prediction of the expected range of values for reporting individual x-rays.

The process capability (from Chapter Five):

$$\sigma = \overline{S}/c_4 \text{ or } = 8.6 / 0.979 = 8.78$$

$$\text{Minimum} = \overline{\overline{X}} - 3\sigma = 21.4 + 3 * 8.78 = -4.8 \text{ hrs.}$$

$$\text{Maximum} = \overline{\overline{X}} + 3\sigma = 21.4 - 3 * 8.78 = 47.8 \text{ hrs.}$$

The frequency plot of the individual turnaround times (Figure 13.12) shows some skewness in the times to the high side. This leads to the negative value for the lower capability limit. The upper capability limit (maximum) indicates that the turnaround time for all routine x-rays can meet the 48-hour standard.

Start time: After developing a flow diagram of the scheduling and preparation process for CT scans, the improvement team met with the staff and radiologists that did the scans and brainstormed some ideas for improvement. Over a two-week period they

FIGURE 13.12   Frequency Plot for Turn-Around Times

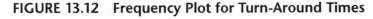

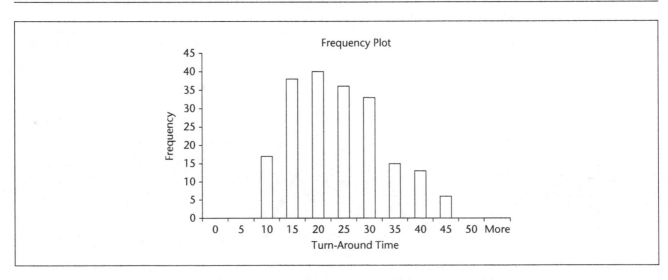

FIGURE 13.13   Updated X̄ and S Charts for CT Scan Start Times (Actual – Scheduled)

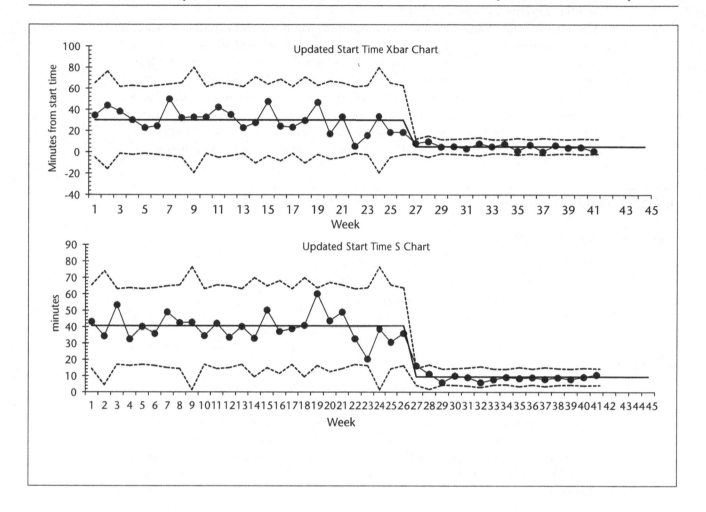

tested changes in both scheduling and the process to prepare patients for the scan. After a number of iterations they agreed to three-month tests of the new protocols. Figure 13.13 shows the updated X̄ and S charts for the starting time after the three months. Then initial limits were extended and finally, after seeing signals of special causes, the limits were recalculated using the subgroups during the test period for the new protocols. The improved process had start times that averaged less than five minutes from the scheduled time with much less variation than before the changes.

At the radiology department meeting, the improvement team presented the results of their three projects using the Shewhart charts for each of the key project measures. Everyone was impressed and proud of their ability to develop and implement changes in their department that led to better-performing systems and thus better health care for their patients. The discussions focused on holding the gains for these three projects and selecting other areas to work on during the next six months.

Leadership Issues

1. The department management team has done a good job of focusing their improvement efforts on a few key projects every six months. The use of Shewhart charts for key

measures helps everyone in the department to understand the impact of the changes and buy into the success.

2. The idea for the change for the turn-around project came from studying a special cause on the chart for the turn-around times. If a department will use Shewhart charts to display management data that is routinely collected, many opportunities for learning will present as signals show up for specific circumstances that arise.

3. It is important for the department managers to understand the nature of the changes that the improvement teams are working on. The key change for the turn-around time was to schedule the right number of staff to match demand. Sustainability will require managers to continue to monitor demand and be prepared to adjust staff accordingly.

CASE STUDY C: REDUCING POST-CABG INFECTIONS

Key Points for This Case Study

1. Developing appropriate Shewhart charts for count data
2. Aggregate data may obscure special cause that is revealed through disaggregation, rational subgrouping, and stratification
3. Stratification and subgrouping strategies

Situation

XYZ Health System is a two-hospital system. The system's post–Coronary Artery Bypass Graft (CABG) infection rate had averaged .06 infections per CABG. The system does about 1,200 CABGs per year between its two facilities. A systemwide improvement effort is about to start to control pre- and post-surgical blood glucose levels. They'd like to make sure they are able to tell whether this new protocol results in improvement. See Table 13.2 for their post-CABG infection and CABG workload data prior to testing the new protocol.

Questions

1. What type of Shewhart chart would you choose for these data and why?
2. Why would it be useful to create this Shewhart chart before beginning new protocol?

Analysis and Interpretation

The team selected a U chart tracking the rate of post-CABG infections each month (number of infections/number of CABGs). They chose a U chart (Figure 13.14) because the data are *attribute data*, they were counting *each post-CABG infection*, and the *subgroup size (number of CABGs performed) varied* each month.

We often have a choice as to how we view attribute data. The team chose to view the attribute data as count (counting each occurrence—each post-CABG infection). They could have chosen to view the data as classification (classifying each CABG case as having had an infection or not). If one post-CABG case had two infections and we were approaching the data as classification we would note that one case had infection present and ultimately get a percentage of our CABG cases that had an infection. If we have a choice between viewing the data as count or classification, count data would count both infections and ultimately get a rate of infections per CABG. Count data will tend to be more helpful in our learning because we get a better view of the magnitude of the occurrences.

Table 13.2   CABG Infection Data Prior to Improvement Project

Month	Number of Infections	Number of CABG Performed
June 07	11	101
Jul	2	104
Aug	7	98
Sep	4	81
Oct	3	96
Nov	6	80
Dec	9	85
Jan 08	7	98
Feb	9	94
Mar	5	131
Apr	9	101
May	3	126
Jun	0	88
Jul	3	93
Aug	9	103
Sep	4	82
Oct	10	105
Nov	3	63
Dec	8	94
Jan 09	3	90
Feb	4	73

FIGURE 13.14   CABG Infection Data Prior to Improvement Project

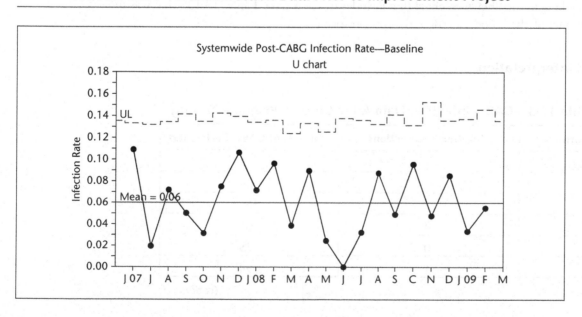

The team thought it would be useful to make a Shewhart chart with their existing data before they started the new protocol for three reasons:

- They had historical data and it seemed easy and prudent to try to learn from it.
- They wanted to understand whether their system was stable at the aggregate level, or whether anything unusual had had an impact on their post-CABG infection rate. Ideally before beginning an improvement we'd like to know that our process is stable. If it's not stable we'd like to learn from the special cause and take appropriate action to stabilize the process.
- Historical data graphed on a Shewhart chart allows us to better tell whether our change(s) resulted in improvement. If changes are an improvement we'll see special cause to the good on the Shewhart chart.

Sometimes it's impossible to get data for a "before improvement" Shewhart chart. Sometimes getting "before" data is possible but would take so much energy no one is willing to work on improvement anymore! Improvement happens when we are willing to test changes using the Model for Improvement. Question Two of the Model for Improvement asks, "How will we know a change is an improvement?" Although we'd have a higher degree of belief that our changes are improvements with a "before" Shewhart chart, it would be counterproductive to let the lack of such a Shewhart chart stop us from working on improvement.

Situation

The baseline Shewhart chart at Figure 13.14 reveals that the system is stable for the last 21 months with a mean rate of .06 infections per CABG (or 6 per 100 CABGs). The team planned to track the infection rate as they began using the protocol by continuing to plot each month's aggregate infection rate on this Shewhart chart.

Questions

3. How would you handle the limits on the Shewhart chart as data are added monthly (Table 13.3)?
4. Looking at the Shewhart chart that includes this new data (Figure 13.15) what was the impact of the blood glucose reduction protocol?

Analysis and Interpretation

Table 13.3 CABG Infection Data After Glucose Protocol Testing

Month	Number of Infections	Number of CABG Performed
M 09	7	102
A	0	89
M	2	108
J	4	101
J	0	75
A	1	94

(continued)

Table 13.3   Continued

Month	Number of Infections	Number of CABG Performed
S	2	81
O	0	54
N	2	89
D	3	84
Jan 10	3	69
F	4	100
M	6	77

FIGURE 13.15   CABG Infection Data After Testing Glucose Protocol

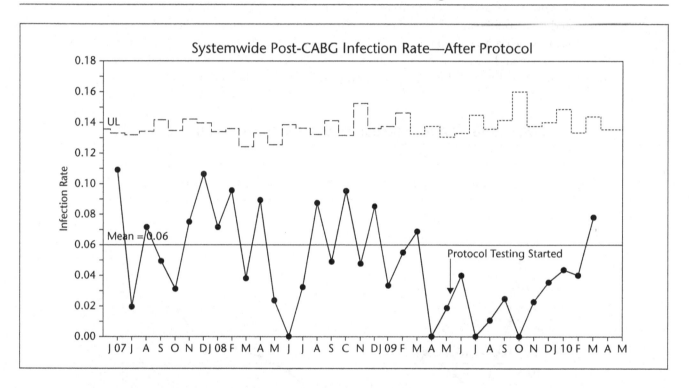

The team knew that the limits could be calculated with as few as 12 data points. (Chapter Four provides guidance for making and revising limits). Limits calculated with fewer than 20–25 data points should be considered "trial limits." Once made, they are "frozen" and extended into the future. They are recalculated when 20–25 data points become available. Once 20–25 data points are available and the system showed that it was stable, the team could make initial limits and extend the mean and limits into the future as a dotted line. This allows them to compare the new data to the previous performance of the process.

The team decided that the 21 data points (21 months) they had before testing the new glucose protocol was around 20–25 and could be used to calculate limits for the system "before the change." Their system was stable so they extended their mean into the future, used the extended mean in obtaining the limits and recorded their data each month after protocol testing was begun.

The impact of the blood glucose reduction protocol can be seen in Figure 13.15. The team determined that the blood glucose protocol improved the post-CABG infection rate because they saw a special cause to the good; shift of eight consecutive points below the system's mean after they started the protocol.

The team had learned a lot about making this protocol work. They had been diligent about continuing to track their data after they saw improvement to see whether they were maintaining the improvement. By March 2010 the team decided that they had enough data to calculate trial limits for the "after glucose protocol" process to see whether it was stable (see Figure 13.16).

Situation

The XYZ system was excited about their post-CABG infection rate improvement. They were a bit worried, however, about the apparent increase in the infection rate recently. Even though the rise was not a special cause, the team was concerned with the pattern. The team knew that aggregated data could conceal special cause. They decided that their next Shewhart chart should stratify the data by hospital and display both hospitals on the same Shewhart chart. That way they could see whether either hospital was special cause when compared to the other hospital. See Table 13.4 for their data and Figure 13.17 for their graph.

FIGURE 13.16   CABG Infection Data After Protocol with Trial Limits

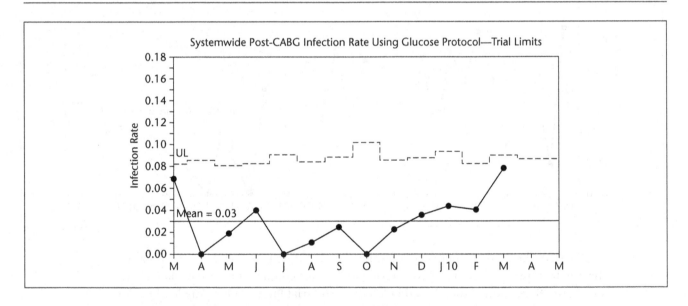

Table 13.4   CABG Infection Data After Protocol Stratified by Hospital

Month	Hospital	Number of Infections	Number of CABG Performed
Mar 09	A	5	69
A	A	0	61
M	A	2	71
J	A	3	73
J	A	0	56

(continued)

Table 13.4   Continued

Month	Hospital	Number of Infections	Number of CABG Performed
A	A	0	65
S	A	1	58
O	A	0	32
N	A	1	60
D	A	2	59
J 10	A	2	48
F	A	3	62
M	A	6	49
Mar 09	B	2	33
A	B	0	28
M	B	0	37
J	B	1	28
J	B	0	19
A	B	1	29
S	B	1	23
O	B	0	22
N	B	1	29
D	B	1	25
J 10	B	1	21
F	B	1	38
M	B	1	28

FIGURE 13.17   CABG Infection Data After Protocol Stratified by Hospital

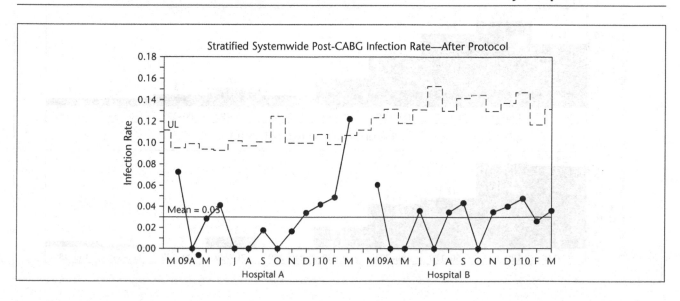

The team discovered that Hospital A had special cause with March 2010 being outside the upper limit. The big question now was what was the reason for the special cause at Hospital A in March? The team involved process experts to identify possible reasons for the special cause. They first thought that Hospital A had changed the way they collected or recorded their data in March. They even wondered whether Hospital A had made a data entry error. The team found no change in Hospital A's measurement method nor any data entry error. Next the team considered whether Hospital A had recently stopped using the blood glucose control protocol. When they checked they found the protocol being used very consistently.

The medical director was asked to share the data with the three physicians in the group practice at Hospital A. He asked them what might have caused the special cause signal in infection rates in March. The only difference the physicians could identify was that Dr. L harvested veins from the leg using a continuous incision from groin to ankle whereas the other two physicians were using an "interrupted" technique with small intermittent incisions down the leg. The physicians noted that although this was a difference among the physicians, it was a long-standing difference. It wasn't something they had just started in March.

The team still hadn't found the source of special cause in Hospital A in March. The process experts put their heads together and developed the following additional theories:

- That Hospital A might be experiencing longer "cut-to-close" time recently and, as result, more infections
- That the special cause in infection rate at Hospital A was due to other differences among the physicians

The team was able to get cut-to-close times for each of Hospital A's CABG cases between March 2009 and March 2010. They created two histograms at Figure 13.18

FIGURE 13.18 Stratified Histograms: Common Versus Special Cause Time Frames

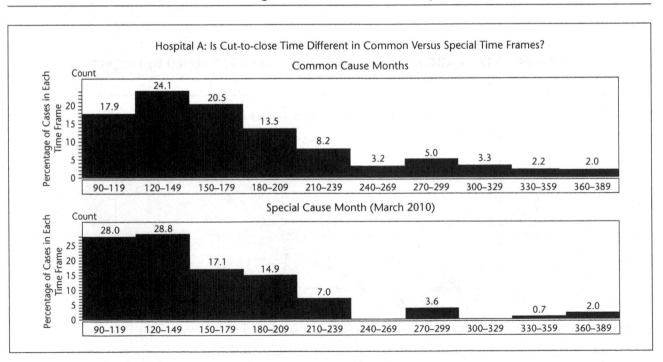

comparing the distribution of cut-to-close times for the common cause months (March 2009 to February 2010) to the distribution in the special cause month (March 2010). Each histogram displayed the percentage of the cases that fell in each surgical time zone rather than the number of cases falling in each time zone. The team did this because they were comparing 12 common cause months with many cases to one special cause month with far fewer cases. Studying the percentage of cases falling in each time category made the common cause and special cause time frames easier to compare directly.

Question

5. What does the histogram reveal about the cut-to-close time during the special cause month when compared to the common cause month?

Analysis and Interpretation

The team didn't find that the percentage of cases with a long cut-to-close was greater during the special cause month than it had been for the common cause months. The theory that cases were taking longer in March and therefore resulting in more infections was not borne out by the data.

The team then studied the data to explore the differences among physicians at Hospital A. They wanted to see whether any of the three physicians' infection rates were special cause when the three were viewed as a system. They created a Shewhart chart rationally subgrouping infection rates by each of the three physicians per quarter. Then they viewed all three physicians' infection rates on one chart (Table 13.5 and Figure 13.19).

Creating a Shewhart chart with the minimum 12 data points recommended for calculating limits takes a lot longer when data are charted at quarterly rather than monthly intervals. Usually we'd like to learn about process performance faster than at quarterly

Table 13.5   CABG Infection Data After Protocol Subgrouped by Physician

Quarter	Physician	Number of Infections	Number of CABG
2–09	K	2	69
3	K	0	66
4	K	1	50
1–10	K	1	50
2–09	S	1	64
3	S	0	55
4	S	1	45
1–10	S	2	50
2–09	L	1	72
3	L	0	58
4	L	1	56
1–10	L	8	59

FIGURE 13.19   CABG Infection Data After Protocol Subgrouped By Physician

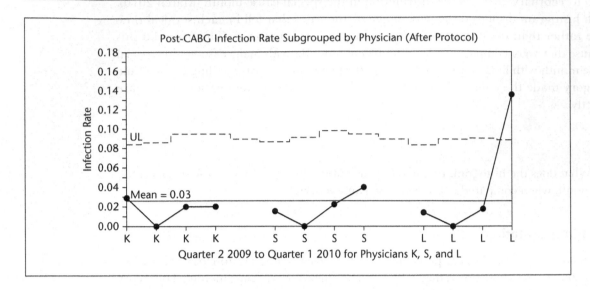

intervals. In this case however, charting each physician's post-CABG infection rate monthly would have resulted in a Shewhart chart with a lot of zeros. If a Shewhart chart shows us 25% or more of the data points as zero, the chart becomes less effective for learning. By using a larger subgroup size we have a greater likelihood of avoiding time frames with zero infections. In this particular hospital, grouping the monthly data into quarterly data allowed them to have enough opportunities for infections so that not more than 25% of the quarters had zero proportion infections.

The team discovered that Dr. L's infection rate was special cause when compared to the system's performance (all three physicians). The team wondered why. The team wondered whether Dr. L's post-CABG infections during the special cause time frame were related to a particular infectious organism. They reviewed the medical records for each of Dr. L's post-CABG infections. Seven out of eight of Dr. L's post-CABG infections in the most recent quarter were one organism, Methicillan Resistant Staphylococcus Aureus (MRSA). MRSA can easily be harbored in the nose and carried without the carrier's knowledge. It's effectively treated with a nasal antibiotic ointment. The infection control nurse spoke with the medical director and asked to obtain a nasal culture from Dr. L to see whether he did harbor MRSA. The medical director insisted that he could not ask the physician to have a nasal culture. He did promise that he would share the information with Dr. L immediately.

The team believed that as soon as Dr. L saw the data he would self-treat with antibiotic ointment. They decided to continue to monitor the quarterly infection rates for each physician to see whether the rates were changing. The team started to study the special cause in Hospital A in April. It took them a while to identify the potential MRSA problem. Dr. L didn't find out about the MRSA until the beginning of May. The team hoped that his data for the second quarter of 2010 would show improvement in his post-CABG infection rates. The data, in Table 13.6, and Shewhart chart in Figure 13.20 are shown for the next two quarters. Dr. L's current infection rate had returned to below the upper limit rapidly after the medical director shared the MRSA information with him. Dr. L had no post-CABG infections at all during the most recent quarter.

Table 13.6   CABG Infection Data After Protocol Subgrouped by Physician with Additional Data

Quarter	Physician	# Infections	# CABG
2–09	K	2	69
3	K	0	66
4	K	1	50
1–10	K	1	50
2	K	2	48
3	K	1	42
2–09	S	1	64
3	S	0	55
4	S	1	45
1–10	S	2	50
2	S	1	43
3	S	1	55
2–09	L	1	72
3	L	0	58
4	L	1	56
1–10	L	8	59
2	L	4	43
3	L	0	56

FIGURE 13.20   CABG Infection Data After Intervention with Physician L

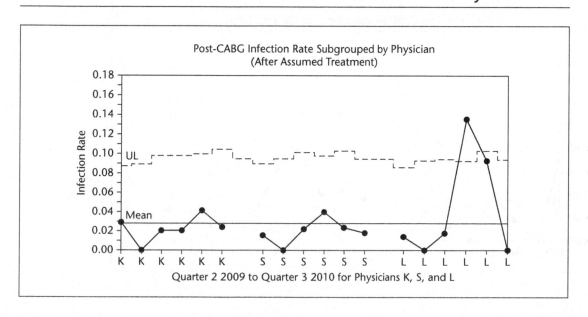

The team knew that continuing to track the impact of changes on the system by monitoring the aggregate level Shewhart chart was an integral part of holding on to improvements made by adapting and adopting the glucose protocol. The team learned that their system still was stable at the aggregate level by creating the chart in Figure 13.21.

The team had learned quite a bit from the special cause in their system. They had corrected the special cause and their post-CABG infection rate was now stable. They decided to continue to monitor the impact of their glucose protocol changes using their Shewhart charts.

Leadership Issues

1. Management needs to be aware that highly aggregated data may obscure special cause. Stratifying the data by hospital helped this organization learn about the special cause in Hospital A that was hidden in the aggregated data.
2. Clinical leadership in this case was faced with data indicating that Dr. L may harbor MRSA yet was unwilling to obtain a culture to verify this. Harboring MRSA may well be embarrassing; it is not a professional or personal fault. The physician may have been embarrassed to be asked for a culture; the team was frustrated and felt let down when leadership didn't support their request for a culture. As a result, the team is still not really certain that their MRSA theory was correct and they are less excited about working to make improvements in the system.
3. Shewhart charts using rational subgrouping techniques, such as subgrouping the infection data by physician, can help us learn where we may want to focus.
4. Shewhart charts used to monitor clinical aspects of care can aid physicians and other members of the health care team in identifying detrimental special cause in clinical outcomes and in learning from these special causes.

FIGURE 13.21   CABG Infection Data Post Protocol Indicating Sustained Improvement

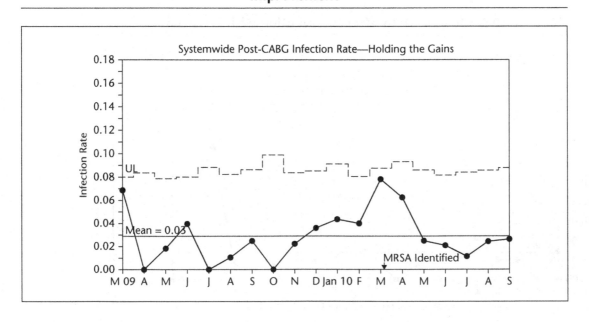

CASE STUDY D: DRILLING DOWN INTO PERCENTAGE OF C-SECTIONS

Key Points for This Case Study

1. Viewing data using a Shewhart chart can help us learn whether the variation we are observing in the process is inherent in our system the way it's currently designed (common cause) or whether something unusual (special cause) has entered our system.
2. The drill down approach described in Chapter Nine can be used by small, as well as large, organizations.
3. The value of displaying multiple organizational units or multiple physicians on one Shewhart chart.
4. The value of rational subgrouping and stratification.
5. The drill down approach can be a useful framework for starting to learn from aggregate data.
6. The need to plot data quarterly when monthly data are too few to be useful.
7. The kind of process performance we would have to have if the UCL was to never exceed 17% (the percentage that would get the organization an unwanted letter from the payer!).

The Background

This small rural hospital received a letter from their major payer informing them that their percentage of C-sections for 2004 was unacceptable. The percentage for 2004 was much higher than their 2003 percentage and it exceeded the payer's acceptable maximum annual percentage of 17%. The hospital was required to respond to the payer with their plan to correct this situation. The pertinent hospital staff and leadership didn't think 2004 "felt" any different from 2003. The director of nursing had just learned about Shewhart charts and the Drill Down Pathway (Figure 13.22) and wondered whether the hospital staff could, by using Shewhart charts, learn about their system's performance and find ways to improve that performance.

This small community hospital is independent. They have one OB unit with two OB physicians, Dr. A and Dr. Z. Data are collected and aggregated quarterly because they have too few deliveries for monthly data to be useful. Each quarter they report the data you see in Table 13.7. By the time they were notified by the payer of their unacceptable percentage of C-sections, they had additional data for the first three quarters of 2005. They decided to include these data on their Shewhart charts.

Questions

1. Using the Drill Down Approach (Figure 13.22) and their data (Table 13.7), what is the first chart you would make to begin to learn from the C-section data? Why make this Shewhart chart?
2. Had the percentage of C-sections changed significantly in 2004 (that is, was 2004 special cause when viewed on the Shewhart chart at Figure 13.23)?

FIGURE 13.22   The Drill Down Pathway

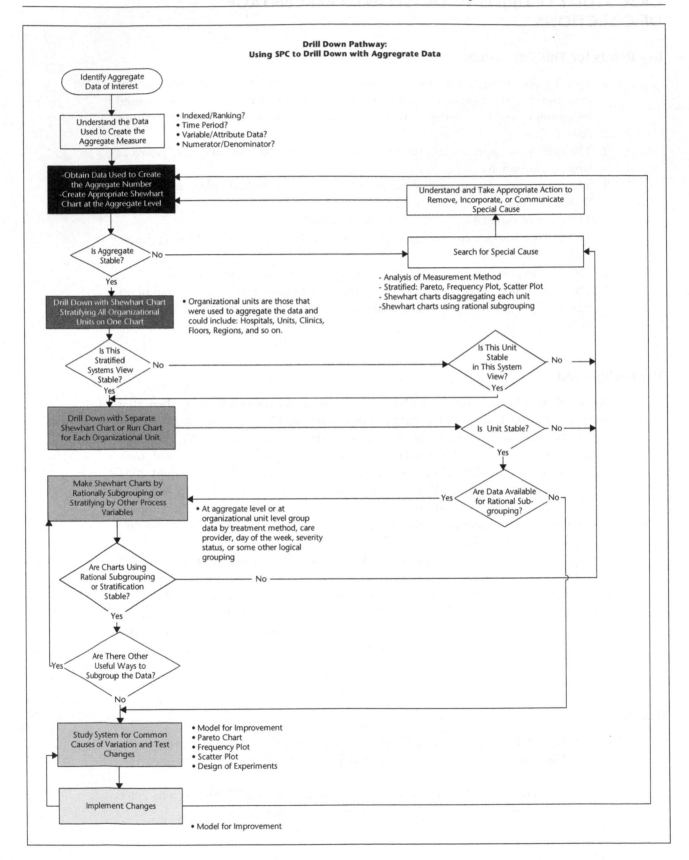

Table 13.7 C-Section Data

Qtr	Total C-Sections	Total Deliveries		By Dr.	C-Sections	Deliveries
1/00	3	32		Z	2	21
				A	1	11
2/00	3	43		Z	3	24
				A	0	19
3/00	9	36		Z	5	22
				A	4	14
4/00	3	36		Z	2	21
				A	1	15
1/01	6	35		Z	3	19
				A	3	16
2/01	5	33		Z	3	15
				A	2	18
3/01	5	56		Z	3	34
				A	2	22
4/01	6	37		Z	4	20
				A	2	17
1/02	5	22		Z	4	12
				A	1	10
2/02	5	27		Z	2	18
				A	3	9
3/02	5	35		Z	5	22
				A	0	13
4/02	3	30		Z	2	13
				A	1	17
1/03	5	27		Z	4	15
				A	1	12
2/03	7	39		Z	5	21
				A	2	18
3/03	7	53		Z	1	32
				A	6	21
4/03	10	58		Z	7	28
				A	3	30
1/04	5	27		Z	2	16
				A	3	11
2/04	9	31		Z	6	18
				A	3	13

(continued)

Table 13.7 Continued

Qtr	Total C-Sections	Total Deliveries		By Dr.	C-Sections	Deliveries
3/04	9	33		Z	6	19
				A	3	14
4/04	5	33		Z	4	21
				A	1	12
1/05	1	27		Z	1	18
				A	0	9
2/05	4	28		Z	2	15
				A	2	13
3/05	7	24		Z	7	14
				A	0	10

FIGURE 13.23   P Chart of Aggregate Percentage of C-Section Deliveries

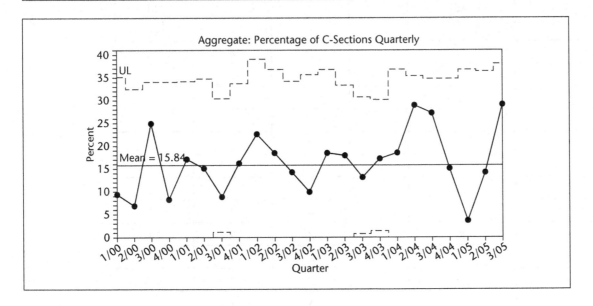

Analysis and Interpretation

The Drill Down Approach suggests a Shewhart chart of the *aggregate-level* C-section data as the first Shewhart chart we would make (See Figure 13.23). This Shewhart chart would be a P chart because the data are attribute data, the attribute data are classifying deliveries as being by C-section or not, and the subgroup size (the number of deliveries each quarter) is different from quarter to quarter.

Why make an aggregate-level Shewhart chart? The purpose of the aggregate-level Shewhart chart is to determine whether, at this systemwide level, the system is stable. (Note that this is also the level at which the payer is viewing the hospital's performance.) If the aggregate-level Shewhart chart reveals that the system is not stable, we'd want to investigate the special cause, determine what was different about the system when the special cause occurred compared to the system when it showed no special cause, and take appropriate action. Did we change the way we collected the data? Did we change our C-section protocol? That said, aggregate-level Shewhart charts will very often show that the system is stable. We'll see this because the aggregate data are often so highly aggregated, with many pieces of data rolled together, that variation is hidden by combining different organizational units, different providers, and different treatment methods. If the system is stable at the aggregate level we often have an opportunity to unmask the variation and learn some more by drilling down into the data.

The second question asked if the percentage of C-sections had significantly changed in 2004. The aggregate level Shewhart chart that this hospital made (Figure 13.23) shows no evidence of special cause. None of the quarters in 2004 are special cause when viewed on the Shewhart chart.

Questions

3. The Drill Down Approach suggests that the next drill down step is to make a chart displaying all organizational units on the same Shewhart chart. Could this hospital do this?
4. This hospital did have data collected in a way that allowed them to rationally sub-group the percentage of C-sections by physician. Why did they choose to make one Shewhart chart with both physicians on it? What do you learn when looking at their results (Figure 13.24)?
5. Using the Drill Down Approach, what would you do next after studying Figure 13.24?

Analysis and Interpretation

Each organization needs to consider their organizational structure when applying the Drill Down Approach. This hospital doesn't have multiple organizational units. They are a single hospital with only one OB unit, so they can't display multiple organizational units on one chart.

FIGURE 13.24   Percentage of C-Section Stratified and Sequenced by Physician

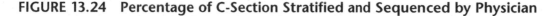

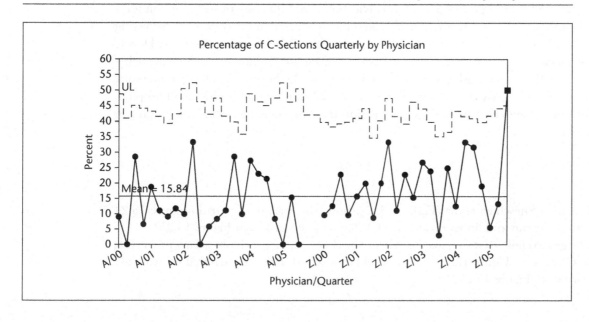

Depending on organizational structure and the way the data was collected we may not be able to use every step of the Drill Down Approach. In many cases this simply means we move on to the next step in the Drill Down Approach. Sometimes we may identify an opportunity to improve the way we collect the data that will enable us to do an even more complete job of drilling down in the future.

Question Four asked why they chose to make a Shewhart chart with both physicians on the same chart. After recognizing that they couldn't drill down by organizational unit, this hospital moved on to the next step in the Drill Down Approach, *rational subgrouping by other than organizational unit* to learn about causes of variation in the system. Their theory was that the difference in the percentage of C-sections was due to different physicians. They did have the C-section data by physician, so each quarter they could chart the percentage of C-sections for each physician. They chose to put both physicians on one Shewhart chart because they wanted to find out whether one of the physicians was special cause *compared to the other physician*. They could then analyze the chart to see whether one physician's percentage of C-sections was special cause when compared to the other physician by using the rules for interpreting a Shewhart chart.

The Shewhart chart in Figure 13.24 shows that Dr. Z's proportion of C-sections was special cause in the most recent quarter charted; her percentage of C-sections that quarter exceeded the upper control limit. Notice that the aggregate-level Shewhart chart (Figure 13.23) didn't reveal this quarter as special cause. By aggregating even just these two physicians' data the data were smoothed enough to mask the special cause. By drilling down we may uncover special causes and gain opportunities to learn.

The Drill Down Approach indicates that the next step should be to investigate the special cause related to Dr. Z's proportion of C-sections in the most recent quarter. A useful question to ask when we see special cause is "What was different about the process during the special cause time frame?" A special cause signal could be the result of a change in the process we use to collect the data or a change in our operational definition. This happens fairly often in health care. Using the Drill Down Approach we're encouraged to check this out right away. If a change in operational definition is the reason for the special cause signal we can either return to the original way we defined the data or, if this isn't possible, annotate the chart so that we are aware of the change in operational definition and its impact on our data.

Of course, a change in operational definition is not the only possible reason for a special cause signal. Something unusual could have occurred in the process of delivering babies too! In this C-section case the special cause virtually leapt out at everyone. During the special cause quarter Dr. Z delivered two sets of high-risk twins, each requiring delivery by C-section. This had never happened before in the hospital's collective memory. These two C-sections were enough to send a special cause signal in this small hospital. The hospital decided that there was no action that they needed to take based on this special cause.

Questions

6. The next Shewhart chart (Figure 13.25) shows the Shewhart chart in Figure 13.24 with the mean and limits recalculated. What do you learn from Figure 13.25?
7. The group chose next to make a separate Shewhart chart for each physician's proportion of C-sections (Figure 13.26). What would these charts help us learn that we wouldn't learn from Figure 13.25?

FIGURE 13.25 Percentage of C-Section by Physician with Special Cause Removed

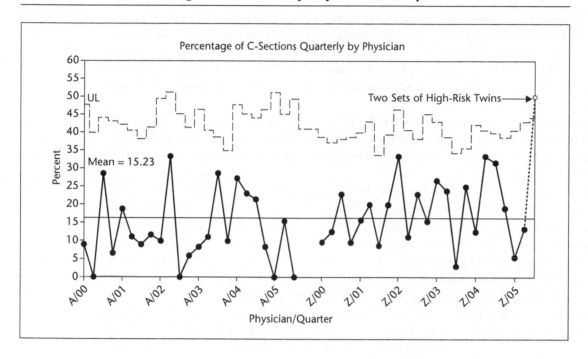

FIGURE 13.26 Percentage of C-Section Shewhart Chart for Each Physician

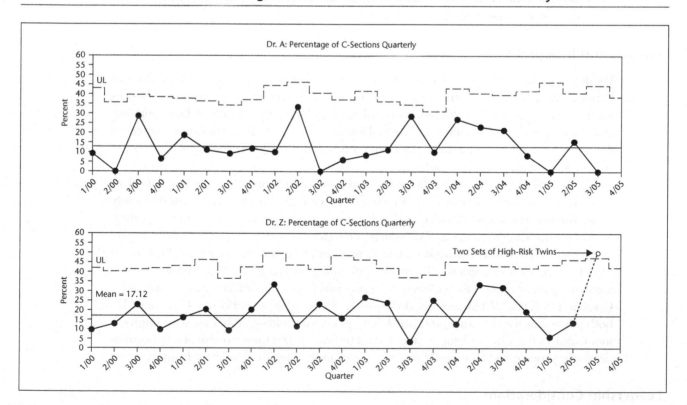

Analysis and Interpretation

This hospital investigated the special cause found on the control chart at Figure 13.25. After learning from the special cause and taking appropriate action (in this case no action) they decided to leave the special cause data point on the chart so that everyone would know it happened but to remove it from the calculation of the mean and limits to find limits that more accurately reflected their process. (Chapter Four provided additional guidance for making and revising limits.)

Figure 13.25 now shows that neither physician is special cause to the other; they don't stick out statistically to the good or to the bad. The percentage of C-sections shows only common cause variation in the system. This means that the variation is inherent given the way the process is designed.

With Figure 13.25 we know that both physicians are common cause, statistically stable, when viewed together on one control chart. But that doesn't mean that they are stable in and of themselves when viewed separately. Each chart in Figure 13.26 represents a single physician's percent of C-sections only. The mean and control limits are calculated using only the data produced by that physician and represent solely the variation in his or her practice. The chart that results allows us to see whether each physician is statistically stable in his or her own practice. Each of the Dr.'s charts in Figure 13.26 shows only common cause. They are each different in their mean and control limits but each stable in his or her own proportion of C-sections. This means that their outcome is a predictable result of the process they each use. If they want our outcomes to significantly improve then they're going to need to study and redesign their delivery process.

Question

8. Using the Drill Down Approach what might this hospital do next to continue to learn and improve their percentage of C-Sections?

Analysis and Interpretation

We now know that 2004 was not special cause. The C-section levels observed in 2004 could happen again and result in more payer dissatisfaction and perhaps negative consequences for the organization! They did have a special cause in Dr. Z's percentage of C-sections but after investigating and learning, the hospital found no way to improve the process based on this special cause. Does that mean there is no way to improve the percentage of C-sections? Are we stuck with what we have?

The Drill Down Approach helps us see that we aren't stuck. We now go to work to understand the common causes that influence C-sections. This hospital started to study their common cause system by creating a Pareto chart of the reasons cited in the medical record for deciding to perform a C-section. This Pareto chart is at Figure 13.27.

This started a lively discussion. How do they define "failure to progress?" What about the cases where no reason was listed for performing a C-section? What about the cases involving patient request for a C-section, or previous C-section, or failed vaginal birth after C-section (VBAC)? What protocol do we use to decide when to perform a C-section? Do both physicians use the same protocol? Is it as good as it could be? What ideas for improvement could we get by studying protocols used by others? Did these present any opportunities for improvement? How could we test these changes using the Model for Improvement?

Leadership Considerations

1. Drilling down into aggregated data is something we need to do to be able to learn and to transition from data for accountability to data useful for improvement. Placing multiple

FIGURE 13.27   Pareto Chart of Documented Reasons for C-Sections

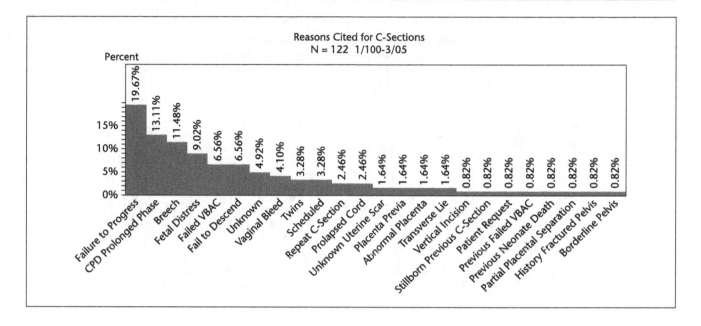

organizational units on one chart in order to learn whether any units are special cause to the rest of the system represents a potentially valuable learning opportunity. This can be very frightening to people who work in the various units. Rational subgrouping placing multiple practitioners on the same Shewhart chart can engender even more emotion. If management is going to be successful in helping people use these data as an opportunity for learning and improvement, it will need to be steadfastly committed to using the data for improvement. Avoiding blame and recrimination will be essential to clinical and financial improvement.

2. Creating a Shewhart chart with 20–30 data points takes much longer when data are charted at quarterly rather than monthly intervals. Usually we'd like to learn about process performance faster than at quarterly intervals. In this case however, we see that charting the proportion of C-sections each month results in a Shewhart chart with a lot of zeros (Figure 13.28).

If a Shewhart chart contains 25% or more of the data points as zero, the chart becomes much harder to learn from. The upper control limit is very wide. Look at the difference between the control limits using quarterly data and those using monthly data (Figure 13.29).

By using a larger subgroup size we have a greater likelihood of avoiding time frames with zero C-sections. (See Chapter Five for more guidance.) We could combine two months' workload together and plot the proportion of C-sections every other month. In this particular hospital, grouping the monthly data into quarterly data allowed them to have enough opportunities for C-sections that they didn't have any quarters with zero proportion C-sections.

Another issue illustrated by this case study is the opportunity to determine how our process would have to perform if we really had to make sure that we didn't exceed the payer's limit of 17% annual C-sections. While we are looking at C-sections on our Shewhart chart quarterly to learn whether our system has special cause or solely common cause

FIGURE 13.28 Monthly Aggregate Percentage of C-Section

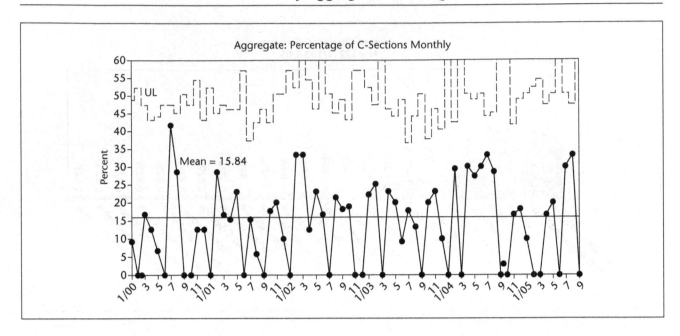

FIGURE 13.29 Monthly Compared to Quarterly Aggregate Percentage of C-Section

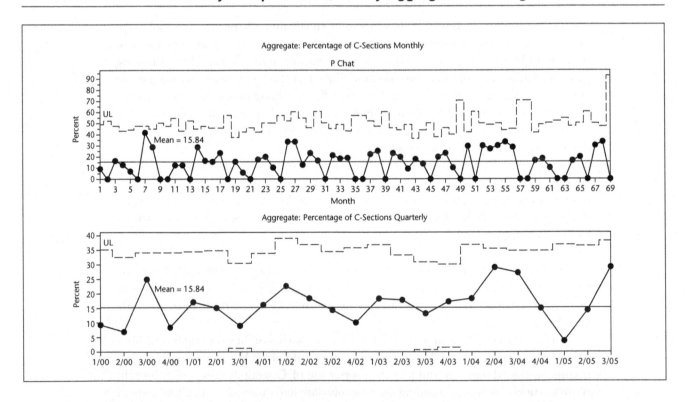

variation, the payer is looking at our data annually to see whether we exceed 17% annual C-sections. Let's say a small hospital had 138 deliveries in 2004 and an average percentage of C-sections of 15.84%. Given these data we can calculate an upper control limit as high as 25.2%. If we don't do something we are going to have some years where our annual average percentage of C-sections exceeds 17% with our common cause system. We probably can't change the number of deliveries at our hospital so we need to reduce the C-sections. The question becomes "What average proportion of C-sections do we need to achieve to ensure that we don't have a year whose average exceeds 17%? In other words, to have an upper control limit that is less than or equal to 17%?" The P chart formula follows:

$$\sigma\rho = \frac{\sqrt{\overline{p} * (100 - \overline{p})}}{n} = \frac{\sqrt{* (100 -)}}{n} = \underline{\hspace{2cm}}$$

$$UL = \overline{p} + (3 * \sigma\rho) \qquad LL = \overline{p} + (3 * \sigma\rho)$$

The P chart uses subgroup size (the denominator) as part of the way it calculates the upper and lower control limits. Using the P chart formula we can keep our number of deliveries the same but plug in different average proportions of C-sections and calculate what our upper control limits would be with different average percentages of C-sections. It turns out that if we want to have an upper control limit of 17% with a volume of deliveries at 138 per year we have to have an average of 9.5% C-sections per year. A level of 9.5% of C-sections necessary to achieve an upper control limit of 17% a year would be far under the health care average. This average percentage of C-sections is so low it might actually concern us. Are we performing all the C-sections we really need to perform?

It's not reasonable to expect a small hospital to never exceed 17% C-sections for an attribute measure like C-sections. Achieving an upper control limit of 17% is a function of their average proportion of C-sections and the volume of deliveries at that facility. Large hospitals delivering many babies will have a much easier time attaining an upper control limit of 17% or less than will small hospitals because of the impact of their larger volume of deliveries alone. This may be important to understand and communicate when working with others in our profession.

CASE STUDY E: ACCIDENTAL PUNCTURE/LACERATION RATE

Key Points for This Case Study

1. Using comparative report card data as a starting point for improvement
2. The importance for learning of moving from an aggregate report card score to the original data used to create that score
3. The use of the Drill Down Pathway to guide learning from aggregate data
4. Developing appropriate Shewhart charts for count data
5. Subgrouping and stratification strategies

Background

Hospital F was compared to seven other hospitals in its peer comparison group and received a report card detailing its performance and that of its peers (see Table 13.8). Several ratings were "high" for hospital F and caused concern among the hospital leadership team. Accidental Punctures/Lacerations during Procedure (APL) was one of the areas of concern. The hospital leadership team was not clear about how to use the report card findings. Most of the leaders wanted to appoint a responsible person and task them to spread the word and

Table 13.8 Clinical Quality Measures Comparative Summary

Excerpt—Inpatient Care: Medicare Population A and B from 2/2005 to 1/2006									
Dimension	Measure	Hosp. A	Hosp. B	Hosp. C	Hosp. D	Hosp. E	Hosp. F	Hosp. G	Hosp. H
Volume	Total Cases	4,987	7,812	11,101	8,542	9,658	7,421	4,822	6,798
Utilization	Cost Per Case	0.86	1.23	0.92	1.17	1.04	0.96	0.93	1.2
	ALOS	0.92	1.1	0.87	1.06	0.98	0.86	0.99	1.04
Clinical Care	Mortality	0.71	0.83	1.1	1.03	1.4	0.74	0.88	1.01
	Accidental Puncture and Laceration	1.16	0.84	1.27	1.09	1.17	**1.64**	0.92	1.34
	Cardiac Complications Resulting from a Procedure	0.84	1.16	1.09	0.87	0.74	0.59	1.11	1.04
	Postoperative Infections	0.98	1.43	0.67	0.89	0.9	0.87	1.16	0.82

All data are indexed. Index = actual divided by expected. An index of < 1.00 is favorable. All data case mix adjusted and grouped using grouper.

correct the problem. Others said the entire report card should be ignored because they were sure it didn't reflect reality. The leadership team decided that, now that they were aware of a potential problem, they wanted to work toward improvement. The question was "How?" One leader pointed out that the hospital didn't know whether something had happened recently to result in the poor APL rate or whether the rate had always been high. Another person pointed out that outcomes were the result of a process or processes of clinical care; did the hospital know which clinical processes needed to be changed? Did they know how the clinical process needed to be changed? After more discussion the vice president of Quality Improvement suggested that this situation might be a good one in which to use a formal drill down pathway that they had just learned about. (See Figure 13.30.)

Questions

1. The Drill Down Pathway starts with the step "identify the aggregate data of interest." It had already been decided that APL was the aggregate score of interest. The next step is to "understand the measure." What does 1.64 APL mean?
2. Why is it important to move from 1.64 APL to the monthly raw data? See Table 13.8 for the raw data.
3. Using the Drill Down Pathway:

   - What type of Shewhart chart is appropriate for these data?
   - What is the first Shewhart chart you would construct?
   - What actions might you take if you found evidence of special cause on this first Shewhart chart?

FIGURE 13.30   The Drill Down Pathway

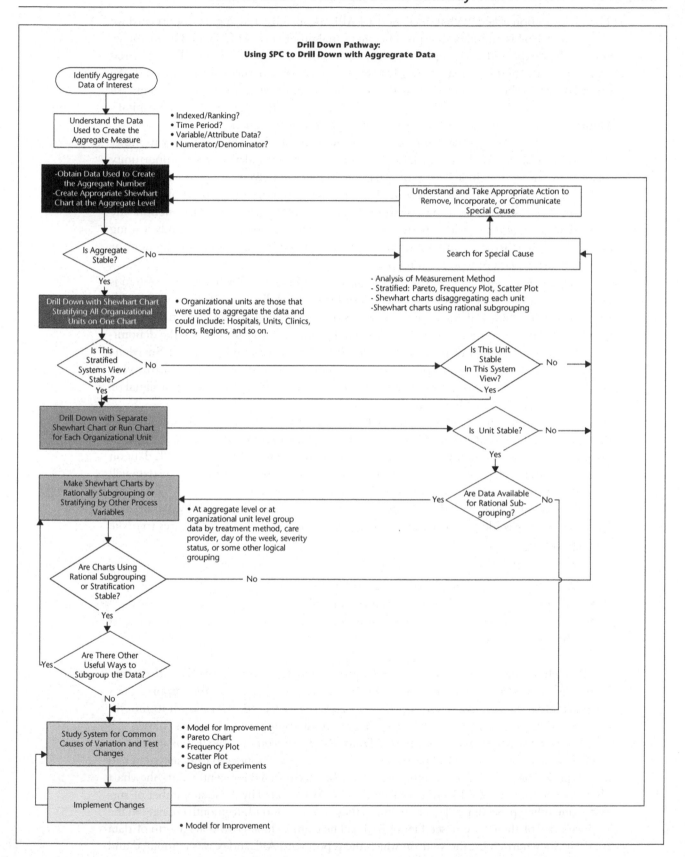

Analysis and Interpretation

The first question asked "What does the 1.64 APL mean?" By studying the report card we can see that 1.64 is an index. It represents the actual number of APL divided by the number of APL "expected" for hospital F. Anything less that 1.00 means fewer APLs occurred than expected; anything greater than 1.00 means more APLs occurred than expected. We don't know whether "expected" was the same last year, or what it will be next year. We also see that the data were collected over a one-year time frame, were for the hospital's Medicare population only, and were case-mix and severity adjusted.

Question 2 asked why it is important to move from the indexed to the raw monthly data. Table 13.9 shows their raw data. The index of 1.64 may alert us to an opportunity for improvement. The index score of 1.64 however, doesn't give us any indication about how to improve the situation. Did something unusual happen, causing most of the APLs to occur in one short time frame, or were the APLs spread fairly evenly throughout the year? If we can get the basic puncture data over time (each month) we can study it using a Shewhart chart to see if anything unusual has occurred in our system or whether our system is just consistently performing poorly.

The use of an indexed value 1.64 also makes it difficult to tell whether our system is changing over time. Even if we had the indexed value of APL for last year as well as this year, we wouldn't know if the difference between them was due to a change in the actual number of APLs (the numerator) or due to a change in the "expected" APLs (the denominator). If we can get the raw data over time (each month) we can study it using a Shewhart chart to see if the APLs we're producing each month are unusually different this year compared to last. If this year's monthly data are unusually different we will see a signal of special cause on the Shewhart chart.

The indexed value 1.64 also only tells us about our Medicare population because this is the database that all comparison hospitals had in common. If hospital F wants to improve APLs they probably want to do so for all populations. They collect APL data on all procedures for all populations; why not use it all for learning? Getting the raw data will help us study the whole system, not only the Medicare population.

A key point is that an indexed value from a scorecard may be a useful wake-up call. But once we've decided to answer the call, it takes more fundamental measures to make much progress.

Question 3 asked:

- What type of Shewhart chart is appropriate for these data?
- What is the first Shewhart chart you would make?
- What actions might you take if you found evidence of special cause on this first Shewhart chart?

A U chart was appropriate because the puncture data were attribute data; they were counting each APL, they could have more APLs than surgeries and the opportunities for punctures (the subgroup size or number of surgeries) varied from month to month. (Chapter Five provides guidance on selecting the most appropriate Shewhart chart.)

The first Shewhart chart that the Drill Down Pathway recommended was an aggregate-level view (all procedures and all patients over time). The team wondered if their system had always performed this way or whether something big had affected it recently. This Shewhart chart plotted the rate of APLs [the total number of APL divided by the total number of surgeries (including procedures)] each month so they could see month-to-month changes in the performance of their system (see Figure 13.31). The team included two years' worth of data on their Shewhart chart, the year on which the report card APL index was computed and all of the months since. They used this much data because they knew that control limits are

Table 13.9   APL Raw Data

Mo	Tot Surg	Total Punc	Site A # Surg	Site A # Punc	Site B # Surg	Site B # Punc	Site C # Surg	Site C # Punc	Total Lap. Surg	# Punc. In Laps	Total Open Surg	# Punc. in Open Surg	Total Sch. Surg#	Punc. In Sch. Surg	Total Em. Surg	# Punc. In Em.
Jan 04	754	48	202	15	351	25	201	8	494	30	260	18	500	28	254	20
Feb	589	35	170	5	290	19	129	11	280	22	309	13	421	28	168	7
Mar	688	28	193	8	334	13	161	7	471	20	217	8	590	22	98	6
Apr	901	35	303	9	361	16	237	10	546	28	355	7	762	24	139	11
May	712	24	205	6	369	11	138	7	481	19	231	5	600	20	112	4
Jun	803	37	233	9	411	19	159	9	402	26	401	11	712	33	91	4
Jul	687	38	212	12	295	17	180	9	480	26	207	12	553	28	134	10
Aug	713	34	199	9	403	16	111	9	460	26	253	8	600	26	113	8
Sep	681	35	186	10	302	14	193	11	398	27	283	8	537	30	144	5
Oct	809	28	220	7	419	12	170	9	512	17	297	11	664	19	145	11
Nov	869	45	267	14	442	24	160	7	559	34	310	11	730	39	139	6
Dec	647	42	231	17	299	19	117	6	444	31	203	11	527	31	120	11
Jan 05	798	46	226	13	404	25	168	8	358	22	440	24	648	40	150	6
Feb	687	37	211	12	346	18	130	7	420	29	267	8	590	29	97	8
Mar	801	38	246	11	354	17	201	10	497	30	304	2	626	28	175	10
Apr	826	45	227	13	415	21	184	11	509	33	317	12	700	33	126	12
May	729	30	236	10	332	13	161	7	477	23	252	7	610	26	119	4
Jun	780	34	282	11	388	17	110	6	499	22	281	12	652	29	128	5
Jul	836	36	250	13	426	16	160	7	507	27	329	9	710	27	126	9
Aug	698	29	208	8	354	14	136	7	400	19	298	10	601	26	97	3
Sep	807	44	279	15	367	23	161	6	472	30	335	14	690	34	117	10
Oct	747	31	221	9	406	14	201	8	444	22	303	9	620	27	127	4
Nov	760	71	249	24	375	32	136	15	460	40	300	31	652	52	108	19

FIGURE 13.31 Aggregate APL Rate per Surgery

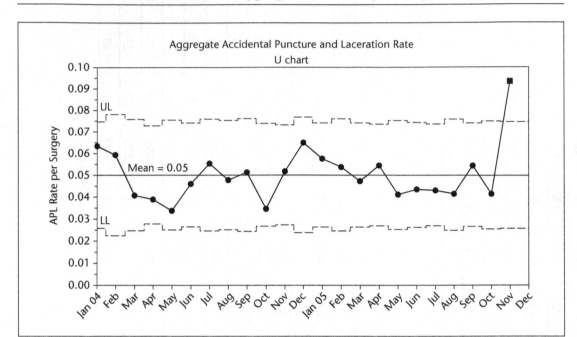

considered "trial limits" when made with fewer than 20 data points. Control limits become more accurate if they can use 20 or more data points. (See Chapter Four for guidance on when to create and revise limits.) Also, since report card data tend to be old, they wanted to be sure to include their more recent data in order to learn about the current performance of their system

The team did see something impacted their entire system in this big picture Shewhart chart. The Drill Down Pathway (Figure 13.30) suggested they investigate the special cause by checking for a change in the measurement method or by comparing the special cause time frame to the common cause time frame using a stratified Pareto chart, stratified histogram, or stratified scatter plot to see the differences in causal factors (types of procedures, types of errors, and so forth). The team discovered that the method used to define and record information on APL had been "clarified" in the most recent month. The new guidance wasn't very clear and caused people to duplicate entries. The hospital decided to return to their original data collection guidance. They considered recollecting all of the data for November using the original measurement guidance, but decided they couldn't afford the amount of chart review this would require. They noted the special cause on their Shewhart chart and did not use November's data in calculating the mean or limits for their chart (Figure 13.32).

Questions

4. What Shewhart charts would you next make to drill down by organizational unit? Looking at Figure 13.33, is any one site special cause to the hospital as a system? Looking at Figure 13.34, what's your conclusion about each site?

5. The next step in the Drill Down Pathway is rational subgrouping. Looking at the data you have available (Table 13.9), what charts could you make using rational subgrouping? Looking at Figures 13.35 and 13.36, what do you learn from these Shewhart charts? Where could you go next in your study of APL?

6. What data don't you have that you would like to have to develop rational subgrouping?

FIGURE 13.32 Aggregate APL Rate per Surgery with Special Cause Data Excluded

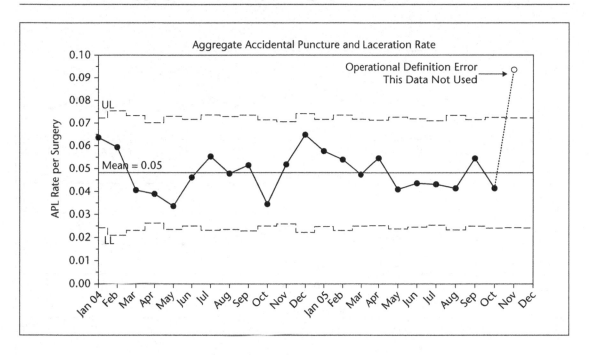

FIGURE 13.33 APL Rate Disaggregated by Site

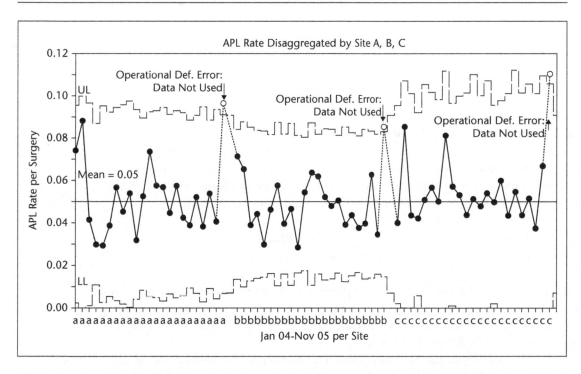

Analysis and Interpretation

The next step in the Drill Down Pathway was to create one Shewhart chart with all three organizational units on it. The mean came from all the data on the chart. The limits then were calculated using the system mean and the data for each month. The team studied Figure 13.33 and concluded that no one site was special cause to the rest of the hospital as a system.

FIGURE 13.34   Separate Shewhart Charts of APL Rate for Each Site

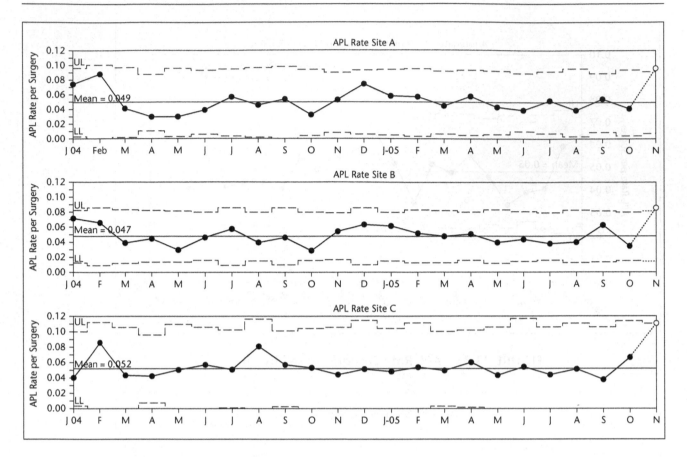

Figure 13.34 showed the team that nothing unusual was happening at any of the three sites with regard to how many APLs it produced per surgery/procedure (no special cause signals on of the charts). Between Figures 13.33 and 13.34 the team now knew that no site was unusually different from the other sites and that each site's performance was stable.

The next step in the Drill Down Pathway is rational subgrouping. With the data readily available (Table 13.9) the team decided they could compare APL in:

a. Scheduled versus emergency surgeries/procedures
b. And laparoscopic versus open surgeries/procedures

With each of these rational subgrouping pathways the team also had to decide how they wanted to stratify the data—how they wanted to sequence it on the Shewhart chart. They decided to show all the monthly scheduled data for the two years, then all of the monthly emergency data for the two years.

The team learned from the Shewhart chart that neither scheduled nor emergency APL rates were special cause when viewed as a system. There was no unusual difference between them. Emergency APL rates showed wider limits than did scheduled surgeries/procedures due to the smaller volume of emergency surgeries/procedures at this hospital (effect of subgroup size on U chart).

The team also realized that the data allowed them to rationally subgroup laparoscopic versus open surgeries/procedures APL rates (Figure 13.36). In doing this the team learned

FIGURE 13.35 **Rational Subgrouping Scheduled Versus Emergency Surgery APL Rate**

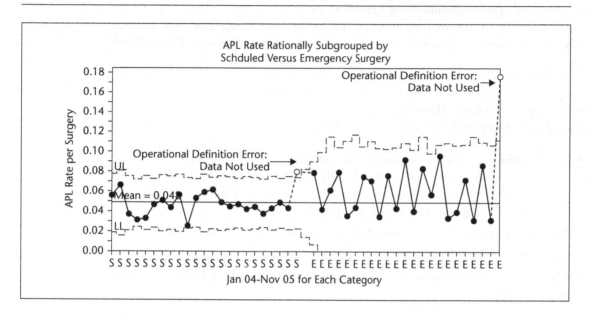

FIGURE 13.36 **Rational Subgrouping Laparoscopic Versus Open Surgery APL Rate**

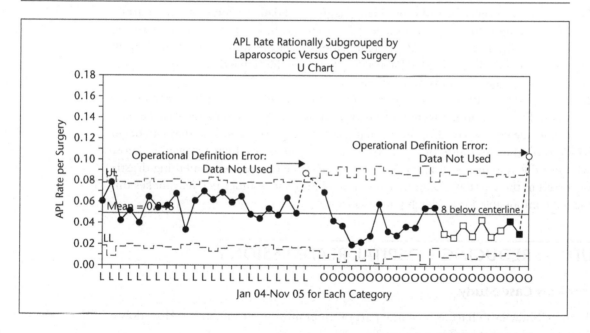

that the rate of APLs in open surgeries/procedures was unusually different (special cause of a run of 8 or more consecutive points on the same side of the center line) from the laparoscopic rates. APL rates in laparoscopic and open surgeries were not part of the same system.

Where could you go next in your study of APL? The team decided that they had found a place to focus. Using the Drill Down Pathway the team decided to search for the source of the special cause. Why is the APL rate for open surgeries so much lower than that for laparoscopic surgeries? This was a good time for the process experts to speak up and propose some theories about the differences. They decided to try to get procedure codes and use a stratified Pareto chart comparing the APLs for procedure codes for open surgeries/procedures to the APLs for laparoscopic surgeries/procedures to see which procedures that could be done either way accounted for the difference.

Since some procedures are only done by one method (solely open or solely laparoscopically), they also decided to see whether they could get the data for four other Pareto charts:

- The laparoscopic procedures with the highest *number* of APLs
- The laparoscopic procedures with the highest *rate* of APLs
- The open procedures with the highest *number* of APLs
- The open procedures with the highest *rate* of APLs

Question 6 asks what data do you wish you had for rational subgrouping? The team could think of several more useful ways to rationally subgroup the data. They then had to weigh the cost of getting the information and the time they had available for further study. Some of the rational subgrouping ideas discussed included:

Which operating room or treatment room was used?

Which physician performed the surgery/procedure?

What time of day the laparoscopic procedures with the highest number of APLs are occurring?

Leadership Considerations

1. Report cards, scorecards, and other highly aggregated data are increasingly a part of health care management environment. A key to using these report cards for learning lies in leadership insisting that their organizations focus inward on improving clinical care processes. To do this leadership needs get and use the actual data—not the report card score—in their improvement efforts.
2. Leaders need to insist on seeing more than one lump of data such as the APL rate for last year. They should insist that anyone reporting health care data display the data over time (ideally weekly or monthly, or, if they must, quarterly) so that they can begin to focus on the capability of their system for key outcomes. Leaders need to know whether the system's performance is stable over time or whether something drastic occurred in their system. Data that are lumped into one number per year makes this virtually impossible for leadership to discern.

CASE STUDY F: REDUCING HOSPITAL READMISSIONS

Key Points for This Case Study

1. Using a Shewhart chart as a central part of an improvement initiative ("How do we know if a change is an improvement?")
2. Analyzing classification data with variable subgroup size
3. Illustrating guidelines for updating and reporting Shewhart control limits
4. Using Shewhart charts for continued monitoring of improvements

Background

A health plan with an elderly patient population was looking for ways to improve their health care system. Care of patients with congested heart failure (CHF) was one of their large expense categories. They formed a team to investigate ways to improve care and reduce costs. After meeting with senior leaders and reviewing existing data, the team used the Model for Improvement to focus their improvement effort:

What are we trying to accomplish?

Improve the system of care for CHF patients to reduce hospital readmissions by at least 50% (a possibility based on literature and benchmark data).

How will we know that a change is an improvement?

Establish a Shewhart chart of CHF readmissions for the past two years (1996–1997). Extend the limits and compare the current performance to the historical data.

What changes can we make that will lead to improvement?

Do a literature review and visit an organization that is using population focused health improvement methods for CHF patients.

Operational Definition: For this study a CHF readmission was defined as an admission to the hospital for any reason by a previously diagnosed CHF patient in the health plan.

Questions

1. What type of Shewhart chart is appropriate for the readmission data? How much historical data should be used to establish a Shewhart chart (Figure 13.37)?
2. How do you improve a system when all of the variation is attributed to common causes?

Table 13.10 shows readmission data gathered for the two previous years (1996–1997). The data in Table 13.10 were used to construct the following P chart (Figure 13.37):

FIGURE 13.37   P Chart of Hospital Readmissions for CHF

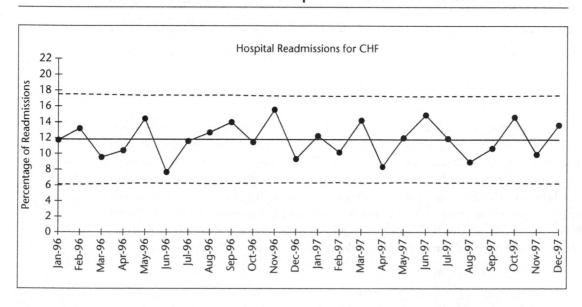

Table 13.10   Hospital Readmissions for CHF Data

Subgroups	Current Number of diagnosed CHF Patients	Number of CHF patients with a hospital readmission during the month	P Statistic (percentage readmissions)
Jan-96	290	34	11.72
Feb-96	288	38	13.19
Mar-96	293	28	9.56
Apr-96	298	31	10.40
May-96	305	44	14.43
Jun-96	300	23	7.67
Jul-96	302	35	11.59
Aug-96	299	38	12.71
Sep-96	300	42	14.00
Oct-96	305	35	11.48
Nov-96	308	48	15.58
Dec-96	310	29	9.35
Jan-97	310	38	12.26
Feb-97	314	32	10.19
Mar-97	309	44	14.24
Apr-97	311	26	8.36
May-97	316	38	12.03
Jun-97	315	47	14.92
Jul-97	310	37	11.94
Aug-97	312	28	8.97
Sep-97	308	33	10.71
Oct-97	307	45	14.66
Nov-97	302	30	9.93
Dec-97	300	41	13.67

The team investigated ideas to reduce the CHF readmission rate (the statistic is a percentage, but the team and others called it a rate). From the P chart of the historical data, they realized that a fundamental change in their care system was required to achieve the team's aim of a 50% reduction in readmissions. The hospital leadership team had convinced them that other organizations had been able to cut the readmission rate in half by using preventive care methods. The team visited an organization that had reduced their CHF readmission rates by instituting regular nursing contact with elderly patients to reinforce adherence to their physician's orders and to identify early warning signs (for example, use of a nurse manager). Meetings with the organization indicated that they could potentially reduce their current rates by 50% and lower the total costs (inpatient plus outpatient) for care of their CHF population.

They team planned a series of PDSA Cycles to test, adapt, and implement the use of a nurse manager for CHF patients.

PDSA Cycle 1: Develop the concept of a nurse manager for use with the current CHF population. Have the plan reviewed by the nursing staff, physicians treating CHF patients, and the finance department for feasibility and cost-effectiveness.

PDSA Cycle 2: Test the concept of a nurse manager with the 50 patients of two physicians for two months (January and February 1998). Adapt the plan as needed. Determine a reasonable caseload for a nurse manager.

PDSA Cycle 3: Implement the concept for all CHF patients (target, March 1998).

While completing these cycles, the team continued to plot CHF readmission data each month (Figure 13.38).

Question 3: How do you use a Shewhart chart to test for the effect of changes to a health care system (Figure 13.38)?

Question 4: When should limits for a Shewhart chart be updated? How do you decide which data to use (Figure 13.39)?

The team was able to implement the use of nurse case managers with all CHF patients by May 1998. When they observed the special cause on the chart in June 1998, they concluded that their use of the nurse case managers had reduced the readmission rate. The team decided to continue plotting monthly data and then calculate trial limits using data from June 1998 through May 1999. These data gave them the

FIGURE 13.38   P Chart of Hospital Readmissions for CHF with Special Cause

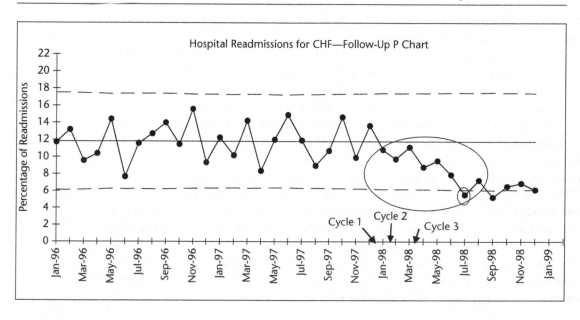

FIGURE 13.39   P Chart of Hospital Readmissions for CHF with Updated Limits

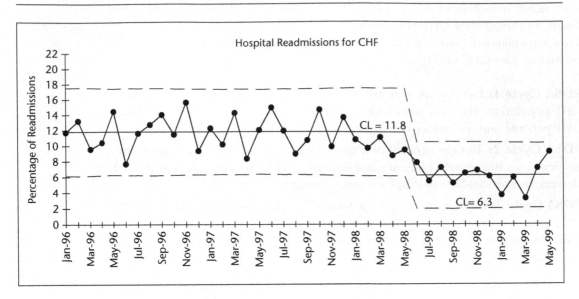

recommended minimum of 12 subgroups that represent the process after full implementation of the use of case managers.

Question 5: How do you use Shewhart charts to report the results of an improvement initiative (Figure 13.40)?

The chart in Figure 13.40 shows the data through May 1999 and the revised limits. The team presented this chart to management in June 1999 and celebrated their success in this improvement initiative. They had been able to reduce the readmission rate from 11.8 to 6.3%.

Analysis and Interpretation

1. *What type of Shewhart chart is appropriate for the readmission data? How much historical data should be used to establish a Shewhart chart?*

The CHF readmission data fit the definition of classification attribute data. The data had been historically collected by the health plan each month. The number of active patients diagnosed with CHF and the number of patients with one or more readmissions were recorded. So each active CHF patient could be classified as having or not having a readmission during the month. Ideally, the control limits for the P chart should be calculated with 20–30 subgroups, so the team used data for the most recent two years (24 months) to construct Figure 13.37.

2. *How do you improve a system when all of the variation is attributed to common causes?*

The initial P chart indicated that all of the variation in the monthly CHF readmissions could be attributed to common causes of variation. The existing system was stable relative to this measure. The organization could expect readmissions to continue at about 12% per month with any given month varying from 6% to 18%. The Shewhart chart makes it clear that a fundamental change to the current system must be made to reduce the readmission rate (for example, percentage of readmissions). So the team looked outside their system for ideas that could lead to improvement.

3. *How do you use a Shewhart chart to test for the effect of changes to a health care system?*

The teams tested a change (use of a nurse manager to contact CHF patients after discharge) in January 1998 and completely implemented the change by April. They extended the center line and the formula for the control limits calculated from the 1996–1997 data for the next 12 months (Figure 13.38). Each month, the current CHF patient population was used to calculate the limits from the UCL and LCL formulas, and the percentage for the month was plotted. A point below the lower control limit in July 1998 and eight consecutive points below the center line (January through August) indicated a special cause. The team attributed the improvement to the use of the case managers. Their knowledge of the change, the expected improvement, and the signals of a special cause on the Shewhart chart led them to the conclusion on the effectiveness of the case manager on CHF readmission rates.

4. *When should limits for a Shewhart chart be updated? How do you decide which data to use?*

By August 1999, the team was convinced that the use of a CHF case manager had resulted in a significant improvement in readmissions rate. Based on their understanding of the time lags in implementation and the data on the Shewhart chart, they agreed that the data beginning in June 1999 should be used to develop the P chart to characterize the readmission rate for the improved system. They were anxious to calculate the new limits, so they agreed to wait for the minimum of 12 months and calculate trial limits. Figure 13.38 shows the updated limits (center line = 6.3%; control limits of about 2% to 10.5%). The CFO was asked to determine the financial impact of the improvement and the team quickly reported the results to management and celebrated their success.

5. *How do you use Shewhart charts to report the results of an improvement initiative?*

The team used the P charts in Figure 13.38 and 13.39 to document their accomplishment of the team aim (in June 1999). Both charts were included in a presentation to the leadership team. But in September, the medical director reported that somehow the new system was not working as expected. She said that readmission rates were above 13% in August. One of the managers agreed to investigate and determined the following:

- Beginning in April 1999, one of the CHF case managers was asked to temporarily fill in for other nurses on vacation. She had to temporarily curtail her calls to CHF patients. When the case manager went on paternity leave for two months in June, his position was not replaced. The temporary assignments continued for the first case manager all through the summer. When the third case manager went on vacation in July, very few contacts were being made with the CHF patients.
- The managers agreed to fix the problem when the case manager returned from paternity leave in September, but he was assigned to a team preparing for a certification visit when he returned. He did not resume the planned CHF case management activities until November.

After reviewing these findings, the leadership team made changes in job descriptions, staffing levels, and ongoing measurement to permanently sustain the improvements made by the CHF improvement team. In July 2000, the medical director updated the Shewhart chart to summarize the results of the improvement initiative for the leadership team. The revised center line and control limits (to characterize the improved process) were calculated using the data from June 1998 through March 1999 and from January through June 2000, a total of 17 subgroups. She felt this best represented the time periods when the effect of case management could be completely observed. The chart shown in Figure 13.40 was prepared a year after the team completed their work.

FIGURE 13.40 P Chart of Hospital Readmissions for CHF One Year Post Improvement

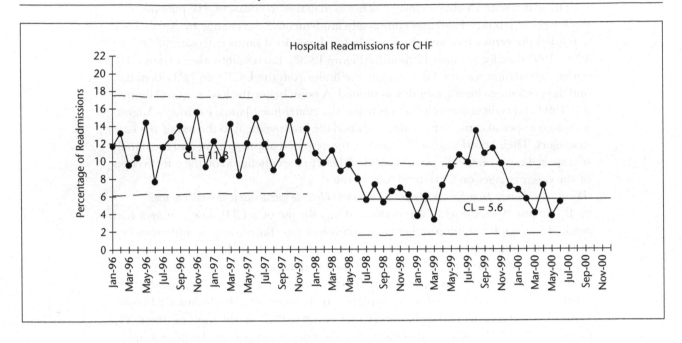

FIGURE 13.41 Use of Shewhart Charts to Monitor Process After Improvement

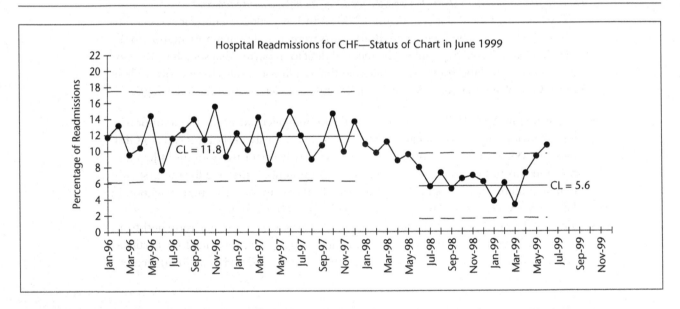

Leadership Considerations

1. Improvement teams should be encouraged to use Shewhart charts to help answer the question *how do we know that a change is an improvement?* But the use of the chart should not end when the team has completed their work. Continued use of Shewhart charts on key measures by the management team is an important way to maintain the gain of improvement efforts. If the management team had continued to monitor the Shewhart chart in Figure 13.38, they would have learned about the loss of the case manager by June 1999 (special cause) rather than three months later (see Figure 13.41).

2. The change that the CHF team implemented had a very positive impact on readmission rates. But the change required additional resources. Whenever additional staffing resources are a part of an improvement, the results are very susceptible to staffing problems that continually arise in health care organizations. Are there ways to obtain the same results without full-time case managers? The various components of the work of the case manager should be documented and then alternative ways to deliver them considered. For example, could CHF patients be taught self-management techniques that would allow them to do for themselves what the case manager was contributing to their health care? The management team should encourage improvement teams to look further after their initial successes.

3. Don't get in a hurry to celebrate improvements. Wait until the changes settle down in the revised system so the long-term impact can be determined.

CASE STUDY G: VARIATION IN FINANCIAL DATA

Key Points for This Case Study

1. Using control charts to study financial data
2. Using $\overline{X}$ and R or S charts for continuous data
3. Use of subgrouping strategies
4. Use of scatter diagram to help learn about common cause variation
5. Selecting the best measure to learn about a process

Situation

A physicians group that supported the community hospitals was trying to find some opportunities to improve its financial situation. The accounting department for the group collected information on charges for all of the doctors in the organization. The head of the group asked the department to study the variation in the charges to see if they could gain some insights that could be exploited. The analyst in the accounting group initially focused on charges where the principal diagnosis was pneumonia. Data on charges were obtained for all cases in 2006 (157 cases for the 17 physicians). When organizing the data on each pneumonia case, the analyst recorded the physician, the number of codiagnoses, and the length of stay associated with each case. Figure 13.42 shows a run chart for the pneumonia charges data. The irregularly spaced horizontal scale is due to seasonal variation in volume of pneumonia cases.

Questions

1. What information can be learned from the run chart of the pneumonia charges data? Have charges increased over the past year?
2. What type of Shewhart chart should be developed for these data?
3. How do you test theories about differences in physicians?

Analysis and Interpretation

The basic rules of a run chart do not indicate any unusual patterns (6 consecutive points above or below the center line, a trend of 5 points up or down). There is no indication that charges have changed during the year. There are 3 or 4 values that appear high but they are not separated from the other values enough to be conclusive.

FIGURE 13.42   Run Chart of Pneumonia Charges (All Physicians in Practice)

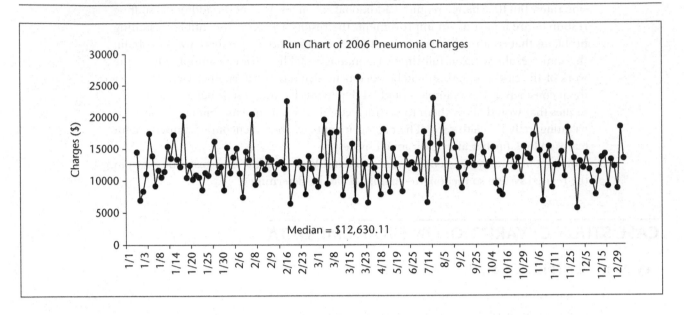

FIGURE 13.43   I Chart of Pneumonia Charges (All Physicians in Practice)

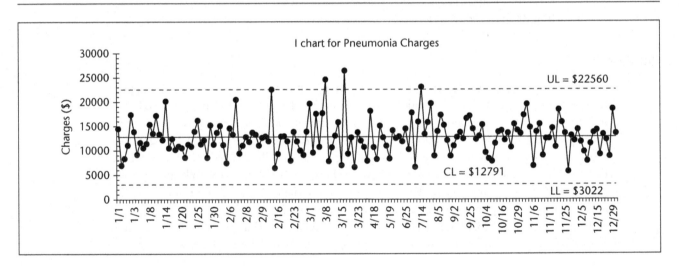

To develop a Shewhart chart, first note that the data are continuous (amount of money in dollars). One value is reported for each case, so an I chart could be developed (Figure 13.43).

The I chart indicates that three of the high values seen on the run chart are indications of special causes. Two of the values occurred in March and one in July. One theory suggested for these special causes was that some new physicians joined the practice in both March and July and they could be responsible for the unusual charges.

Question 3 asked how to test theories about differences in physicians. The data on the X chart can be reordered by physician to get an indication of variation between physicians. How should the 17 physicians be ordered? Because a theory about the special causes was related to experience, the physicians were ordered by years of experience with the physicians group (A = experienced to Q = new). Figure 13.44 shows the reordered I chart.

FIGURE 13.44 I Chart of Pneumonia Charges (All Physicians in Practice)—Reordered Data

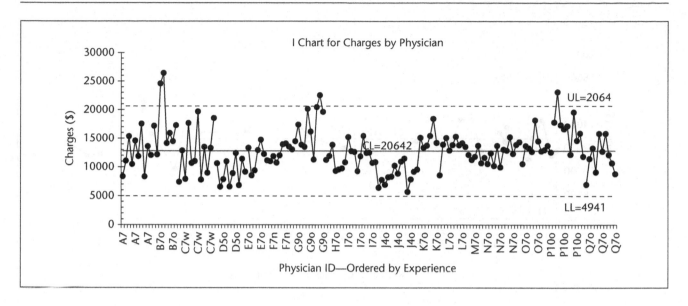

This I chart indicates numerous special causes. The two high values in March were both charges for patients of physician B who had been with the organization for many years. The high value in July was a patient of physician P who had joined the organization in June 2006. But there were numerous runs of 8 or more points above and below the center line associated with different physicians. There does not appear to be a general trend across the chart. So there is no support for the theory that physician experience has an impact on the charges.

Additional Questions

    4. Why is it difficult to interpret the I charts in Figures 13.43 and13.44?
    5. What other types of charts could be used to examine these data?

Analysis and Interpretation

The run charts are difficult to study with 157 data points on a single chart. General patterns and trends can be observed, but when many special causes are present (Figure 13.44), it becomes difficult to develop a strategy to identify them. Changes in average levels are more easily observed on the I chart than changes in the amount of variation.

For continuous data, $\overline{X}$ and S (or $\overline{X}$ and R) charts are appropriate to study variation when enough data are available and the data can be organized into rational subgroups. Instead of the pure time-ordered I chart, an $\overline{X}$ and R chart can be constructed by grouping equal numbers of consecutive data points into subgroups. A subgroup size of 4 or 5 is generally recommended for $\overline{X}$ and R charts. Figure 13.45 shows $\overline{X}$ and R charts based on subgroups of 5 consecutive cases (the last two data points were not used).

What about the I chart ordered by physician? When the data are subgrouped by physician, the number of data points per physician ranges from 5 to 12. When the subgroup sizes vary, an $\overline{X}$ and S chart is the appropriate choice. Figure 13.46 shows this set of charts.

FIGURE 13.45 $\bar{X}$ and R Chart for Pneumonia Data Ordered by Date of Diagnosis

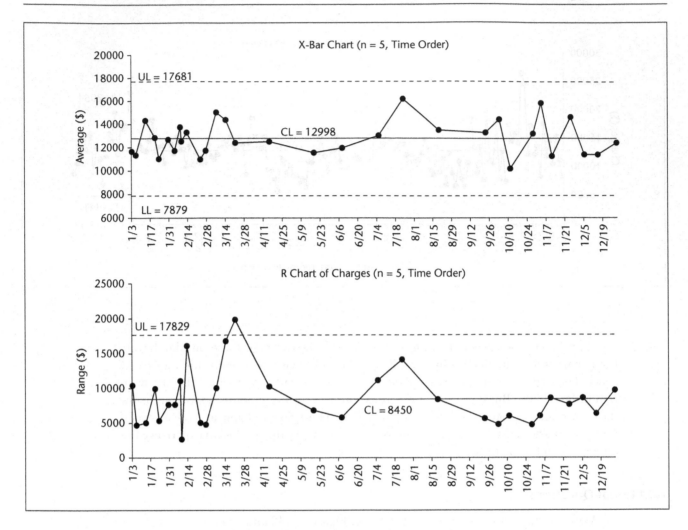

The charts in Figue 13.46 indicate special causes on both the $\bar{X}$ and S charts. Studying the $\bar{X}$ chart, physicians B and P tend to be associated with high charges while the average charges for physician J are lower than the others in the system. For the S chart, the variation for physicians B and C appears greater than the other physicians in the system. The head of the physicians' group planned to meet with these individual physicians to look for some insights into the special causes. But the average standard deviation in the pneumonia charges for a physician in the system was $2,818 (= 22% of the total charges). Why were the charges not more consistent?

Additional Questions

6. In addition to learning from the special causes, how can one learn about the common causes of variation in the charges? Are there other factors that should be considered when interpreting the variation in the charges? How can the effect of these factors be examined?

7. How could other factors be incorporated into the control charts for charges?

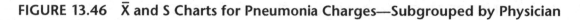

FIGURE 13.46   X̄ and S Charts for Pneumonia Charges—Subgrouped by Physician

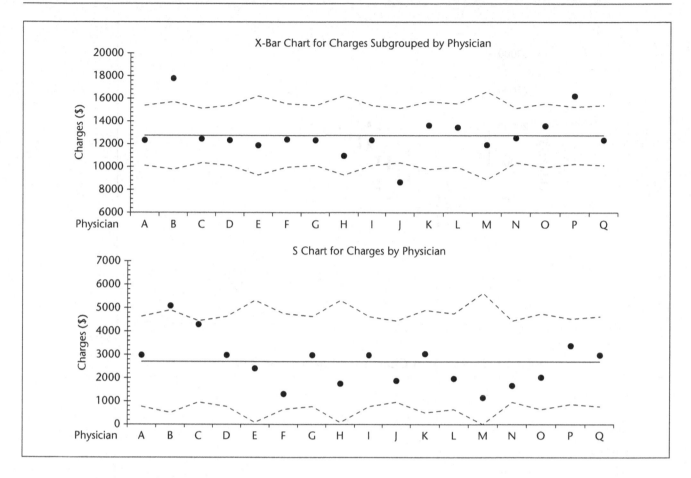

Analysis and Interpretation

Question 6 asked about some other factors contributing to the common cause of variation. When the charges data was originally collected, the analyst also recorded the length of stay in the hospital and the number of co-morbidities (other important conditions diagnosed, 0, 1, 2, or greater than 2) for each case. As the number of days is a measure of time (length of stay) a scatter plot can be used to study the relationship between length of stay and charges. Figure 13.47 shows this scatter plot.

The scatter plot indicates a strong positive relationship between charges and length of stay. After a base charge of about $5,700 for the first day, there is a linear increase in the charges for each additional day the patient stays in the hospital. Much of the variation in total charges can be attributed to the length of stay (the coefficient of determination, $R^2 = 0.73$, indicates 73% of the variation in the charges can be explained by the length of stay).

Question 7 asked how to incorporate other factors into the control charts for charges, Because there is a strong linear relationship with length of stay, the variation in the charges should be adjusted for days of stay before studying the effect of other factors (such as physicians). One way to do this is to transform the charges data to charges per day by dividing the total charges by the number of days for each case. Figures 13.48, 13.49, and 13.50 show the same charts presented earlier for the charges per day measure: run chart; X̄ and R chart subgrouped by consecutive five days; and X̄ and S chart subgrouped by physicians.

FIGURE 13.47   Scatter Plot for Charges and Days

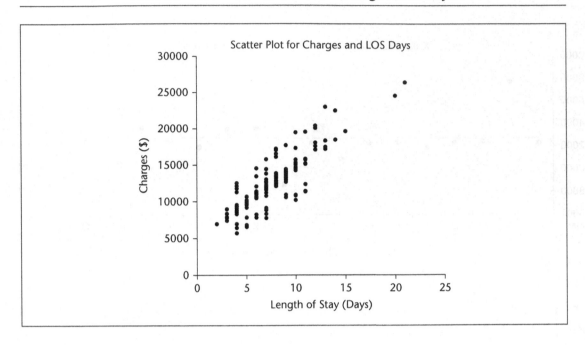

FIGURE 13.48   Run Chart for Charges per Day

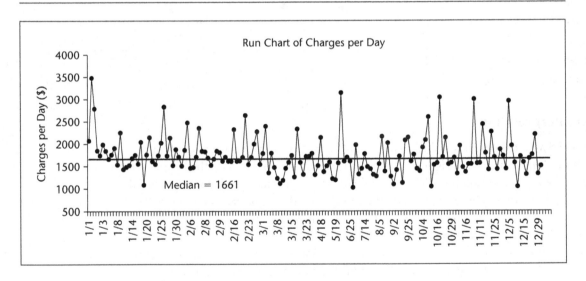

The charts for charges per day are quite different from the charts for total charges. The patterns on the run chart indicate slightly higher charges during January and February than during later in the year. There appear to be eight to ten unusually high values spread throughout the year.

The $\overline{X}$ and R chart indicate that the variation is stable. There is a special cause (high average) in the $\overline{X}$ chart for the first subgroup of data (confirming the pattern on the run chart).

The $\overline{X}$ and S chart subgrouped by physicians had some differences from the charts for total charges. Relative to the rest of the physicians, physician D was still low and physician P was still high. The charges per day for physicians B, J, and O were also low. On the S chart, physician C had more variation in charges per day than the other physicians.

FIGURE 13.49   X̄ R Chart for Charges per Day

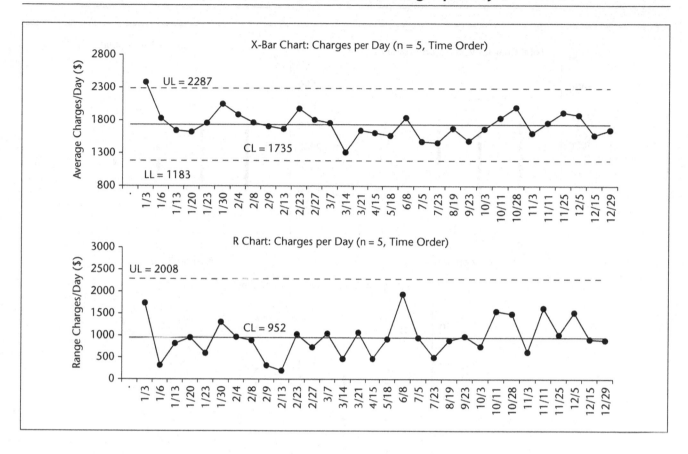

FIGURE 13.50   X̄ S Chart for Charges per Day by Physician

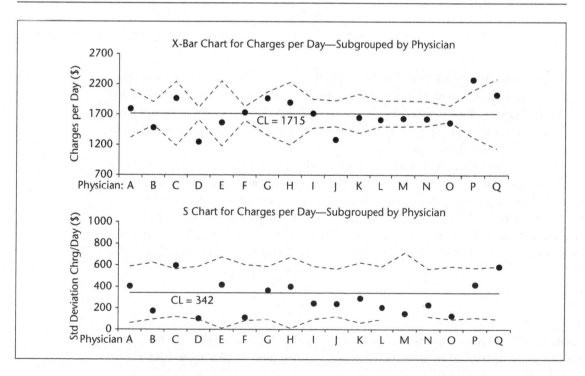

FIGURE 13.51 Scatter Plots for Comorbidities Versus Days and Charges

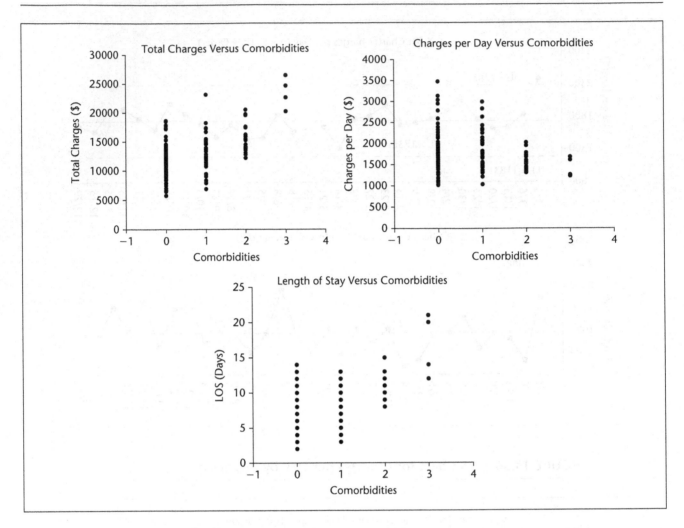

The average standard deviation was $342.42 (= 20% of the average charges per day). On a percentage basis, the variation still had not been significantly reduced by this transformation of charges. The accounting group team decided to investigate the effect of comorbidities on the charges. Figure 13.51 shows scatter diagrams for the comorbidities versus total charges and charges per day.

From these scatter plots, it is clear how multiple diagnostic conditions (comorbidities) affect the length of stay in the hospital. After the charges are adjusted for length of stay (calculating charges per day), there is no relationship to the number of comorbidities.

See table in Table 13.11 with averages for each of the measures and each level of comorbidities. The physician manager was going to share these data when he talked to the physicians that were associated with special causes on the $\bar{X}$ and S charts for charges per day.

SUMMARY

Run charts, control charts, and scatter plots were used to study variation in charges for pneumonia patients treated by a physician group. Scatter plots were used to understand

Table 13.11   Scatter Plots and Data for Comorbidities Versus Days and Charges

Number of Comorbidities	0	1	2	3 or more
Number of Cases	92	40	21	4
Charges ($)	7.00	7.73	10.00	16.75
LOS (Days)	11611.32	12905.38	15716.84	23433.44
Charges per Day ($)	1760.66	1778.50	1585.73	1444.71

relationships of variables in the financial database. When there is a large amount of data, $\bar{X}$ and R or S charts are preferred for identifying special causes. An individual chart (I chart) includes both average and variation issues in a single chart. The $\bar{X}$ charts separate these two issues for study.

Special causes were noted in the control charts subgrouped by physician. Before investigating the special causes, it is useful to have a basic understanding of the common cause factors affecting the measure of interest. For the pneumonia charges, the measure "charges per day" was appropriate for the different complexities of the patients (comorbidities).

Leadership Considerations

Run charts and control charts are effective tools to study variation in financial data. Health care managers should be encouraged to use the methods to display financial measures in regular monthly and quarterly reports.

Shewhart Chart Selection Guide

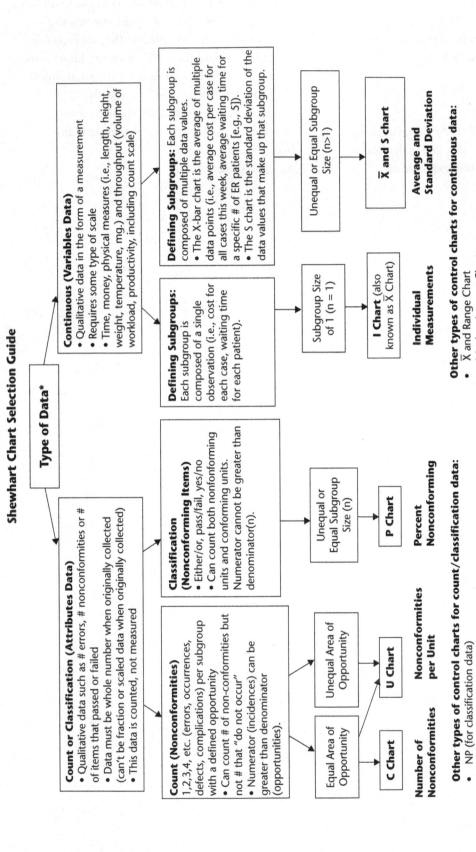

Type of Data*

Continuous (Variables Data)
- Qualitative data in the form of a measurement
- Requires some type of scale
- Time, money, physical measures (i.e., length, height, weight, temperature, mg.) and throughput (volume of workload, productivity, including count scale)

Count or Classification (Attributes Data)
- Qualitative data such as # errors, # nonconformities or # of items that passed or failed
- Data must be whole number when originally collected (can't be fraction or scaled data when originally collected)
- This data is counted, not measured

Defining Subgroups: Each subgroup is composed of multiple data values.
- The X-bar chart is the average of multiple data points (i.e., average cost per case for all cases this week, average waiting time for a specific # of ER patients [e.g., 5]).
- The S chart is the standard deviation of the data values that make up that subgroup.

Defining Subgroups: Each subgroup is composed of a single observation (i.e., cost for each case, waiting time for each patient).

Unequal or Equal Subgroup Size (n>1)

$\bar{X}$ and S chart

Average and Standard Deviation

Subgroup Size of 1 (n = 1)

I Chart (also known as $\bar{X}$ Chart)

Individual Measurements

Other types of control charts for continuous data:
- $\bar{X}$ and Range Chart
- Moving Average Chart
- Median and Range Chart
- Cumulative Sum (CUSUM) Chart
- Exponentially Weighted Moving Average (EWMA)
- Standardized Control Chart

Classification (Nonconforming Items)
- Either/or, pass/fail, yes/no
- Can count both nonconforming units and conforming units. Numerator cannot be greater than denominator(n).

Count (Nonconformities)
1,2,3,4, etc. (errors, occurrences, defects, complications) per subgroup with a defined opportunity
- Can count # of non-conformities but not # that "do not occur"
- Numerator (incidences) can be greater than denominator (opportunities).

Unequal or Equal Subgroup Size (n)

P Chart

Percent Nonconforming

Unequal Area of Opportunity

U Chart

Nonconformities per Unit

Equal Area of Opportunity

C Chart

Number of Nonconformities

Other types of control charts for count/classification data:
- NP (for classification data)
- T Chart [time between rare events]
- Cumulative sum (CUSUM) Chart
- G Chart [cases between rare events]
- Standardized Control Chart
- P' and U' Charts

*A run chart may be used with any type of data. It is often the starting point for viewing data over time when little data are yet available.

Detecting Special Cause

1. A single point outside the control limits.

2. A run of eight or more points in a row above (or below) the center-line.

3. Six consecutive points increasing (trend up) or decreasing (trend down).

4. Two out of three consecutive points near (outer one-third) a control limit.

5. Fifteen consecutive points close (inner one-third of the chart) to the center-line.

Using Shewhart Charts to Give Direction to Improvement Projects

Select a Key Measure Related to the Aim of the Improvement Effort

Develop an Appropriate Shewhart Chart for the Measure

Is the System Stable Relative to this Measure?

Yes

Change the System (Remove Common Cause(s))
Responsibility (ordered by importance)
1. Management
2. Technical Experts

Identify Common Cause(s)
Tools Methods:
• Planned Experimentation
• Rational Subgrouping
Responsibility (ordered by importance)
1. Technical experts
2. Supervisors
3. Workers in the system

No

Learn from and Act on Special Cause(s)
Responsibility (ordered by importance)
1. Local supervision
2. Technical experts
3. Management
4. Workers in the system

Identify Special Cause(s)
Tools Methods:
• Shewhart Charts
• Cause and Effect Diagram
• Rational Subgrouping
• Planned Experimentation
Responsibility (ordered by importance)
1. Workers in the system
2. Supervisors
3. Technical experts

Some Chart Selection Examples

Area	Application	Measure	Possible Subgroup Strategy	Chart
Overall	Chronic care	Number in registry	Month/specific disease/provider	I
	Satisfaction	Employee satisfaction score	Employee categories	
	Financial	Revenue ($)	Month/unit/provider/DRG	I
		Accounts receivable	Week/payer	
Long Term Care	Workload	Number of resident days	Month/unit/payer	I
		Number of medication doses	Day/shift/staff category	I
	Quality care	Hours of social activity	Week/resident/sex/age	$\bar{X}$ S
Behavioral Health	Workload	Number of client visits	Day/provider/type visit/location	I
	Satisfaction	Client rating of provider	Month/client category/diagnosis	I
	Care process	Days sobriety	Program/patient characteristics	.
ED	Access	Percentage left without being seen	Month/day of week/shift/ethnic group	P
	Care process	Percentage given ACE inhibitor	Day/shift/provider/shift	P
Surgery	Care process	Percentage antibiotic on time	Week/provider/day	P
	Care process	Percentage antibiotic D/C in 24 hr.	Week/provider/service	P
	Care process	Percentage ASA level 3 patients	Month/provider/procedure	P
	Timeliness	Percentage on-time start	Day/location/provider	P
Surgery	Safety	Total number of complications	Number of surgeries of a constant subgroup size (e.g., sample of 50 surgeries for each subgroup)	C chart
		Number of complications per 100 surgeries	All surgeries this month (when the number of surgeries varies each month)	U chart
Lab	Accuracy	Total number of bacteria in sample	Total centimeters tested per subgroup always the same (e.g., 2 cm each subgroup)	C chart

Lightning Source UK Ltd.
Milton Keynes UK
UKOW05f2332230118
316694UK00003B/10/P